T0261248

NSCA's Guide to Sport and Exercise Nutrition

Second Edition

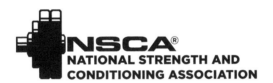

NSCA®
NATIONAL STRENGTH AND
CONDITIONING ASSOCIATION

Bill I. Campbell, PhD, CSCS, FISSN

Editor

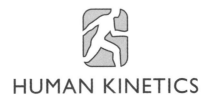

HUMAN KINETICS

Library of Congress Cataloging-in-Publication Data

Names: Campbell, Bill I., 1975- editor. | National Strength & Conditioning
  Association (U.S.)
Title: NSCA's guide to sport and exercise nutrition / Bill I. Campbell,
  PhD, CSCS, FISSN, editor.
Description: Second edition. | Champaign, IL : Human Kinetics, [2021] |
  Includes bibliographical references and index.
Identifiers: LCCN 2020018519 (print) | LCCN 2020018520 (ebook) | ISBN
  9781492593515 (paperback) | ISBN 9781492593522 (epub) | ISBN
  9781492593539 (pdf)
Subjects: LCSH: Athletes--Nutrition. | Sports--Nutritional aspects.
Classification: LCC TX361.A8 N38 2021 (print) | LCC TX361.A8 (ebook) |
  DDC 613.202/4796--dc23
LC record available at https://lccn.loc.gov/2020018519
LC ebook record available at https://lccn.loc.gov/2020018520

ISBN: 978-1-4925-9351-5 (print)

This publication is written and published to provide accurate and authoritative information relevant to the subject matter presented. It is published and sold with the understanding that the author and publisher are not engaged in rendering legal, medical, or other professional services by reason of their authorship or publication of this work. If medical or other expert assistance is required, the services of a competent professional person should be sought.

The web addresses cited in this text were current as of May 2020 unless otherwise noted.

Senior Acquisitions Editor: Roger W. Earle; **Managing Editor:** Miranda K. Baur; **Copyeditor:** Bob Replinger; **Indexer:** Rebecca L. McCorkle; **Permissions Manager:** Dalene Reeder; **Graphic Designer:** Denise Lowry; **Cover Designer:** Keri Evans; **Cover Design Specialist:** Susan Rothermel Allen; **Photographs (interior):** © Human Kinetics; **Photo Production Manager:** Jason Allen; **Senior Art Manager:** Kelly Hendren; **Illustrations:** © Human Kinetics; **Printer:** Sheridan Books

Printed in the United States of America   10 9 8 7 6 5 4 3 2 1

The paper in this book is certified under a sustainable forestry program.

Human Kinetics
1607 N. Market Street
Champaign, IL 61820
USA

United States and International
Website: US.HumanKinetics.com
Email: info@hkusa.com
Phone: 1-800-747-4457

Canada
Website: Canada.HumanKinetics.com
Email: info@hkcanada.com

E7924

Tell us what you think!
Human Kinetics would love to hear what we
can do to improve the customer experience.
Use this QR code to take our brief survey.

NSCA's Guide to Sport and Exercise Nutrition

Second Edition

Contents

Introduction

The field of sport nutrition is continuing to grow at a rapid pace. One needs to look no further than the rate at which record-breaking athletic performances are occurring or the ever-expanding scientific investigation into the effects that nutrition has on performance, health, and body composition. Whether you are a weekend warrior, an elite athlete, or a first-time gym member—this book will help you improve your performance by applying the latest scientific findings in your own training and exercise programs.

The *NSCA's Guide to Sport and Exercise Nutrition, Second Edition*, is intended to be a complete resource for sport nutrition professionals, students, educators, and researchers. The chapters are designed to provide both foundational and applied information in the areas of nutrition, exercise, and human performance.

This book discusses how food and sport supplements interact with the body's biological functions. Pertinent research is cited to highlight specific nutrient intakes that have been shown to improve exercise and sport performance. Additionally, information on assessing an athlete's nutritional status and developing a plan based on this assessment is presented. Taken in its entirety, the book will give you a better understanding of how food that is ingested is metabolized, stored, and oxidized for energy. Further, research is presented that has demonstrated how the proper selection of these nutrients can improve performance.

This updated second edition brings several intriguing and contemporary sport nutrition issues to the forefront. Recent developments into the mismatch of energy expenditure and caloric intake (exercising too much and not eating enough) can lead to a host of detrimental health and performance outcomes. This condition, referred to as relative energy deficiency in sport (RED-S), is comprehensively discussed in the first chapter. We have known for decades that carbohydrate feeding during moderate-intensity aerobic endurance exercise can delay fatigue and improve performance. Is it possible that simply rinsing the mouth with a carbohydrate-containing solution can have the same effects as actually consuming it? This fascinating area of research—carbohydrate mouth rinsing—is fully discussed in chapter 3. New sections on popular dietary supplements, including insect protein, preworkout supplements, and protein and amino acids are also highlighted. These new content areas are just part of the recent updates for this second edition.

The *NSCA's Guide to Sport and Exercise Nutrition, Second Edition* is divided into 11 chapters. The first chapter jumps right in to examine energy balance and the implications that undereating and overeating can have on performance. Next, important information is presented in terms of assessing an athlete's nutrition status using some of the most popular software and smartphone apps available today. The next several chapters discuss the macronutrients (carbohydrate, protein, and fat). Specifically, these chapters examine how these nutrients are metabolized, stored, and oxidized for energy. Recommendations based on scientific evidence are given in terms of ingesting these macronutrients to improve aerobic, anaerobic, and resistance training performance. Fluids are discussed next; specific sections discuss the fluid needs of younger and older adults and the effect that hydration can have on performance. Micronutrients and their role in metabolism and exercise are considered. The next several chapters discuss specific nutrition techniques and nutritional ergogenic aids that have been shown to improve aerobic endurance, strength, and power performance. The latest findings in the realm of nutrient timing are presented, as are the best practices for taking all the information presented in the book, applying it during a consultation with an athlete, and subsequently developing the athlete's plan.

A considerable amount of information can be covered under the umbrella of sport nutrition. We hope that you will gain better understanding of how food, supplements, and their interactions with the body's biological systems can enhance the health and performance of your athlete, client, or team.

Chapter 1

Energy Expenditure and Body Composition

Ann Brown, PhD, CISSN

Of the many physical attributes that can be modified, body composition is of paramount importance for most athletes regardless of the sport they participate in or their sex. Most athletes have one of two goals when attempting to change their body composition:

- Increase lean muscle mass (i.e., skeletal muscle)
- Decrease fat mass

A desire to improve body composition may be due to a wish to improve athletic performance, although many athletes and fitness enthusiasts seek to improve body composition for aesthetic reasons alone. In addition to its effect on performance and appearance, excessive body fat, particularly visceral (i.e., abdominal) fat, likely plays a role in the development of deleterious conditions such as heart disease, insulin resistance, non-insulin-dependent diabetes, sleep apnea, certain cancers, and osteoarthritis (8, 43, 50, 55, 63, 79, 85, 89).

Athletes, though, tend to be interested in the consequences of excessive body fat related to sport performance; in most sports, the inability to maintain optimal body composition can negatively influence the athlete's performance. For example, increased body fat without a concomitant increase in lean muscle mass may decrease acceleration, jumping ability, and overall

The author would like to acknowledge the significant contributions of Paul La Bounty and Jose Antonio to this chapter.

power in activities in which body weight needs to be moved through space. In sports that require a high power–to–body weight ratio (e.g., gymnastics), excess body fat is not desirable. Therefore, athletes often devote significant effort to improving or maintaining body composition. Body composition can be modified through diet, exercise, nutritional supplements, various drugs, and surgery. This chapter focuses on two basic nutritional strategies that can affect body composition: hypercaloric diets to gain weight (with an emphasis on lean muscle mass accretion) and hypocaloric diets with the goal of decreasing body weight, particularly body fat. In addition, the chapter discusses relative energy deficiency in sport (RED-S), a syndrome previously known as the female athlete triad. RED-S has been introduced as a more comprehensive term to include a larger demographic suffering from deleterious effects of energy deficiency.

Energy Balance

One of the ways that people can achieve weight loss and fat loss is by modifying nutritional intake, primarily the amount and type of calories consumed. The easiest way for athletes to change their body composition is to alter the energy balance equation. The energy balance equation, when in equilibrium, states that energy intake (i.e., food consumption) equals energy expenditure through normal metabolic processes and activity or exercise. When in a state of energy balance, a person is consuming a **eucaloric diet**. A eucaloric diet is a diet that includes the number of daily calories needed to maintain existing weight, achieved by consumption of the number of calories equal to an individual's **total energy expenditure**. Total energy expenditure (TEE) is the total number of calories expended throughout the day including basal metabolic rate, thermic effect of food, and physical activity. TEE can vary depending on a person's body size, gender, body composition, genetics, and physical activity level.

Because of fluctuations in body weight, the energy balance equation is not always in perfect balance. If more food is consumed than calories are expended, a positive energy balance is created and weight gain is likely to occur. Conversely, if fewer calories are consumed than needed for normal daily activities and metabolism, an energy deficit is created (figure 1.1). A diet inducing an energy deficit is termed a hypoenergetic or hypocaloric diet. A diet inducing a positive energy balance is known as a hyperenergetic or hypercaloric diet.

Thermic Effect of Food

Total caloric intake, as well as the macronutrient ratio of ingested nutrients, plays a role in weight gain and loss. The energy released from the catabolism of carbohydrate, protein, and fat is approximately 4, 4, and 9 kcal per gram, respectively (47). Often overlooked, however, is that the process of

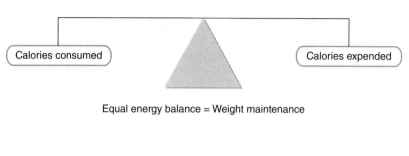

Equal energy balance = Weight maintenance

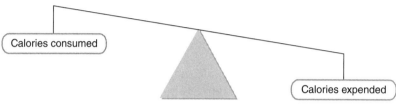

Negative energy balance (more calories are expended) = Weight loss

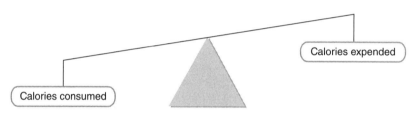

Positive energy balance (more calories are consumed) = Weight gain

FIGURE 1.1   The energy balance equation.

digesting, absorbing, transporting, and storing the various macronutrients is associated with the expenditure of energy (i.e., calories). This process, known as the thermic effect of food or diet-induced thermogenesis (DIT), causes a release of energy in the form of heat. The thermic effect of food actually increases a person's metabolism above the normal baseline energy expenditure for a period of time (possibly several hours) after a meal (77).

Because of the thermic effect of food, each macronutrient produces less net usable energy for the body after it is ingested (as compared with its energy content on the training table before a meal). Furthermore, certain macronutrients require more energy than others (i.e., have a higher thermic effect) to be digested, absorbed, transported, and stored. Specifically, the thermic effect of the caloric content of fat, carbohydrate, and protein is approximately 0% to 3%, 5% to 10%, and 20% to 30%, respectively (77). In other words, fat has a relatively low thermic effect, protein has the highest thermic effect, and carbohydrate is in the middle. Some scientists would like to revamp the current food labels to reflect the actual net calories that are gained after subtraction of the calories required to digest and store the macronutrients (i.e., net metabolizable energy) (47). If the current system were changed, the energy balance equation would be more accurate and meaningful (47).

Keeping the thermic effect of food in mind is important when formulating a nutritional plan to enhance weight gain or weight loss, because all calories are not the same biologically. For example, if a person consumed 300 kcal of extra protein every day for a year as opposed to 300 kcal of extra sucrose (i.e., table sugar) for the same length of time, it could be theorized that the effect on weight gain would not be the same because of the differing thermogenic properties of these macronutrients. When athletes embark on a hypocaloric diet to lose body weight, they will invariably lose some lean muscle mass. By increasing the proportion of protein ingested during a hypocaloric diet, the athlete realizes two benefits. First, the higher protein content will help preserve lean muscle mass, and second, more calories will be burned because of the high thermogenic properties of protein.

Deleterious Effects of Energy-Restricted Diets

Athletes in weight-restricted sports such as mixed martial arts, wrestling, boxing, gymnastics, figure skating, and diving may need to lose body weight or improve body composition or both. Reasons for wanting to lose weight may range from enhancing performance to qualifying for a lower weight class or may involve aesthetic considerations. Regardless of why an athlete desires to lose weight, the athlete or trainer should focus on losing excessive body fat and attempt to minimize the loss of lean muscle mass.

An important phenomenon to consider is that when a person loses body fat, lean muscle mass typically decreases concomitantly. In fact, one study demonstrated that after six weeks of consuming a very low-calorie diet, obese subjects lost approximately 11.5 kg (25.3 lb) (26); of that weight, however, approximately 63% was from fat and the remaining 37% was from lean muscle mass. Other studies using short-term caloric-restricted diets have also reported varying losses of lean muscle mass (34, 78, 84, 90). In rare instances, an athlete may want to lose both muscle and fat (e.g., a very lean elite wrestler needing to drop into a lower weight class). For the most part, however, loss of fat, not lean muscle, is the primary goal. In these cases, some muscle may need to be sacrificed to achieve the goal.

Hypocaloric Diets

When athletes need to lose weight, one of the first things they often do is adopt an energy-restricted diet **(hypocaloric diet)**. A hypocaloric diet is described when fewer calories are consumed than are needed to maintain existing body weight. Hypocaloric diets can modestly or severely reduce total calorie intake. On the extreme end of dieting, some people adopt diets commonly referred to as **very low-calorie diets** (VLCD). With athletes, depending on the sport, performance can begin to suffer if caloric intake becomes too low.

The VLCD as defined by the National Heart, Lung, and Blood Institute is a specific type of diet containing less than 800 kcal/day (77, 81). Generally, the diet consists of relatively large amounts of dietary protein (70-100 g/day or 0.8-1.5 g/kg of "ideal body weight"), relatively modest carbohydrate (80 g/day), and minimal fat (15 g/day) (77, 81). The VLCD, however, generally meets 100% of the Recommended Dietary Allowance (RDA) of all essential vitamins and minerals (77, 81). These diets are often consumed in a liquid form (56) and are generally advocated only for people who are obese (body mass index [BMI] ≥30) and are working with a physician, psychologist, dietitian, or exercise physiologist (77, 81).

Typically, VLCDs are 12 to 14 weeks in duration; a diet consisting of whole foods is then slowly reintroduced over the next two to three months to stabilize the person's weight (77, 81). The average weight loss on a VLCD is approximately 1.5 to 2.5 kg (~3-5 lb) per week for an average weight loss of 20 kg (44 lb) after 12 to 16 weeks (56). But maintaining this reduction in weight is not easy, as seen in a study in which 113 men and 508 women adhered to a VLCD for 12 weeks (as part of an overall 26-week weight-loss program) and lost approximately 25.5% and 22.6% of their original weight, respectively (87). All participants were followed up two years later, and only 77.5% of the men and 59.9% of the women had maintained losses of 5% or more of body weight (87).

A similar type of diet, the **low-calorie diet** (LCD), allows approximately 1,000 to 1,500 kcal/day of whole foods. Tsai and Wadden (83) conducted a meta-analysis on the effectiveness of the VLCD and the traditional LCD regarding weight loss. The authors concluded that initial weight loss was greater with the VLCD. But in contrast to what had been shown in an earlier meta-analysis (1), Tsai (83) and Wadden (87) concluded that after a year's time, the actual weight loss with the VLCD was not significantly different from that achieved with the traditional LCD. These authors reported that the earlier meta-analysis had not actually compared VLCD and LCD studies head to head but had "extrapolate[d] information across investigations, in which only one or the other diet was used" (p. 1289). Equally important, Tsai (83) and Wadden (87) noted the conclusion of the National Heart, Lung, and Blood Institute's expert panel that the LCD should be advocated over the VLCD. From a practical standpoint, an LCD is much more realistic for most people to adhere to on a day-to-day basis.

Because of the deleterious effects of energy-restricted diets on lean muscle mass as already discussed, VLCDs are not recommended for athletes (except very rarely in weight-restricted sports when making weight is a critical issue). If VLCDs are prescribed for athletes, performance may be severely limited because a drastic reduction in overall kcals decreases glycogen stores in skeletal muscle (20, 34). Furthermore, VLCDs have been reported to decrease both absolute strength and muscular endurance (26).

These potentially harmful effects may diminish the ability to train intensely and adequately recover from exercise. Of these two types of diets, an LCD is a better approach for athletes attempting to lose weight. Because the caloric deficits are not as severe, lean muscle mass is better maintained, and glycogen levels, although compromised, would not be as depleted and would not affect training intensity to the same extent as with a VLCD regimen.

High-Carbohydrate, Low-Fat Diets

Regarding weight loss, the optimal ratio of carbohydrate to protein to fat has been debated for some time, and consensus is currently lacking. Relatively high-carbohydrate, low-fat diets have been popular in athletic populations for years. But these diets, particularly in nonathletic populations, have lost some of their popularity over the last few years because of the introduction of various high-protein, low-carbohydrate diets.

Studies lasting 12 months or less suggest that low-carbohydrate diets may be more advantageous than high-carbohydrate diets for short-term improvements in body composition (10) (high-protein diets are discussed later in the chapter). The current long-term data (>12 months) suggest that weight loss is similar in those consuming low-fat, high-carbohydrate diets and those consuming higher-protein, lower-carbohydrate diets (42). Debate continues as to the type of carbohydrate in the diet (i.e., high glycemic index, high glycemic load, low glycemic index, or low glycemic load) that is optimal for weight loss.

Although a handful of weight-loss studies have involved athletes and trained people (28, 46), in most cases these studies have used overweight or obese nonathletic subjects. Thus, much of the research information pertaining to weight loss can be extrapolated only to athletic populations. Many studies using relatively high-carbohydrate, low-fat hypocaloric diets have manipulated the type of carbohydrate consumed to determine its effect on weight loss. In 2004, the CARMEN study (Carbohydrate Ratio Management in European National diets) revealed that people who consumed either a low-fat, high simple carbohydrate diet (LFSC) or a low-fat, high complex carbohydrate diet (LFCC) lost similar amounts of both body weight and fat mass (0.9 and 1.8 kg [2.0 and 4.0 lb], 1.3 and 1.8 kg [2.9 and 4.0 lb], respectively) while maintaining lean muscle mass (69).

Similarly, Sloth and colleagues (72) demonstrated that when everything was equal except for the type of carbohydrate consumed (low or high glycemic index), people had lost approximately the same amount of body weight (−1.9 and −1.3 kg [−4.2 and −2.9 lb], respectively) and fat mass (−1.0 kg [−2.2 lb] and −0.4 kg [−0.9 lb]) at the conclusion of the 10-week study. Furthermore, the two groups lost approximately the same amount of lean muscle mass (i.e., −0.8 kg [−1.8 lb]) (72). Das and colleagues (18) obtained comparable results for weight loss and body composition with diets consisting of either a low (40% carbohydrate, 30% fat, 30% protein) or high (60% carbohydrate, 20% fat, and 20% protein) glycemic load. The authors reported that at the end of the study no significant differences were seen between the two groups in body weight, body fat, resting metabolic rate, hunger, or satiety. After 12 months, the percent changes in body weight were –7.81% and –8.04% and in body fat were –17.9% and –14.8% in the low and high glycemic load groups, respectively (18). Results for weight loss were similar in another study comparing hypocaloric diets while varying the type (low vs. high glycemic index) of carbohydrate ingested (70).

Conversely, de Rougemont and colleagues (68) reported that in a five-week study, people in the group that ingested a low glycemic index diet lost significantly more weight (–1.1 vs. –0.3 kg [–2.4 vs. –0.7 lb]) than the group that consumed a high glycemic index carbohydrate diet. Regarding fat loss, neither group lost a significant amount of fat (0.17 vs. 0.04 kg [0.37 vs. 0.09 lb]) during the five-week intervention, and no significant difference was seen between the groups (68). Bouche and colleagues (8) also demonstrated in a five-week study that a low glycemic index diet compared with a high glycemic index diet led to a significant decrease in fat mass (0.7 kg [1.5 lb]), as well as a statistical trend toward gaining lean muscle mass, without actually changing body weight.

Although not all research agrees, note that other positive effects of a low glycemic index diet have been reported. Specifically, an increase in satiety (4), an improvement in lipid profile (decreased low-density lipoprotein and total cholesterol) (68), and enhanced insulin and glucose control (12, 67) have been observed with a low- versus a high-glycemic diet. Athletes often are encouraged to ingest high-glycemic carbohydrate to enhance glycogen resynthesis after exercise, which may also have an effect on weight loss and lean muscle mass changes during a period of dieting. Unfortunately, much of the published research in this area is conflicting. Thus, more research is needed to allow conclusions about whether a high or a low glycemic index diet is more efficacious for improving body composition and weight loss in an athletic population.

Fat ingestion remains an area of scientific investigation, and at this point specific recommendations regarding fat intake remain elusive. Concerning body composition, Strychar (76) has reported that a reduction in overall fat ingestion in a weight-loss program is beneficial, but the optimal percentage is not fully agreed on by scientists. Nevertheless, the 2009 position stand of the American Dietetic Association, Dietitians of Canada, and the American College of Sports Medicine on nutrition and athletic performance gives some guidance pertaining to fat intake (67). One point made in the position is that "Fat intake should be sufficient to provide the essential fatty acids and fat-soluble vitamins, as well as contribute energy for weight maintenance" (p. 709). Another is that "Fat intake should range from 20% to 35% of total energy intake. Consuming ≤20% of energy from fat does not benefit performance" (p. 710). Fat is an important part of athlete's diets because it is a source of energy, fat-soluble vitamins, and essential fatty acids (67). For more information on fat intake and athletic performance, refer to chapter 5.

In conclusion, hypocaloric diets such as VLCD and LCD can lead to significant weight loss. These diets, however, are not generally advised for athletes because performance and recovery may suffer dramatically (20, 34). Hypocaloric diets that are relatively high in carbohydrate and low in fat have been shown to decrease body fat and improve body composition. But the optimal amount of fat in the diet to promote weight loss is still unclear. Furthermore, whether high- or low-glycemic carbohydrate or the glycemic load affects weight loss remains debated. People engaging in high-intensity training have different needs than sedentary or minimally active adults. Specifically, intense activity is primarily fueled by skeletal muscle carbohydrate (which is burned for energy during the process of glycolysis). For this reason, those engaged in high-intensity training need higher levels of carbohydrate in the diet.

High-Protein Diets

High-protein diets, often with concomitant carbohydrate restriction, have gained a lot of attention and become quite popular as a means to lose weight, improve body composition, curb hunger, and improve certain blood lipid profiles and insulin sensitivity (3, 9, 26, 35, 59). Published research findings demonstrate that diets higher in protein most likely aid in weight loss because of the satiating and thermic effect of protein (10). In fact, Johnston and colleagues (38) demonstrated that the thermic effect of a meal containing relatively high protein (30% of energy as complex carbohydrate, 10% as simple sugar, 30% as protein, and 30% as fat), on average, was nearly two times greater than that of a high-carbohydrate meal containing equal calories (i.e., isocaloric) (50% of energy as complex carbohydrate, 10% as simple sugar, 15% as protein, and 25% as fat).

An additional suggestion is that people who consume higher-protein diets are more likely to eat less at subsequent meals because of the satiating effects of protein (32). Specifically, eating a high-protein meal has resulted in consuming 12% (5) and 31% (44) fewer calories at the next meal. One reason that higher-protein diets may be more satiating than high-carbohydrate diets is that protein, as opposed to fat and carbohydrate, is a relatively strong stimulator of the satiating gastrointestinal hormone cholecystokinin (CCK) (38). Elevated CCK levels have been shown to inhibit food intake in both rats and humans (9).

Researchers in Denmark showed that when participants on a high-protein diet (46% carbohydrate, 25% protein, 29% fat) or a high-carbohydrate diet (59% carbohydrate, 12% protein, 29% fat) ate ad libitum (i.e., as much as they wanted), those on the high-protein diet consumed significantly fewer calories over the course of the study (71). Moreover, the high-protein diet group lost significantly more weight than the participants on the high-carbohydrate diet. Specifically, participants on the high-protein and high-carbohydrate diets lost 8.9 and 5.1 kg (19.6 and 11.2 lb) of body weight and 7.6 and 4.3 kg (16.8 and 9.5 lb) of fat, respectively (71). Layman and colleagues (45) examined the effects of two different hypocaloric (~1,700 kcal/day) isoenergetic diets with varying carbohydrate-to-protein ratios on body composition. One of the diets had a carbohydrate-to-protein ratio of 3.5 (providing 68 g protein per day), and the other had a carbohydrate-to-protein ratio of 1.4 (providing 125 g protein per day). The two diets resulted in similar weight loss, but the diet that contained a greater percentage of protein led to greater fat loss, better lean muscle mass preservation, and ultimately improved body composition (45).

According to Brehm and D'Alessio (10), among studies lasting up to 12 months, randomized, controlled trials repeatedly demonstrate that high-protein diets are comparable, and possibly superior, to low-protein diets when it comes to weight loss, preservation of lean muscle mass, and improvement in several cardiovascular risk factors. Therefore, diets that moderately increase protein and modestly restrict carbohydrate and fat may have beneficial effects on body weight and body composition (9, 26).

As Kushner and Doerfler (42) point out in a review, long-term data continue to indicate that total weight loss does not differ significantly between low-carbohydrate dieters and low-fat dieters. Therefore, although not all research agrees, high-protein, low-carbohydrate diets may be better for weight loss and body composition in the short term, but long-duration studies suggest that the traditional lower-fat, higher-carbohydrate diets may be just as effective. Although diets higher in protein and lower in carbohydrate seem promising, scientists point out that the long-term effects of a high-protein diet on overall cardiovascular and metabolic health need to be studied (42). To date, however, most "high-protein" studies that evaluated the potential effects on cardiovascular risk profile actually show an improvement or reduced risk in comparison with traditional Western diets.

In conclusion, diets moderately higher in protein and slightly lower in carbohydrate appear to be beneficial when it comes to weight loss and improving body composition. Furthermore, increasing protein intake during weight loss at varying calorie intakes will prevent a negative nitrogen balance, which may also help lessen the loss of lean muscle mass and ultimately resting metabolic rate (74). Adequate carbohydrate intake, however, is also critical for several aspects of athletic performance and high-intensity exercise. Therefore, with physically active individuals, advocating a drastic decrease in carbohydrate intake is often unwise because this may adversely affect muscle glycogen stores and performance (16). Hypocaloric diets that restrict carbohydrate intake are probably not prudent during the competitive season if the sport relies on heavy carbohydrate usage, as do long- and middle-distance running, swimming, basketball, wrestling, and others. Variations of these diets, however, may be beneficial in promoting weight loss for athletes in the off-season. An important point is that weight loss should take place in a competitive athlete's off-season when possible. Because competitive performance is not a part of the off-season, attaining an ideal body weight and body composition through changes in dietary intakes at this time will not directly affect competitive performance.

Combining Diet and Exercise for Weight Loss

The research on whether the combination of aerobic exercise and a hypocaloric diet leads to (statistically significant) improvements in body composition versus a calorie-restricted diet alone remains somewhat equivocal. Nieman and colleagues (58) demonstrated that aerobic exercise (i.e., walking at 60%-80% of maximal heart rate) plus an energy-restricted diet did not lead to greater weight loss than a hypocaloric diet alone in obese individuals. Similarly, 30 minutes of moderate-intensity cycling performed three times a week for 16 weeks by sedentary men did not lead to greater improvements in body weight or body composition than a calorie-restricted diet alone (17). Kraemer and colleagues (40) have also reported that neither weight loss nor percent body fat during moderate caloric restriction was enhanced by the addition of aerobic exercise. Several other studies have also shown that the addition of aerobic exercise to a hypocaloric diet did not significantly enhance body composition or weight loss above that observed with dieting alone (17, 18, 21, 69).

Tips to Decrease Body Fat

1. If possible, attempt to reduce body fat in the off-season or pre-season.
2. Keep a record of all food and drink intake (record the amount and type of food consumed and feelings, times, and places associated with food intake).
3. The easiest way to decrease body fat is to alter the energy balance equation (i.e., create a negative energy balance).
4. For most athletes, reduce calories by approximately 500 per day (or ~20% below maintenance calories).
5. Reduce caloric intake by reducing the number of calories derived from fat in the diet. Maintain or slightly increase protein intake (protein recommendations are 1.8 to 2.7 g per kilogram body weight per day) when following a hypocaloric diet.
6. Assess body composition frequently to confirm that weight lost is coming from stored body fat and not lean muscle mass.
7. Make weight loss gradual to ensure maximum fat loss and preservation of lean muscle mass. For most athletes, a loss of 1 pound (0.45 kg) per week is optimal.

Unfortunately, many researchers making this comparison did not control energy deficits. In other words, in some of the investigations, the diet plus exercise group created a greater energy deficit than the diet-only group. Thus, it is difficult to make accurate comparisons from and interpretations of these studies or to draw conclusions about whether diet alone or diet plus exercise is superior for weight loss and body composition improvements. One study, however, by Redman and colleagues (64), did control energy deficits. Participants were randomized into one of three groups for six months:

- A control group placed on a weight maintenance diet
- A group placed on a 25% calorie restriction
- A group placed on caloric restriction (12.5% deficit) and aerobic exercise (12.5% deficit)

The authors reported that both energy-restricted groups lost approximately 10% of their overall body weight, 24% of their fat mass, and 27% of their visceral fat (64). They concluded that exercise plus caloric restriction was just as effective as caloric restriction alone with respect to body composition and fat mass. Both groups lost approximately 2 to 3 kg (~4 to 7 lb) of lean muscle mass, but the groups did not significantly differ from each other (64). The investigators also pointed out that the people who lost the weight with the addition of exercise realized added benefits such as enhanced aerobic fitness and improved cardiovascular health. To realize those health benefits, the recommendation is to combine modest dietary restriction with physical activity.

Resistance training (as compared with aerobic training) combined with a hypocaloric diet may be more promising regarding maintaining lean tissue and decreasing fat mass. After weight loss, people who performed resistance training, but not aerobic exercise, were able to preserve both lean muscle mass and resting metabolic rate (35). Frimel and colleagues (28) also demonstrated preservation of lean muscle mass when a progressive resistance training program was combined with a hypocaloric diet (as opposed to just dieting alone). Demling and DeSanti (19) studied the effects of a 12-week moderate hypocaloric, high-protein diet combined with resistance training on body composition, using two different protein supplements (whey and casein protein hydrosylates), and compared this combination with a hypocaloric diet alone. At the end of the study, all three groups lost approximately 2.5 kg (5.5 lb) of body weight (19). But the individuals using diet alone, diet and exercise plus casein, and diet and exercise plus whey protein decreased body fat from 27% to 25%, 26% to 18%, and 27% to 23%, respectively (19). The average fat loss was 2.5, 7.0, and 4.2 kg [5.5, 15.4, and 9.3 lb] in the three groups, respectively. Equally important, lean muscle mass did not improve in the diet-alone group but increased by 4 and 2 kg (8.8 and 4.4 lb) in the casein and whey groups, respectively (19). The information reported in this study is welcomed by athletes who need to lose body fat. Assuming that all athletes engage in resistance training (as they should) to improve functional strength on the playing field, this study also provides scientific support indicating that resistance training during dieting will assist the athlete in preserving lean muscle mass.

In some studies, however, resistance training combined with aerobic exercise and a hypocaloric diet did not lead to enhanced weight loss or improved body composition over diet alone (39). In addition, a four-week study that added resistance training to a VLCD consisting of approximately 812 kcal/day did not lead to the preservation of lean muscle mass or resting metabolic rate (30). This result, however, is most likely attributable to the fact that the VLCD provided only 40 g protein per day. The minimal amount of protein supplied in the diet was most likely not able to prevent excessive protein degradation (74).

Hypercaloric Diets

On the other end of the spectrum of body composition modification is the need or desire to gain weight, particularly lean muscle mass. If excess calories (i.e., a **hypercaloric diet**) are consumed by untrained individuals, even without resistance training, both fat mass and lean muscle mass accretion can occur (27). Moreover, initial body composition may play a role in the type of weight (fat vs. muscle) that is gained on a hyperenergetic diet. Forbes (27) stated in a review that the weight gain of thin people is composed of 60% to 70% lean muscle mass (in overfeeding studies lasting at least three weeks). Conversely, in obese people, only 30% to 40% of the weight gain was lean tissue.

If gaining lean muscle mass is the primary goal, two things must occur. First, an appropriate stimulus must be exerted on the skeletal muscles to enhance hypertrophy. This objective is generally achieved through performance of a consistent resistance training program. Second, more calories need to be consumed than are expended. The types of calories consumed may also influence the type of weight gained. As a general rule, to optimize lean muscle mass gain while also minimizing fat mass accretion, the increased caloric intake should come predominately from protein–amino acids and carbohydrate, with only minimal increases in fat (particularly saturated fat) consumption.

The combination of an appropriate anabolic stimulus (resistance exercise) and ingestion of adequate substrate (protein) results in a positive nitrogen balance. Positive nitrogen balance occurs when protein synthesis exceeds protein degradation (i.e., breakdown). Remember that for protein synthesis to occur in skeletal muscle, all 20 amino acids (particularly the essential amino acids), in proper amounts, must be present (7, 37). Thus, an adequate supply of amino acids must be consumed in the diet. The sidebar lists some general recommendations for enhancing lean muscle mass. Around 0.1 to 0.7 kg (0.25 to 1.5 lb) a week is a realistic weight-gain goal, although the percentage of actual lean muscle mass that can be gained is highly variable.

Tips to Increase Lean Muscle Mass

1. Consume a hypercaloric diet, approximately 10% to 15% above what is needed to maintain existing body weight.
2. Spread out daily caloric intake over five or six meals.
3. Engage in a consistent resistance training program.
4. Consume approximately 40% to 50% carbohydrate, approximately 30% protein, and approximately 20% to 30% fat. For additional calories, consume high-protein, high-fat foods.
5. Ingest adequate protein every day (~1.4-1.7 g per kilogram body weight per day).

Of all sports, few place as much emphasis on gaining lean muscle mass as bodybuilding. The current literature has clearly demonstrated that to increase lean muscle mass through overfeeding, protein intake should be emphasized as opposed to carbohydrate and fat (46). To optimize gains in lean muscle mass in an athletic population, protein intake should be higher than that recommended for a nonathletic population (2, 14). This recommendation would allow enough protein to optimize muscle growth without sacrificing carbohydrate and fat to allow optimal energy for high-intensity resistance training and adequate testosterone production in the body (43). Protein synthesis requires the use of adenosine triphosphate (ATP), so an energy-deficient diet may decrease protein synthesis. As a result, a slightly hyperenergetic diet, with an increase in energy intake of approximately 15% above what is required to maintain weight, is recommended to optimize muscle protein synthesis (i.e., hypertrophy) (43).

More recently, Campbell and colleagues (15) observed body composition differences among female physique athletes following two different diet regiments (high protein: 2.5 g per kilogram body weight per day and low to moderate protein: 0.9 g per kilogram body weight per day) in conjunction with a resistance training program. Following eight weeks of resistance training and an additional 400 kcals/day, the high-protein group demonstrated increased lean muscle mass when compared with those in the low-protein group. Although fat mass decreased in the high-protein group (−1.1 kg [−2.4 lb]), changes were similar to the low-protein group. These findings (15) further emphasize the recommendation to keep protein intake relatively high for athletes seeking to increase lean muscle mass while participating in a resistance training program.

Timing of the intake of macronutrients around a resistance training session may play a role in muscle hypertrophy and improving body composition. Tipton and colleagues (82) demonstrated that a preworkout intake of a carbohydrate and essential amino acid solution was more efficacious in promoting postworkout protein synthesis than ingesting the same mixture immediately after the session. The same group (80) then compared the effects of whey protein consumed before and after a resistance training bout to determine if the timing of intact, whole proteins would have a similar effect on protein synthesis as in the earlier study. Both the pre- and postworkout whey protein meals increased protein synthesis to an extent that was different, but not significantly so (80). Other researchers have also investigated the timing of protein intake and its effects on maximizing the anabolic stimulus of a resistance exercise bout (6, 54, 62, 65, 73, 75). For a complete discussion on the timing of protein and carbohydrate intake, refer to chapter 10.

How much protein should an athlete consume to promote increases in lean muscle mass? Currently, all experts do not agree. But the International Society of Sports Nutrition published a recent position stand on protein and exercise (36) that included the following findings:

- Vast research supports the contention that individuals engaged in regular exercise training require more dietary protein than sedentary people.

- To maintain a positive protein balance, exercising people should consume 1.4 to 1.7 g per kilogram body weight per day.

- Even higher protein intake (>3.0 g per kilogram body weight per day) may have beneficial effects on body composition, particularly lean muscle mass, when engaging in resistance exercise.

- To attain maximal stimulation of muscle protein synthesis, protein doses should contain a relatively high content of leucine.

- When part of a balanced, nutrient-dense diet, protein intakes at this level are not detrimental to kidney function or bone metabolism in healthy, active people.

A large-scale meta-analysis study encompassing 49 studies and over 1,800 participants found that protein supplementation in conjunction with prolonged resistance training significantly increased measures of muscle hypertrophy—up to a point. The authors reported that the beneficial effects of additional protein reached a threshold when total protein intakes exceeded approximately 1.6 g protein per kilogram body weight per day (51). Campbell and colleagues, however, found that when female physique athletes were supplemented with high protein (2.5 g per kilogram body weight per day), lean muscle mass increased compared with those supplemented with low protein (0.9 g per kilogram body weight per day) while both groups were enrolled in a resistance training program (14). Body fat decreased across the eight-week study, but changes were not different between the protein groups. Similarly, in a female collegiate dance population, in which dancers engaged in daily technique training, those who were supplemented for 12 weeks on a high-protein diet (2.2 g per kilogram body weight per day) improved **body composition index** (BCI) when compared with those consuming a lower-protein diet (0.9 g per kilogram body weight per day) (11). BCI reflects overall changes in body composition to provide a broader understanding of whole-body tissue changes. It is calculated by summing the difference in lean muscle mass from pre to post and fat mass from pre to post:

$$(LMM_{post} - LMM_{pre}) + (FM_{pre} - FM_{post})$$

The body composition changes in the female dancers occurred without significant changes in weight, which is a critical component to consider for an aesthetic athlete population.

The bottom line is that a slight increase in protein consumption does not appear to be harmful in healthy adults and may enhance training adaptations like muscle hypertrophy. Therefore, athletes may consider slightly increasing lean protein consumption when attempting to increase lean muscle mass and improve body composition. As discussed in chapter 4, a protein intake of 1.4 to 1.7 g per kilogram body weight per day is recommended. Athletes attempting to gain lean muscle mass should opt for the upper levels of this range. In conclusion, to increase body weight, athletes must consume a hyperenergetic diet. To emphasize lean muscle mass accretion, however, the hypercaloric diet should be combined with resistance training and a protein intake adequate to support protein synthesis.

Relative Energy Deficiency in Sport (RED-S)

In 2014, the International Olympic Committee (IOC) published a consensus statement introducing a broader, more comprehensive term for the previously known term **female athlete triad**, named **relative energy deficiency in sport** (RED-S) (53). One of the most notable differences between the female athlete triad and RED-S is that both males and females are included in RED-S. The female athlete triad is not only specific to females but also explains the connection between three specific symptoms that are interrelated: energy availability, menstrual function, and bone health. **Energy availability** (EA) is defined as the **energy intake** (EI) minus **exercise energy expenditure** (EEE) relative to lean muscle mass (LMM), and is summarized in the formula below:

$$EA = [EI \text{ (kcals)} - EEE \text{ (kcals)}]/LMM$$

Energy availability can become disrupted either when energy intake is not adequate or when exercise energy expenditure is heightened. RED-S expands on the three etiologies of the female athlete triad to include a wider array of physiological functions that can become impaired by **low energy availability** (LEA). Here is a list of some of the health consequences of RED-S:

- Immunological
- Gastrointestinal
- Cardiovascular
- Psychological (can either precede RED-S or be the result of RED-S)
- Growth and development
- Hematological
- Metabolic
- Endocrine
- Bone health
- Menstrual function

RED-S goes one step further to include potential performance effects from LEA. Here is a list of some of these potential effects:

- Decreased endurance performance
- Decreased muscle strength
- Decreased glycogen stores
- Depression
- Irritability
- Decreased concentration
- Decreased coordination
- Impaired judgement
- Decreased training response
- Increased injury risk

Therefore, new terminology was suggested to provide a more all-encompassing and accurate term for what was previously known as the female athlete triad. This proposal, however, created much initial controversy (24), leading to an IOC update in 2018 that provided updates on the scientific evidence of health and performance decrements of LEA (52). Additionally, debate continues about the energy availability threshold and whether one cutoff point can truly be applied to everyone. The current threshold for LEA is less than 30 kcal per kilogram lean muscle mass per day, which approximately equals average resting metabolic rate. A sliding scale range, however, may be more practical and appropriate to predict menstrual disturbances as opposed to one threshold value (23).

The female athlete triad and RED-S both stem from LEA or inadequate energy sources to support proper physiological functions for daily life and optimal athletic performance. The introduction of RED-S sought to provide a more comprehensive understanding of the deleterious effects that inadequate energy can have on the body as well as to be inclusive of the male population (31, 61, 86). Although most research in LEA has been conducted in a female population, males too have been reported to exhibit symptoms of LEA (47, 80). Sports that emphasize leanness or low body weight often have the greatest prevalence of athletes with LEA. Male athletes at greatest risk are those participating in gravitational sports (ski jumping), weight-class sports (wrestling), and non-weight-bearing sports (cycling). These athletes are at heightened risk for RED-S regardless of risk for disordered eating or eating disorders. Additionally, a variety of factors are thought to contribute to LEA in male athletes (13):

1. Body weight and composition cycling
2. Prolonged inadequate EI to meet high demands of exercise energy expenditure
3. Changes in training volume or intensity
4. Participation in strenuous aerobic endurance events

It is well established that LEA has detrimental effects on the female endocrine system, although the complex hormone interactions are still being investigated. It is primarily thought that LEA disrupts the gonadotropin-releasing hormone release in the hypothalamus, which further disrupts luteinizing hormone and follicle-stimulating hormone, both of which are necessary for proper release of estrogen and progesterone (29). This change in hormone release can lead to **amenorrhea**, the complete absence of menstruation. It is unknown what role the duration and severity of LEA play in disrupted menstrual function in the female population. Endocrine dysfunction in the male population has been studied much less in regards to LEA duration and severity when compared with females. Reduced luteinizing hormone as well as testosterone have been identified previously in different groups of male aerobic endurance athletes, although findings have not been consistent (25, 41, 49). Research has previously established a strong connection between altered menstrual function and decreased **bone mineral density** (BMD) in a female population. BMD is a measurement of density, which reflects the strength of bones. BMD is also an important predictor for whether a person is at risk for fracture in the future. Altered menstrual function and BMD place the female athlete at greater risk for bone stress and fracture injuries. Even short-term LEA has shown decreases in bone marker turnover in both males and females (5, 53). Athletes that engage in non-weight-bearing activity (i.e. swimmers, cyclists, jockeys) are at greater risk for decreased BMD because of the absence of mechanical loading in their sports.

Suggested treatment strategies for menstrual function restoration include weight gain, particularly through adequate protein and carbohydrate intake to restore glycogen and facilitate LH release (48). Weight gain may also support improved bone formation contributing to greater BMD, although full bone recovery may not always be possible. BMD can be greatly improved with mechanical loading, and therefore non-weight-bearing athletes or those with low BMD should implement resistance training at least two or three days per week (57). Dietary changes can also help to improve BMD. Vitamin D levels in the blood should be between 32 and 50 ng/ml with approximately 1,500 to 2,000 IU/day of vitamin D (33). If BMD is low, both dietary and exercise programming should be investigated further to optimize bone health for athletes.

Because of the previously discussed physiological health consequences of RED-S, a reasonable conclusion is that athletic performance can become impaired as a result of LEA. Performance is thought to become impaired by LEA through multiple indirect mechanisms such as impaired recovery, disruption of glycogen stores and suboptimal muscle protein synthesis (2, 72). Those participating in sport in a state of LEA are also at a high risk for illness and injury, which would directly affect performance if the athlete is not healthy enough to participate in training or competition. Woods and colleagues (88) demonstrated that with increased training load and no change in energy intake, reduced training recovery was observed, which the authors concluded could partially explain the deterioration in 5 km (3.1 mi) time-trial performance. Although evidence supports the notion that LEA can impair athletic performance, further intervention research is warranted to improve understanding of the variety of performance consequences as they relate to RED-S.

Reported Physiological Consequences of Low Energy Availability

1. Metabolic: Decreased resting metabolic rate (−111 ± 116 kcal) occurred following a four-week period of intensified training load with no subsequent increase in energy intake in elite rowers (88).

2. Cardiovascular: Endothelial dysfunction and abnormal lipid profiles have been previously reported in female athletes presenting with amenorrhea (66).

3. Gastrointestinal: In severe cases of LEA with diagnosed eating disorders, various alterations have been reported including sphincter function, delayed gastric emptying, and constipation (60).

4. Immunological: Respiratory tract infections, body aches, and head-related symptoms were reported in Australian Olympic athletes with LEA (25).

5. Psychological: Drive for thinness score is an indicator of energy deficiency and related to ineffectiveness, cognitive restraint, and bulimic tendencies (22).

Professional Applications

When attempting to optimize body composition, athletes seek either to increase lean muscle mass or to lose body fat. Although a plethora of scientific studies provide details on how to lose or gain body weight, some of these approaches are not appropriate for athletes. For instance, athletes who ingest a hypocaloric diet (eating fewer calories than needed) will lose weight, but a significant proportion of the weight lost will be from lean tissue if the protein intake is not sufficiently adjusted and if the resistance training program is not maintained. Additionally, athletes would place themselves at risk for RED-S if participating in a hypocaloric diet, which may result in a variety of detrimental health and performance outcomes. Similarly, a hypercaloric diet (eating more calories than needed) will cause weight gain, and a large proportion of the weight gain may be in the form of body fat if the athlete's resistance training and conditioning programs are not adjusted accordingly.

Athletes attempting to lose weight can do one of two things—either increase their physical activity or decrease their caloric intake. Assuming that athletes are already engaged in weight training, sport skills training, and conditioning, the option of increasing physical activity must be balanced against the risk of exhibiting symptoms of overtraining syndrome. Therefore, decreasing caloric intake is often recommended for athletes wishing to lose weight. This method must be done carefully, however, because decreasing energy intake may place the athlete at greater risk for overtraining, losing hard-earned lean muscle mass, and RED-S. To maximize fat loss and prevent the loss of lean muscle mass, dieting athletes must participate in a consistent resistance training program. In addition, as calories are reduced, the reduction should come primarily from carbohydrate and fat, and protein intake should not be limited to a large extent. Although this approach will help maximize fat loss and preserve lean muscle mass, training intensity and exercise performance may suffer because of the reduced carbohydrate intake. For this reason, weight-loss programs should be undertaken in the off-season (so that competitive performance is not sacrificed) whenever possible.

Athletes attempting to gain weight (in the form of lean muscle mass) should adhere to two simple rules: (1) Follow a consistent resistance training program and (2) consume more calories than are expended. These two simple rules serve as the blueprint for gaining lean muscle mass. More specifically, the increased caloric intake should come predominately from protein and carbohydrate, with only minimal increases in fat. This intake will optimize gains in lean muscle mass while minimizing fat mass accretion. To what extent should calories be increased above maintenance levels? Approximately 15% above maintenance levels is a good place to begin. For instance, if a female basketball player wishes to gain lean muscle mass and her caloric intake is 2,100 kcal to maintain her current weight, then the advice would be to increase her caloric intake to 2,415 kcal. But body composition should be monitored during this time to make sure that weight gain is manifesting itself primarily as lean muscle mass, not body fat. In addition to changes in caloric intake, creatine monohydrate supplementation has been shown to promote significant gains in lean muscle mass and its use should be considered.

Summary Points

- When attempting to lose weight (in the form of body fat), athletes and physically active people should decrease caloric intake but keep protein intake at 1.8 to 2.7 g per kilogram body weight per day.

- When athletes are attempting to gain weight (in the form of lean muscle mass), ingesting approximately 15% calories above maintenance levels is a good place to begin.

- Whether the goal is to lose body fat or increase lean muscle mass, athletes need to follow a well-designed, consistent resistance training program.

- Whether the goal is to lose or gain weight, changes in body composition should be monitored so that the dietary plan and resistance training program can be adjusted if undesirable changes are occurring (i.e., weight loss is occurring with too much loss of lean muscle mass; weight gain is occurring with too much gain of body fat).

- Chapters 2 and 11 discuss how to determine nutritional needs and how to develop a nutrition plan.

- RED-S is a syndrome that describes the many consequences of low energy availability including menstrual function, bone health, cardiovascular health, metabolism, immunology, mental health, and gastrointestinal health. RED-S is inclusive of both males and females and includes performance consequences because of changes in physiology.

Chapter 2

Nutritional Needs Analysis

Marie A. Spano, MS, RD, LD, CSCS, CSSD

Before working with an athlete to develop an individual nutrition plan, the sport nutrition professional must assess the athlete's current body composition, weight history, diet history, and current diet. In addition, current lab work or bone density scans are valuable tools that can aid in developing a plan tailored specifically to the athlete.

Weight and weight history both provide a glimpse into an athlete's nutrition status and any weight struggles they may have or may have had in the past. An accurate body composition measure, however, tells a lot more than the scale does. By tracking body composition changes over time, the sport nutrition professional can determine if the athlete is maintaining or moving toward a body composition range that is both healthy and beneficial for their specific sport. Body composition changes can help the professional assess if the athlete is gaining, maintaining, or losing lean muscle mass.

In addition to assessing body composition, the sport nutrition professional needs to analyze the athlete's diet. The best way to do this is to have the athlete keep a detailed food record for a minimum of three days by writing down what they consumed after each meal and snack. An accurate, detailed food record can be analyzed through use of a number of nutrition programs to gauge average intake of both macronutrients and micronutrients from food.

Measuring Body Composition

Coaches and athletes alike often place at least some emphasis on **body composition** (an assessment of fat mass as compared with lean muscle mass), especially in sports in which speed and aerobic endurance are critical for success (e.g., running), sports with weight classes (e.g., wrestling), and aesthetic sports (figure skating, gymnastics, diving, and so on). Because measures of body composition can affect how athletes feel about their bodies (potentially promoting eating-disordered behavior), as well as how a coach designs an athlete's workout program, accurate tools must be used to measure body composition and a professional well versed in body composition must interpret the results (in the context of health and the athlete's sport) for the athlete.

Research settings use many methods of body composition: dual-energy X-ray absorptiometry (DEXA), underwater weighing, skinfold calipers, bio-electrical impedance analysis (BIA), dilution techniques, air displacement plethysmography (Bod Pod), near-infrared interactance, ultrasound, magnetic resonance imaging (MRI), and magnetic resonance spectroscopy (MRS). These differing techniques vary in the body components measured, which may include fat, lean muscle mass, bone mineral content, total body water, extracellular water, total adipose tissue and its subdepots (visceral, subcutaneous, and intramuscular), skeletal muscle, select organs, and ectopic fat depots (15). Field measures commonly used include body mass index (BMI), skinfolds, and BIA because these tools are most convenient.

Laboratory Measures

Laboratory measures for assessing body composition are typically more accurate than field measures but also more costly and time consuming; therefore, they are used in the lab rather than in a field setting. The **Bod Pod**, an egg-shaped device that an athlete sits in for assessment of body composition, uses air displacement plethysmography to measure body density (from mass and volume). The Bod Pod obtains body weight from a weighing scale and obtains body volume by first measuring the interior of the empty chamber and then taking this measure again with the person inside. Densitometric principles are used to derive body composition measures from body density (18). This method divides the body into two compartments, fat and lean muscle mass. The dense, lean muscle mass compartment consists of protein, water, mineral, and glycogen, whereas the fat compartment consists of fat.

The Bod Pod is noninvasive and easy to use, and the measurement takes about 5 minutes. The Bod Pod offers other benefits:

- It is comfortable for the person being measured (unless the person is claustrophobic).
- Operation does not require a technician license.
- The machine is mobile (can be rolled to other locations).
- It can accommodate people up to 7 feet tall (2.1 m) and 550 pounds (250 kg).

As a relatively newer technology, Bod Pod has been compared with other, well-established methods of measuring body composition. In a study comparing Bod Pod with DEXA, 160 men (32 ± 11 years) had their body composition measured with both machines. Percent body fat measures were 19.4 ± 6.8 and 21.6 ± 8.4 for DEXA and the Bod Pod, respectively. The two methods were highly correlated, but the mean difference of 2.2% was significant ($p<0.01$). The difference between the two instruments was also greater as body fatness increased (1). This study showed that differences will exist depending on the method used to assess body composition. Therefore, if an athlete is being tested with different measures over time, measured differences in body composition may not be completely accounted for by increases or decreases in body fat.

In a group of Division I female collegiate track and field athletes ($N = 30$), Bod Pod measures were compared with hydrostatic weighing, DEXA, and skinfold calipers. In this study, Bod Pod significantly overestimated body fat in comparison with hydrostatic weighing, and Bod Pod values also differed significantly from those obtained by DEXA. Body fat measured by skinfolds did not differ significantly from body fat measured by Bod Pod. If skinfold values do not differ significantly in this population, using this method would be a more cost-effective way to measure body composition than Bod Pod (4). Another study found the use of skinfold calipers equivalent to Bod Pod. In this study, percent body fat values as obtained by Bod Pod were validated against hydrostatic weighing in 30 high school boys. Body fat was also measured with near-infrared interactance, BIA, and skinfold calipers and compared with hydrostatic weighing. Both near-infrared interactance and BIA produced significant constant error and total error. Bod Pod produced acceptable total error values but significantly higher constant error than hydrostatic weighing, indicating that it is an acceptable choice for measuring body composition but no better than the use of skinfold calipers (20).

Dual-energy X-ray absorptiometry (DEXA) works by emitting X-rays (containing low radiation dosage) at two discrete energy levels, which are collimated into a beam and directed into the body posteriorly to anteriorly (14). DEXA is based on the basic principle that a beam of X-rays passed through a complex material attenuates the beam in proportion to the composition, thickness, and individual components of the material. Therefore, when energy from an X-ray source passes through the human body, it experiences greater reduction in intensity when it interacts with bone than it does with soft tissue (14). DEXA is quick, noninvasive, accurate, and reproducible. As with all methods of assessing body composition, DEXA has benefits and drawbacks. For instance, athletes can have wide fluctuations in body water because of large sweat losses and underhydration. Any fluctuation like this in body water will show up as lower lean muscle mass on DEXA (and other measures of body composition) because lean muscle mass is composed of 70% to 75% of total body water (7). In addition, rapid weight loss leads to a decrease in glycogen content. Carbohydrate is stored with 1.5 to 3 g of water as glycogen in the liver and muscle. By depleting glycogen stores, lean muscle mass will be lower, thereby increasing body fat percent (7).

Regardless of the method used to assess body composition in athletes, changes in body composition, along with body weight, must be monitored over time when altering an existing nutrition or exercise program. By measuring body composition, along with body weight, the coach or trainer can effectively determine what type of weight (i.e., muscle, fat, or water) is being lost or gained.

Field Methods

Field methods for assessing body composition are those that are portable and easy to use for assessment of several people in a short time. How do these measures compare, and what are the major differences between them? Sport nutritionist professionals use several common field measures. Body mass index is a simple calculation:

$$\text{weight in kilograms} / \text{height in meters}^2$$
$$([\text{weight in pounds} / \text{height in inches}^2] \times 703)$$

The resulting number categorizes the person as underweight, normal weight, overweight, or obese. Body mass index is a convenient way to measure obesity rates in a population but should not be used by itself to categorize an individual. Table 2.1 lists the BMI categories.

The National Health and Nutrition Examination Survey (NHANES), a survey research program started in 1959 and directed by the Department of Health and Human Services (a federal government agency), measures BMI in the physical examination component of the survey (both physical exams and interviews are used). The NHANES assesses the health and nutrition status of adults and children in the United States and tracks changes over time to determine the prevalence of disease and risk factors for disease (22).

Measuring BMI is noninvasive and requires only an accurate scale and stadiometer (for measuring height). The downside to BMI is that it does

TABLE 2.1   Classifications of BMI

Classification	BMI (kg/m^2)
Underweight	<18.5
Normal range	18.5-24.9
Overweight	25-29.9
Obese	≥30

Note: This chart has been simplified to show the major categories.

Adapted from World Health Organization. BMI Classification. www.who.int/bmi/index.jsp?introPage=intro_3.html

not assess actual body composition or distinguish between fat and muscle tissue. Because muscle has greater density than fat and weighs more than fat per volume of tissue, BMI tends to overestimate body fat levels in muscular people (31). It can also overestimate body fat in individuals with large body frames (21). For example, a professional running back who is 5 feet 9 inches (1.75 m) tall, weighs 210 pounds (95.5 kg), and has 8% body fat would have a BMI of 31.2. This BMI classifies him as obese. At 8% body fat, however, the athlete is not obese or overfat. The example illustrates a limitation of using BMI in athletes.

Although BMI may overestimate body fat in muscular individuals, it may underestimate body fat in other populations (2, 8). A study conducted using NHANES data showed that BMI cannot accurately diagnose obesity, especially in men and the elderly as well as people with intermediate BMI ranges. Therefore, BMI should only be used to assess population-based rates of obesity and not an individual's status (24). Despite limitations inherent with BMI, it is a useful tool for large population-based studies. Research examining deaths from all causes in 1.46 million adults found that a BMI between 20 to 24.9 is associated with the lowest risk of death in nonsmoking adults. Risk of death increases with increasing levels of overweight and obesity (6). Body mass index is a tool best used to estimate population-based rates of weight correlated to height and not to assess obesity or underweight in single individuals in a clinical setting in the absence of other clinical measures (11).

Trainers and coaches commonly turn to **skinfold calipers** for assessing body composition. Skinfold calipers measure skinfold thickness at various sites on the body. The technician takes measures by grasping a fold of skin and subcutaneous fat with the thumb and forefingers, pulling the fold away from the underlying muscle, pinching it with the caliper, and taking the reading within 2 seconds.

A three-site skinfold is commonly done, and it includes the chest, abdomen, and thigh on men and triceps, suprailiac, and thigh on women (figure 2.1). The five most common sites assessed include triceps, subscapular, suprailiac, abdomen, and thigh (19). Chest and biceps are additional sites that are sometimes used. The skinfold measures (which should be taken two or three times at each site and then averaged) are then incorporated into equations to predict percent body fat. These are the main advantages of skinfold calipers:

- They are easy to use (after the person is well trained in the technique).
- They do not require much time per person.
- They are noninvasive and inexpensive.

The use of skinfold calipers, however, has several disadvantages. These include interperson variability (if body fat is measured by one person and

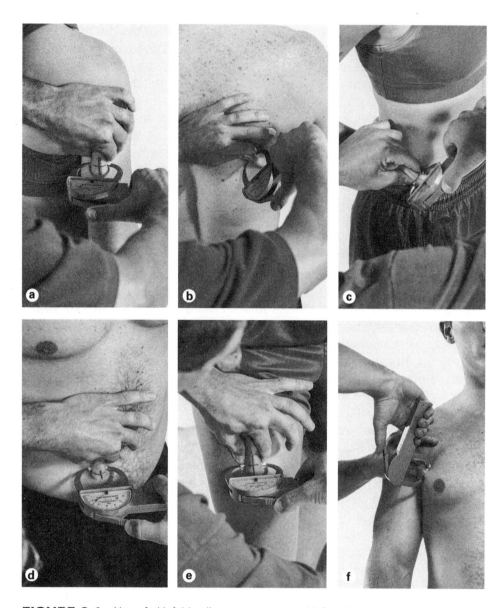

FIGURE 2.1   Use of skinfold calipers to measure skinfold thickness at the *(a)* triceps, *(b)* subscapular, *(c)* suprailiac, *(d)* abdominal, *(e)* upper thigh, and *(f)* chest.

then months later by another person) and less accuracy when less expensive calipers are used. In addition, over 100 different equations are used to estimate body fat from calipers, and people measure different sites among the seven. All these factors can lead to errors in reliability, validity, or both. An accurate measure of body composition using skinfold calipers is within ±3% to 5% error of **hydrostatic weighing** (19).

Hydrostatic weighing (underwater weighing) is a method of measuring body composition whereby the subject is submerged into a tank of water and body composition is determined based on total body density using Archimedes' principle of displacement (the weight of displaced water can be found mathematically). Underwater weighing assumes that the densities of fat mass and lean muscle mass are constant, that lean tissue is denser than water, and that fat tissue is less dense than water (12).

Bioelectrical impedance measures the impedance to the flow and distribution of a radiofrequency, alternating current (5). Both water and electrolytes influence the impedance of the applied current; therefore, BIA measures total body water and then indirectly determines lean muscle mass from this measure (25). Bioelectrical impedance is convenient, cost effective, and quick; and operation requires little knowledge. But this method cannot accurately measure short-term changes in body composition, nor can it accurately assess body composition in obese people (in whom it may underestimate body fat) and very lean people (in whom it may overestimate body fat) (27). Finally, small changes in fluid balance can affect the measurements (25).

Ultrasound

The use of ultrasound to measure fat thickness in humans dates back nearly 50 years (30). Despite the history of ultrasound being used to measure subcutaneous adipose tissue, this technology has not been popularized for assessing body composition until recently (30). Ultrasonography is a noninvasive, quick, and relatively inexpensive alternative for assessing body fat levels (3). Ultrasound technology for body composition works with a probe that transmits a high-frequency (typically 1-5 mhz) sound pulse into the body. These sound pulses reflect, or echo off, tissue interfaces (fat–muscle interface, muscle–bone interface) and back to the probe. The distance from the probe to the tissue boundaries is calculated by measuring the time of each echo's return. The ultrasound screen can display the distances of the echoes, forming a two-dimensional image. Ultrasound technology has been used to estimate body composition in athletic populations. Research has reported that ultrasound technology is comparable with both DEXA (23) and underwater weighing (29).

Recording and Analyzing Food Intake

Before analyzing an athlete's diet, the sport nutrition professional needs to know what the athlete is eating on a daily basis. Methods commonly used to examine what an athlete is eating include dietary recalls and diet records. Although diet records (clients keep a running record of the specific foods and beverages they have consumed, including the amounts of each and how the food is prepared) are preferable to recalls because people often forget what they eat, diet records have limitations as well. The mere act of keeping a diet record makes people change their typical eating habits. In addition, some people are embarrassed by their food or drink consumption and therefore leave out crucial details because of shame. For instance, an American football player who drinks 18 beers on a weekend night might record only 6 of those beers. Another tool that some people use is a camera phone. They snap a picture of their meal and send it to their sport dietitian. A photo, however, does not provide complete details regarding how a food was prepared or the quantities of food consumed. Despite the drawbacks of dietary recalls and food records, these tools are among the best available for helping the sport nutrition professional assess an athlete's dietary intake. Form 2.1 on page 35 is a template that athletes could use for a three-day dietary recall.

Some sport nutrition professionals can examine diet records and quickly spot areas of low intake (e.g., no dairy would signal the likelihood of a shortfall in both calcium and vitamin D). A computerized analysis program, however, can accurately assess every component of the diet.

Food intake is typically analyzed through a food analysis program or with use of a food frequency questionnaire. A food analysis program requires a 24-hour dietary recall, a three-day diet record, or a seven-day diet record (the more days analyzed and averaged, the more accurate the analysis of dietary intake). Food analysis programs can help determine a person's intake of macronutrients, micronutrients, and certain food components such as omega-3 fatty acids. A food frequency questionnaire asks how often a person eats certain foods (how many times per day, week, month, or year, for instance). Researchers commonly use food frequency questionnaires to measure the frequency and total intake of certain foods and correlate intake with disease risk. For instance, epidemiology studies often use food frequency questionnaires to examine how dietary intake relates to risk of chronic diseases such as cancer (28).

A variety of programs, on both computers and phone apps, analyze food intake. Although dietitians can be granted access to their client's food-tracking information, entirely separate and more robust software programs have been developed for dietitians and nutrition researchers to analyze food intake.

Nutrition Tracking Programs for Consumers

The basic programs that are free and that allow people to track their food intake can help an athlete stay within a certain calorie or macronutrient range. Many are free, although some start off free with paid upgrades. Because of advances in technology, the fact that over three-quarters of the U.S. population own a smartphone, and the convenience of smartphones compared with computers—tracking by mobile phones has taken over from web-based programs. Many software programs have benefits, aside from just calculating calorie intake, to keep users engaged, such as charting changes in weight over time, comparing calories burned through physical activity with dietary intake, and providing sample diets for specific calorie levels (1,200, 1,500, 1,800, 2,000, 2,200, and so on).

Smartphone apps are a cost-effective way to promote healthy eating and weight loss. But only a modest number of randomized controlled trials have examined the effectiveness of smartphone apps for weight loss, and none has used athletes. From the research to date it appears that the decrease in BMI from using these apps is modest (10). Although some apps rely on self-entered data from users, which may be incorrect, the accuracy of nutrition measurements on mobile devices is generally good (9).

Despite the upside of food-tracking apps, keep in mind that all rely on the user to produce an accurate log of the type and amount of food consumed. Also, without guidance, consumers need to have a basic understanding of macronutrients and calorie needs. Many programs also have preset macronutrient goals that users need to adjust based on their own needs, which requires an in-depth understanding of nutrition. The best approach is to work with a sport nutrition professional who can help the consumer adjust macronutrients and calories after careful consideration of the person's weight history, goals, food preferences, eating habits, and factors that influence health, athletic performance, and recovery.

Although food tracking can be helpful for many consumers, research suggests that tracking can do more harm than good in those with history of an eating disorder or at risk for an eating disorder. In one study examining the use of the app MyFitnessPal in those with eating disorders, 73.1% of participants said that MyFitnessPal contributed at least somewhat to their eating disorder, and 30.3% said that it contributed very much to their eating disorder. In addition, the more likely a person was to report that usage of MyFitnessPal contributed to their eating disorder, the more likely it was that the person had eating disorder symptoms. Because this study is retrospective and relied on self-reported data, it cannot be used to say that MyFitnessPal causes symptoms of an eating disorder (16). Another study in men found nearly 40% of users perceived MyFitnessPal as a factor contributing to their disordered eating symptoms to some extent. MyFitnessPal users also reported greater psychosocial impairment than nonusers (17). Yet another study with 493 college students found that fitness tracking was uniquely associated with eating disorder symptomatology after adjusting for bingeing and purging behavior in the past month as well as gender (26). In conclusion, it may make sense to screen people for eating disorder symptoms before suggesting they use a calorie-tracking app. Table 2.2 provides a summary of phone apps and computer-based programs for tracking food intake.

TABLE 2.2 Consumer-Based Internet and Mobile-Based Food-Tracking Programs

Program	Internet or mobile app?	Fee?	Capabilities
Lose It!	Mobile app	Basic program is free. Advanced program costs a fee.	The basic program includes the following: Search, scan, or snap a photo to log food intake Calorie tracking Exercise tracking Community access
Fat Secret	Internet and mobile app	No	Food tracking Exercise tracking Community forum Recipes Challenges
MyFitnessPal	Internet and mobile	Basic program is free. The premium program is ad free, contains exclusive content, priority customer support, macronutrient goals, and more.	Food tracking Support and motivation Exercise tracking Community forum
Life Sum	Mobile	Yes	Calorie counter Barcode scanner Exercise tracker Recipes Habit trackers Personalized programs Weight-loss programs
My Plate	Mobile	No	Goal setting Food tracking Support Education
Cron-o-Meter	Internet and mobile	No	Food tracking Exercise tracking Biometrics Forums
Fitday	Internet and mobile	Free	Food tracker Exercise tracker Weight tracker Goal setting
Sparkpeople	Internet and mobile	Free	Food tracker Exercise tracker Goal tracker Recipes Goal setting Challenges Message boards
Calorie King	Internet and mobile	Free	Food tracker Weight-loss programs Recipes Articles

Programs available as of August 2020.

Professional Software Programs

Nutrition professionals in university settings also commonly use software programs for research purposes. The differences between free Internet-based software programs and professional programs may be vast. Professional programs typically have a large database of foods, and they analyze food intake for more than just calories and macronutrient levels. Professional programs can also tally up a client's intake of specific fatty acids, micronutrients, caffeine, and other diet variables. Professional software programs also differ from most free programs in that they provide more detailed, thorough reports that often come in several formats (pie charts, line graphs, and so on). These programs are designed for the nutrition professional or researcher who needs in-depth analysis of a client's or subject's intake.

• **FoodWorks** is a Windows-based software program designed for professionals working in nutrition research, nutrient database development, dietetics, client counseling, fitness and weight control, food service, recipe development, health care, and nutrition education. FoodWorks can analyze meals, recipes, and menu cycles and lets the user choose from four dietary standards: Dietary Reference Intakes (DRIs), dietary values, Canadian RNI, and Food and Agriculture Organization of the United Nations and World Health Organization. FoodWorks also lets clients create diet recalls and submit them to their nutrition professional for analysis. The program offers many different printouts.

• **Dine Healthy 7** (Dine Systems Inc.) is an exercise and dietary analysis software program. The food database contains generic, fast-food, and brand-name items.

• **ESHA Food Processor Standard** analyzes food intake with a food database of over 100,000 foods and provides a variety of graphs and reports including popular foods, ingredients, restaurant items, and recipes. Their database analyzes more than 172 nutritional components including nutrients, amino acids, diabetic exchanges, and MyPlate food groups. Their exercise database includes over 933 activities and reports METs. Food Processor can also be used to analyze recipes. Many professional reports can be printed from the data in Food Processor, which has been in business since 1984.

• **NutriBase** has an extensive food database that includes more than 800,000 foods including more than 148,000 restaurant items, more than 540,000 brand name foods, and the ability to locate more than 500,000 UPC and bar code items. NutriBase can analyze recipes and scale recipes. Meals, recipes, and meal plans are exportable to other NutriBase users. NutriBase has a variety of report options that can be customized to include only specific nutrients, comments, recommendations, and more.

• **Nutritionist Pro Diet Analysis Software** can be used to create diets, analyze a 24-hour recall, and produce a food frequency questionnaire. It can also be used to assess exercise and help clients plan goals, build recipes, and create menus that match goals. It comes with an array of reports.

Keeping a food log or diary can help enhance weight-loss efforts in overweight and obese individuals. In one four-center randomized trial with 1,685 total participants, keeping a daily food record led to twice as much weight loss as not keeping a record (13). Aside from making people accountable for their food intake, food diaries entered into a diet analysis program and reviewed by a nutrition professional can provide in-depth insight into micronutrient intake, which is essential for troubleshooting nutrition-related problems such as anemia and hyponatremia. In addition, a **diet analysis** can help pinpoint areas where an athlete may need to alter intake for health reasons. A diet analysis is a comparison of a person's typical dietary intake with research-based recommendations based on the person's sport and training level as well as the DRIs.

Nutrient analysis programs provide a picture of a person's overall nutrition intake—information that can be examined in relation to health and athletic performance. Analyzing an athlete's diet for a few days every month while tracking weight and body composition changes can help the professional determine what dietary changes are needed to achieve the desired body composition. As a part of this process, working with the athlete to set goals for the nutrition program can be effective. Form 2.2 on page 38 can help athletes identify and track progress on their nutrition goals. Because food fuels athletic performance and an athlete's lean body weight and fat mass affect speed, power, and agility, dietary assessment programs and body composition analysis tools are both useful components in an athlete's training program.

Professional Applications

Before making specific, individualized sport nutrition recommendations to any athlete, the sport nutrition professional should gather as much information as possible. Weight, weight history, dieting history (including disordered eating or eating disorders), body composition, dietary intake, supplement intake, lab values, and a bone density assessment all provide useful information for creating a sport nutrition plan. The following are two examples, using hypothetical athletes, of how a sport nutrition professional would use assessment techniques and an understanding of the athlete's unique situation to develop an effective nutrition plan.

Anthony

A junior transfer football player, Anthony was sent to the sport nutritionist for help with losing weight. Anthony's body composition, as tested by skinfold calipers, was high for a linebacker at 24% (his body fat should be about 15%, according to averages for his position). He was asked to keep a three-day diet record (including one weekend day) and come back to the nutritionist a week later. Running those dietary records through a computerized diet analysis program clearly identified Anthony's problem areas. He consumed 40% of his calories from fat, ate too much fried food, drank quarts of juice every day, and averaged 12 beers on each weekend night. In addition, a plot of his weight history made it evident that his dietary habits had changed in college. Anthony's weight through high school had remained around 220 pounds (100 kg) but had increased steadily in the past two years to his current weight of 245 pounds (111 kg). He said that his mother had cooked all his meals during high school and that everything was planned out back then, whereas now he thought that his days were haphazard; he grabbed food here and there and did not always make the best choices. In addition, Anthony was overwhelmed by the number of food choices on campus—he had the option to eat basically anything, anytime he wanted.

In addition to gaining weight, Anthony mentioned that he felt tired all the time and sometimes reached for an energy drink in the middle of the day for the caffeine and sugar pickup. He knew he should not do this but was at a loss about how to change his lifestyle and diet so that he could feel better. Anthony often stayed up late, until 1 or 2 a.m., yet had a 7 a.m. class three days a week. Operating on little sleep, he went to class and then came home and slept for hours, woke up and consumed an energy drink, and went to practice. After practice, he showered, and twice a week he had night class. after which he ate dinner at about 9 p.m. On the weekends, his sleep and eating schedule was even more erratic. The night before games he tried to go to bed at 11 p.m. but could not fall asleep. On nongame nights he might stay up until 3 or 4 a.m. partying.

The sport nutritionist worked with Anthony to help him see where his lifestyle habits were contributing to poor eating choices. In addition, she covered the effect of alcohol on delaying recovery and potentially hampering his gains in the weight room as well as his daily intake of more than 600 kcal of juice. Anthony agreed to a few simple changes in his schedule, lifestyle, and eating habits, including going to bed by midnight on weeknights, scheduling classes no earlier than 9 a.m. next semester, and sleeping at least 8 hours per night. In addition, Anthony agreed to substitute a low-calorie beverage for the juice, cut his beer intake in half and consume that on only one night per weekend, limit his fried food to one time per week, cut out energy drinks, and work with the strength coach to increase his morning cardio sessions. Although he felt tired at first and had headaches for a few days after cutting out the energy drinks, Anthony continued to work hard to drop the extra body fat he had gained during college. His hard work and dedication paid off in increased playing time.

Samantha

A first-year gymnast named Samantha went to see the sport nutritionist at her university because she was concerned about trying to maintain a low weight to compete on a national level. In addition, she had recently experienced a

(continued)

Professional Applications (continued)

stress fracture in her foot. Measurement of her body composition by DEXA revealed that her body fat was 10% and her bone density was slightly below the average for her age. The sport nutritionist quickly realized that at 10% body fat, Samantha may have menstrual cycle irregularities, but she waited to see Samantha's food recall before making any assumptions. This athlete was fearful of gaining any weight because her coach maintained strict weight and body fat percent guidelines for each athlete on the team. A 24-hour recall revealed that Samantha was eating the same things every single day:

Breakfast—1/2 cup oatmeal

Snack—flavored coffee

Lunch—salad

Snack—fat-free frozen yogurt

Dinner—salad with grilled chicken and diet soda

The sport nutritionist saw several weak points in Samantha's diet. Her caloric intake was way too low (less than 1,000 kcal per day), she lacked most if not all vitamins and minerals (on a low-calorie diet the likelihood of missing vitamins and minerals is even greater), and she fell far short on calcium, vitamin D, and magnesium—all of which are necessary for building bone density and ensuring proper muscle function. Samantha's diet was also short on protein, carbohydrate, and quality fat. At this point, the sport nutritionist was concerned that Samantha could be amenorrhoeic or oligomenorrheic.

After talking with Samantha and getting an idea of her weight history, the sport nutritionist found out that she had weighed 15 pounds (6.8 kg) more in high school, had felt more energetic, and had been doing better at her sport. In addition, when she lost the first 10 pounds (4.5 kg), she stopped her menstrual cycle—putting her at risk for bone loss.

Samantha knew that she could be doing long-term damage to her body but was afraid of losing her scholarship. She said that when she came to school, she had been bigger than all the other gymnasts and that all of them ate very little food and had little body fat. Samantha was concerned that her coach would be unhappy if she gained any weight. She did not think she had an eating disorder per se but could not see how she could get out of her current eating behavior. The sport nutritionist asked Samantha if she would be willing to see a licensed clinical professional counselor in the community, explaining that the counselor regularly worked with clients who had a fear of gaining weight and faced challenges with body image and eating. The sport nutritionist reassured Samantha that she would not tell her coach and that several athletes had worked with the counselor on the same issues. Over the next year, Samantha worked hard at changing her body image and slowly adding calories and nutrients to her diet. Although her issues did not resolve immediately, she continued to work with the dietitian and counselor and was moving in a positive direction.

Summary Points

- Before working with an athlete to develop an individual nutrition plan, the sport nutrition professional should assess (at a minimum) the athlete's current body composition, weight history, diet history, current diet, food preferences and cooking skills.

- A variety of available body composition assessment tools differ in the particular body components measured, including fat, lean muscle mass, bone mineral content, total body water, extracellular water, total adipose tissue and its subdepots (visceral, subcutaneous, and intramuscular), skeletal muscle, select organs, and ectopic fat depots.

- The most common field measure used to assess body composition in athletes is skinfold calipers. After a person is trained, skinfold calipers are easy to use; the method is also quick, noninvasive, and inexpensive.

- Body mass index should not be used as a tool for assessing body composition in athletes; BMI does not assess actual body composition or distinguish between fat and muscle tissue.

- Laboratory measures for assessing body composition are typically more accurate than field measures, but they are also more costly and time consuming and are therefore used in the lab rather than a field setting. Typical lab measures include Bod Pod, DEXA, and underwater weighing.

- By comparing an athlete's diet analysis (as computed from a nutrition software program) with lab work and bone density scans, the sport nutrition professional can assess whether a physician should be involved to prescribe a specific nutrient that the athlete is deficient in (vitamin D or iron, for instance) or whether the sport nutrition professional can help the athlete make up for missing nutrients through dietary intake or dietary supplements.

Three-Day Diet Recall

Instructions: Please be as specific as possible when filling out this form. For example, write down condiments and amounts of foods rather than just a general description. Do not change what you are currently doing because you are keeping a record.

The goal of a three-day recall is to get a good look at what you are currently eating as a starting point for making dietary improvements.

Nondescript example: Cheeseburger and soda

Better example: McDonald's regular-size cheeseburger with lettuce and tomato slices. One packet mayonnaise. 12 ounces of Dr. Pepper.

DAY 1

Date: _____

Meal or snack and time	Food (how prepared and so on)

FORM 2.1

From National Strength and Conditioning Association, *NSCA's Guide to Sport and Exercise Nutrition,* 2nd ed. (Champaign, IL: Human Kinetics, 2021).

DAY 2

Date: _____

Meal or snack and time	Food (how prepared and so on)

DAY 3

Date: _____

Meal or snack and time	Food (how prepared and so on)

From National Strength and Conditioning Association, *NSCA's Guide to Sport and Exercise Nutrition,* 2nd ed. (Champaign, IL: Human Kinetics, 2021).

Goal-Setting Sheet for a Nutritional Plan

Instructions: As you are filling out this form, think about why you want to make a change and what motivates you.

1. My goals are:

   a. _____

      Date I'd like to achieve this by: _____

      Action plan (my plan to reach my goal; this part to be filled out during nutrition consultation): _____

      _____

   b. _____

      Date I'd like to achieve this by: _____

      Action plan (my plan to reach my goal; this part to be filled out during nutrition consultation):_____

      _____

   c. _____

      Date I'd like to achieve this by: _____

      Action plan (my plan to reach my goal; this part to be filled out during nutrition consultation):_____

      _____

2. What is motivating me to make changes to my diet? _____

   _____

3. How will these changes affect my performance and recovery? _____

   _____

4. How will I track my progress? (This part to be filled out during nutrition consultation.) _____

   _____

FORM 2.2

From National Strength and Conditioning Association, *NSCA's Guide to Sport and Exercise Nutrition,* 2nd ed. (Champaign, IL: Human Kinetics, 2021).

Chapter 3

Carbohydrate

JohnEric W. Smith, PhD, CSCS,*D, CISSN

Carbohydrates are compounds consisting of three types of atoms: carbon, hydrogen, and oxygen. As an example, the chemical formula for glucose (the sugar present in the blood as blood sugar) is $C_6H_{12}O_6$. Most human carbohydrate is provided by dietary plant sources. Some dietary carbohydrate, however, is found in animal products, and the liver can make carbohydrate using certain amino acids and components of fats such as glycerol.

Carbohydrates are used throughout the body in a myriad of functions. Energy derived from the catabolism, or breakdown, of carbohydrates ultimately powers many biological processes. Carbohydrates serve as a fuel for all tissues in the body but are critically important because nerve cells rely predominantly on carbohydrate and red blood cells rely solely on glucose. Under normal conditions, the brain uses the blood sugar *glucose* almost exclusively, and the body works to maintain the level of blood glucose within narrow limits to serve this function. Although nerve and red blood cells are critical for cardiovascular functions, muscle recruitment, and oxygen delivery, their carbohydrate requirements are not typically considered in the context of exercise metabolism.

The role of carbohydrate in fueling the contractile elements of muscle during sport and exercise is typically the focus of exercise scientists. Because of the rapid rate at which carbohydrate can be converted into energy, the reliance of skeletal muscle on carbohydrate as a fuel increases as intensity increases from rest to maximal levels (59). The role of carbohydrate in exercise can be observed through performance decrements as carbohydrate stores deplete and performance enhancements when carbohydrate supplementation is introduced.

Another role of carbohydrate oxidation (the breakdown of carbohydrate) is to serve as a carbon primer for fat entry into the Krebs cycle (also known as the tricarboxylic acid cycle). Fatty acid–derived two-carbon *acetyl-CoA*

The author would like to acknowledge the significant contributions of Donovan L. Fogt to this chapter.

(acetyl-coenzyme A) units combine with carbohydrate derivatives in the Krebs cycle, leading to fat oxidation. Without adequate Krebs cycle primers, optimal fat metabolism is not possible.

Types of Carbohydrate

Not all types of carbohydrate have the same form, function, and effect on exercise and sport performance. The basic, single-molecule unit of all carbohydrates is the monosaccharide. The dietary monosaccharides absorbed by humans all have six carbons; although they vary only slightly in chemical configuration, these subtle variations account for important metabolic differences. The number of monosaccharides bonded together provides the basis for classifying carbohydrates and enhances the functionality of carbohydrates in the body. The term *sugar* is commonly used to refer to both monosaccharides and disaccharides such as sucrose (also known as table sugar). The terms *complex carbohydrate* and *starch* are widely used to refer to longer chains, or polymers, of monosaccharides in plants and plant-derived foods like grains, breads, cereals, vegetables, and rice. The following sections discuss the terminology of carbohydrates found in the diet. Athletes need to understand the different types of carbohydrate and how they function in the body—which types quickly restore depleted muscle glycogen, which types maintain blood glucose levels during competition (essential for maintaining force production), and which types promote general health (i.e., cardiovascular and gut health).

Monosaccharides

In humans, the three dietary monosaccharide sugar molecules have similar arrangements of the hexose (six-carbon) chemical formula, $C_6H_{12}O_6$. These sugars are glucose, fructose, and galactose (figure 3.1). Glucose, also known as dextrose or blood sugar, is the most important monosaccharide in humans and the primary one used by human cells. This monosaccharide is readily absorbed from the diet, synthesized in the body from the digestion and conversion of the other monosaccharides, or liberated from more complex carbohydrate molecules called polysaccharides such as starch or glycogen. In addition, the process of **gluconeogenesis** creates glucose in the liver from carbon residues of other compounds such as amino acids, glycerol, pyruvate, and lactate.

After digestion, dietary glucose is absorbed from the small intestine into the blood to serve as an energy source for cellular metabolism, for intercellular storage as glycogen (primarily in the liver and skeletal muscle), or for limited conversion to fat in the liver. Fructose and galactose have slightly different carbon, hydrogen, and oxygen linkages than glucose. Fructose, also known as levulose or fruit sugar, is the sweetest tasting sugar and is found in fruits and honey. Dietary fructose is absorbed from the small intestine into the blood and delivered to the liver for conversion to glucose. Galactose

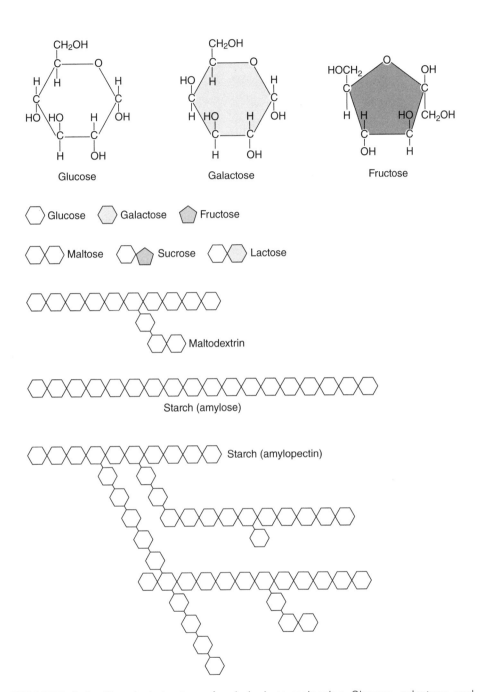

FIGURE 3.1 Chemical structure of carbohydrate molecules. Glucose, galactose, and fructose are monosaccharides. Pairs of monosaccharides form disaccharides such as maltose, sucrose, and lactose, and longer chains form complex polysaccharide molecules such as maltodextrin, amylose, and amylopectin.

Reprinted by permission from A.E. Jeukendrup and M. Gleeson, *Sport Nutrition*, 3rd ed. (Champaign, IL: Human Kinetics, 2019), 3.

exists in nature only in combination with glucose, forming the disaccharide lactose, the milk sugar present only in the mammary glands of lactating humans and animals. As with fructose, the liver converts dietary galactose to glucose. Of the three monosaccharides, glucose is of primary importance, especially for physically active people or for athletes who are training. Once absorbed by the small intestine, fructose and galactose must enter the liver for conversion to glucose, which takes time. In contrast, ingested glucose is much more readily available to the working muscles.

Disaccharides

Disaccharides are structures composed of two monosaccharides. Common disaccharides are shown in figure 3.1. The common disaccharides include a molecule of glucose chemically bound with fructose to forms sucrose, a glucose molecule bound with a galactose to form lactose, and a glucose molecule bound with another glucose monosaccharide to form maltose. Sucrose, or "table sugar," is the most common dietary disaccharide. Sucrose is abundant in most carbohydrate foods but is especially prevalent in highly processed foods. The milk sugar, lactose, is the least sweet disaccharide. Maltose, also called malt sugar, is found in grain products such as cereal and seed foods. Although maltose consists of two glucose monosaccharides, alone it contributes only a small percentage of dietary carbohydrate. Together, mono- and disaccharides are known as the *simple sugars*. These sugars are packaged commercially under a variety of terms. Brown sugar, corn syrup, fruit syrup, molasses, barley malt, invert sugar, honey, and natural sweeteners are all simple sugars.

In the United States, many foods and beverages are sweetened with inexpensive and readily available high-fructose corn syrup (HFCS). HFCS is used to describe corn syrup that has been modified to increase fructose concentration to varying levels. HFCS 42 and HFCS 55 are the most used forms in consumer foods and beverages. The number following HFCS represents the percentage of sugar that is fructose (HFCS 42: 53% glucose and 42% fructose; HFCS 55: 42% glucose and 55% fructose) (50, 77). Because HFCS has similar monosaccharide ratios to sugar beet and sugar cane sucrose, it has a similar "sweetness" while providing cost and manufacturing benefits to food and beverage companies.

Oligosaccharides and Polysaccharides

Oligosaccharides (from the Greek *oligo*, meaning "a few") are composed of 3 to 10 monosaccharides bonded together. The term *polysaccharide* refers to a carbohydrate substance that consists of 10 to thousands of chemically linked simple sugar molecules. Both plant and animal sources contain these large sugar chains. Starch and fiber are the plant sources of polysaccharide, whereas glucose is stored in human and animal tissues as the polysaccharide glycogen.

Starch

Starch is the storage form of glucose in plants, occurring in high concentrations in seeds, corn, and various grains used to make bread, cereal, pasta, and pastries, as well as in vegetables such as peas, beans, potatoes, and roots. Starch exists in two forms (see figure 3.1): (1) amylose, a long, straight chain of glucose units twisted into a helical coil, and (2) amylopectin, a highly branched monosaccharide macromolecule structure. The relative proportion of each form of starch in a plant food determines its dietary characteristics, including its **digestibility**, or the percentage of an ingested food that is absorbed by the body. Starches with a relatively large amount of amylopectin digest well and readily absorb in the small intestine, whereas starch foods with high amylose content digest poorly, thereby slowing the rate at which liberated sugar appears in the blood. The term *complex carbohydrate* is commonly used to refer to dietary starch.

Fiber

Fiber is classified as a structural, nonstarch polysaccharide. The National Academy of Sciences uses three terms to refer to human fiber intakes (36):

- Dietary fiber consists of nondigestible carbohydrate and lignin found in plants, including digestion-resistant starch.
- Functional fiber consists of isolated, nondigestible carbohydrate with beneficial effects in humans (intestinal bacteria can ferment a small portion of some water-soluble dietary fiber producing small-chain fatty acids that are absorbed and are used as fuel for intestinal epithelial cells or white blood cells) (63). Functional fiber is a recent, novel classification of fiber. The term *functional fiber* is used in reference to the health-enhancing effects of fiber. Functional fiber can include not only dietary, nondigestible plant sources but also commercially produced sources of carbohydrate.
- Total fiber is the sum of dietary fiber and functional fiber.

Fibers differ widely in physical and chemical characteristics and physiological action. The cell walls of leaves, stems, roots, seeds, and fruit coverings contain different kinds of carbohydrate fibers (cellulose, hemicellulose, and pectin). Cellulose is the most abundant organic (i.e., carbon containing) molecule on the earth. Dietary fiber sources are commonly referred to as water insoluble or water soluble, although some of these fiber types can be isolated and extracted from foods and marketed as functional fiber sources. Examples of water-insoluble fiber include cellulose and hemicellulose. Wheat bran is a commonly consumed cellulose-rich product. Examples of water-soluble fiber include psyllium seed husk, beta-glucan, pectin, and guar gum—present in oats, beans, brown rice, peas, carrots, corn husk, and many fruits. Dietary fiber provides bulk to the food residues passing

Types and Sources of Dietary Fiber

Types and sources of dietary fiber	
Water-soluble fibers	**Foods rich in water-soluble fiber**
Psyllium	Oats
Beta-glucan	Brown rice
Pectin	Vegetables
Guar gum	Fruits
Water-insoluble fibers	**Foods rich in water-insoluble fiber**
Cellulose	Wheat bran
Hemicellulose	Whole-wheat flour
Lignin	Vegetables
Chitin	Whole grains

through the intestinal tract because it holds a considerable amount of water. Water-insoluble fiber types appear to aid gastrointestinal function and gastrointestinal health by exerting a scraping action on the cells of the intestinal wall, and water-soluble fiber types shorten the transit time needed for food residues to pass through the digestive tract. The sidebar lists examples of soluble and insoluble fiber and food sources of each. Based on *What We Eat in America*, NHANES 2015-2016 (73), the typical adult American diet contains about 18 g of fiber daily. This amount is well under the 38 g for men and 25 g for women recommended by the Food and Nutrition Board of the National Academy of Sciences (36).

Fiber has received considerable attention from researchers and the lay press. Although adequate intake of fiber does not directly affect athletic performance, fiber intake is being promoted because of studies linking high fiber intake, particularly whole-grain cereal fibers, with a lower occurrence of heart and peripheral artery disease, hyperlipidemia (elevated blood lipids), obesity, diabetes, and digestive disorders including cancers of the gastrointestinal tract (52). We now have evidence demonstrating the importance of dietary fiber in the maintenance of healthy gut microbiota diversity, which aides in the reduction of chronic diseases and inflammation associated with a Western diet (44, 51).

Glycogen

Glycogen, a large, branched polymer of glucose units, serves as the body's storage form of carbohydrate. This irregularly shaped, highly branched polysaccharide polymer consists of hundreds to thousands of glucose units linked together into dense granules. The glycogen macromolecule also contains the enzymes that are responsible for, or catalyze, the synthesis and degradation of glycogen and some of the enzymes regulating these processes. The presence of glycogen greatly increases the amount of carbohydrate that is immediately available between meals and during muscular contraction.

The two major sites of glycogen storage are liver and skeletal muscles. The concentration of glycogen is higher in the liver, but because of its much greater mass, skeletal muscle stores more total glycogen (21). Glycogen metabolism in skeletal muscle plays a major role in the control of blood glucose homeostasis by the pancreatic hormone **insulin**, the most important regulator of blood glucose levels. Insulin promotes skeletal muscle blood flow and stimulates glucose uptake, glucose metabolism, and glycogen synthesis in skeletal muscle. Maximizing glycogen stores is important for not only aerobic endurance athletes but also for athletes involved in high-intensity training. Chapter 10 explores some nutritional practices that maximize glycogen resynthesis after exhaustive exercise.

Glycemic Index

The glycemic index (GI) of a carbohydrate source specifies the rate at which glucose levels rise in the blood after consumption of 50 g of carbohydrate in a food compared with the ingestion of 50 g of glucose (8, 38).

$$GI = (AUC_{CHO}/AUC_{GLU}) \times 100$$

where AUC_{CHO} represents the area under the curve for blood glucose following the ingestion of the food containing 50 g of carbohydrate and AUC_{GLU} represents the area under the curve for blood glucose following the ingestion of 50 g of glucose. The glycemic score for a food is largely determined by how quickly ingested carbohydrate empties from the stomach and is absorbed into the blood through the intestinal membrane.

Foods such as brown rice, whole-grain pasta, and multigrain breads have slow absorption rates and a low GI. High-GI foods such as refined table sugar (sucrose) included in many sport drinks and nondiet soft drinks, refined white rice, pasta, and mashed potatoes promote a pronounced, though transient, rise in both blood glucose and insulin production. Complex carbohydrate foods do not always have a lower glycemic response than simple sugar foods because cooking alters the integrity of a starch granule, creating a higher glycemic index. Similar considerations must be given to predicting the glycemic indexes of liquid versus solid carbohydrate sources (14).

Because dietary carbohydrate is a vital component of exercise preparation, performance, and recovery, the carbohydrate requirement for many athletes is increased because of the repetitive nature of their training (16). During periods of intense physical training, an athlete's daily carbohydrate intake requirement may exceed 10 g/kg body weight. Athletes can take advantage of both high- and lower-glycemic carbohydrate foods to optimize performance. For instance, consumption of high-glycemic carbohydrate sources is paramount to maintenance of blood glucose levels during prolonged aerobic endurance exercise (41, 42) and for rapid recovery of muscle glycogen immediately after an exercise bout. But people can eat more slowly absorbed, unrefined, complex carbohydrate to optimize muscle carbohydrate storage between exercise bouts (37). Ingestion of lower-GI carbohydrate prevents dramatic fluctuations in blood glucose while maintaining an extended, low-level blood glucose exposure to the previously exercised muscle during prolonged recovery.

Glycemic Load

In addition to the blood glucose response described by glycemic index, a more detailed method to evaluate the effect of a carbohydrate food on the body is glycemic load. Glycemic load (GL) combines the GI with the amount of carbohydrate contained in a serving of the specific food (24).

$$GL = (GI \times CHO_{FOOD})/100$$

where GI represents the glycemic index of the food and CHO_{FOOD} represents the amount of carbohydrate contained in a serving size of the food in grams. A food with a high GI and a high GL will have a greater effect on blood glucose than a food with the same GI but lower GL because of the larger carbohydrate content of the first food. An example of this can be seen when comparing rice and watermelon in table 3.1. Rice and watermelon both have a GI of 72, classifying them as high-GI foods. A serving of rice (5.3 oz [150 g]), however, provides 42 g of carbohydrate, whereas a serving of watermelon (4.2 oz [120 g]) provides only 6 g of carbohydrate.

The GL is a practical tool that helps people with diabetes select foods that will improve control of circulating blood glucose levels. Although a high-GI food such as rice can lead to large elevations in blood glucose, a serving of watermelon will result in less elevation.

The next section discusses the regulation of carbohydrate in the body, including the maintenance of blood glucose and glycogen synthesis and degradation, as well as aerobic and anaerobic glycolysis.

Carbohydrate Regulation in the Body

Carbohydrate serves as an essential, but limited, fuel source in the body. In the resting state, the liver, pancreas, and other organs help keep blood glucose levels within a narrow range to match the carbohydrate energy needs of the various body tissues. Because the limited stored glycogen in skeletal muscle is a vital energy source during muscle contraction, this carbohydrate source is used sparingly at rest. After a meal, the body stores as much carbohydrate in the form of glycogen as possible while stimulating carbohydrate fuel use to help return the blood glucose level to normal. When in a fasted state, the body mobilizes glucose precursors for gluconeogenesis in the

TABLE 3.1   Glycemic Index and Glycemic Load of Various Foods

Glycemic index (glycemic load)	Food, serving size, carbohydrate	Glycemic index (glycemic load)	Food, serving size, carbohydrate	Glycemic index (glycemic load)	Food, serving size, carbohydrate
HIGH GLYCEMIC INDEX (>70)		**MODERATE GLYCEMIC INDEX (55-70)**		**LOW GLYCEMIC INDEX (<55)**	
102 (23)	Pancakes, buckwheat, 80 g (2.8 oz), 23 g	69 (24)	Bagel, white, 70 g (2.5 oz), 35 g	54 (11)	Potato crisps or chips, 50g (1.8 oz), 21 g
95 (40)	Lucozade (original), 250 ml (8.5 fl oz), 42 g	67 (17)	Doughnut, 47 g (1.7 oz), 23 g	52 (17)	Sweet corn, 150 g (5.3 oz), 32 g
92 (8)	Scones, 25 g (0.9 oz), 9 g	67 (17)	Croissant, 57 g (2 oz), 23 g	52 (16)	Cookies, chocolate, 45 g (1.6 oz), 30 g
88 (23)	Rice bubbles or pops, 30 g (1.1 oz), 26 g	66 (5)	Beer, 250 ml (8.5 fl oz), 8 g	52 (12)	Banana, 120 g (4.2 oz), 24 g
86 (26)	Baked potato, 150 g (5.3 oz), 27 g	65 (9)	Couscous, 150 g (5.3 oz), 14 g	51 (15)	Porridge (wheat and oat), 250 g (8.8 oz), 30 g
83 (16)	Pretzels, 30 g (1.1 oz), 20 g	64 (28)	Raisins, 60 g (2.1 oz), 44 g	50 (13)	Orange juice, 250 ml (8.5 fl oz), 26 g
82 (17)	Puffed rice cakes, 25 g (0.9 oz), 21 g	63 (16)	Coca-Cola, 250 ml (8.5 fl oz), 26 g	49 (10)	Muesli, 30 g (1.1 oz), 20 g
81 (21)	Cornflakes (cereal), 30g (1.1 oz), 26 g	62 (26)	Baguette with butter and jam, 70 g (2.5 oz), 41 g	49 (24)	Spaghetti, white, boiled, 180 g (6.3 oz), 48 g
80 (22)	Jelly beans, 30 g (1.1 oz), 28 g	60 (7)	Bread, white, toasted, 30 g (1.1 oz), 15 g	48 (7)	Baked beans, 150 g (5.3 oz), 15 g
78 (12)	Typical sport beverage, 250 ml (8.5 fl oz), 15 g	59 (10)	Digestives (cookies), 25 g (0.9 oz), 16 g	47 (3)	Carrots, 80 g (2.8 oz), 6 g
75 (11)	Bread, white, wheat flour, 30 g (1.1 oz), 15 g	57 (6)	Ice cream, regular, 50 g (1.8 oz), 10 g	46 (8)	Grapes, 120 g (4.2 oz), 18 g
75 (12)	Weetabix (cereal), 30 g (1.1 oz), 22 g	57 (22)	Blueberry muffin, 70 g (2.5 oz), 39 g	44 (9)	All-Bran (cereal), 30 g (1.1 oz), 20 g
75 (16)	Boiled potato, 150 g (5.3 oz), 28 g	57 (9)	Fruit loaf, 30 g (1.1 oz), 18 g	40 (15)	Rice noodles, boiled, 180 g (6.3 oz), 39 g
74 (21)	Cheerios (cereal), 30 g (1.1 oz), 20 g	56 (24)	Power bar, chocolate, 65g (2.3 oz), 42 g	38 (6)	Apple, 120 g (4.2 oz), 15 g
73 (15)	Iced cupcake, 38 g (1.3 oz), 26 g	56 (23)	Long-grain rice, boiled 150 g (5.3 oz), 42 g	36 (9)	Pizza, margherita, 100 g (3.5 oz), 24 g
72 (9)	Popcorn, 20 g (0.7 oz), 12 g	55 (19)	Snickers bar, 60 g (2.1 oz), 35 g	31 (4)	Milk, full fat, 250 ml (8.5 fl oz), 12 g
72 (30)	Rice, white, boiled, 150 g (5.3 oz), 42 g	55 (10)	Honey, 25 g (0.9 oz), 18 g	30 (5)	Lentils, 150 g (5.3 oz), 17 g
72 (4)	Watermelon, 120 g (4.2 oz), 6 g	55 (9)	Fruit cocktail, canned, 120 g (4.2 oz), 16 g	15 (1)	Tomato, spinach, broccoli, asparagus, 150 g (5.3 oz), 6 g

Reprinted by permission from A.E. Jeukendrup and M. Gleeson, *Sport Nutrition,* 3rd ed. (Champaign, IL: Human Kinetics, 2019), 145; Data from Atkinson, Foster-Powell, and Brand-Miller (2008); Henry et al. (2005); Diogenes GI Database (2010).

liver (hepatic gluconeogenesis) while promoting fat oxidation for energy to preserve carbohydrate fuel.

During exercise and performance, the body increases use of fat and carbohydrate as fuel needs rise. The body begins to use its glycogen stores in the muscle in addition to the circulating glucose in the blood. To maintain blood glucose levels, the liver increases the rate of hepatic glycogenolysis (the breakdown of liver glycogen) and gluconeogenesis. The amount and ratios of carbohydrate and fat used during exercise depends on several factors. Typically, fat is the primary fuel source when at rest and during low-intensity work. As intensity increases, fat use increases until a maximal level is reached around 50% of $\dot{V}O_2$max (59). As intensity continues to increase, carbohydrate provides greater percentages of the fuel needed to meet energy demands. If exercise continues for prolonged durations, glycogen stores decline, resulting in a need to shift back to fat as the significant fuel.

Maintenance of Blood Glucose

The total blood volume of an average adult human is roughly 5 L. Of this total blood volume, adult human blood contains approximately 5 g of glucose. Carbohydrate from food, hepatic glycogenolysis, and gluconeogenesis all help maintain blood glucose levels. During fasting, the latter processes contribute more to blood glucose levels. In this rested state, muscle glucose and glycogen use is extremely low. The balance of the plasma hormones glucagon and insulin has the strongest regulatory effects on blood glucose and tissue glycogen use at rest. When blood sugar falls below normal, the pancreatic alpha cells secrete glucagon, a carbohydrate-mobilizing hormone. Glucagon stimulates gluconeogenesis and glycogenolysis pathways in the liver to bring blood glucose levels back to normal (figure 3.2). When blood glucose levels rise above normal after a meal, the pancreatic beta cells secrete insulin. Insulin removes glucose from the blood by increasing blood flow to insulin-sensitive tissues (primarily skeletal muscle and adipose tissue) and

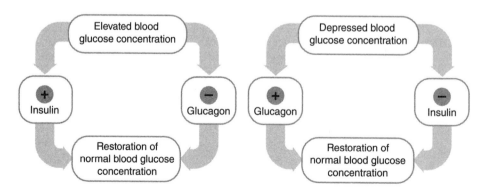

FIGURE 3.2 The roles of the pancreatic hormones insulin and glucagon in the maintenance of blood glucose.

by stimulating diffusion of the sugar molecule into these cell types. Insulin also stimulates cellular energy metabolism from carbohydrate, promotes the storage of glucose as glycogen, and inhibits hepatic and skeletal muscle glycogenolysis and hepatic gluconeogenesis. From a practical standpoint, these systems must work properly to maintain blood glucose levels because aerobic endurance performance declines as blood glucose levels decrease.

Glycogen Synthesis

Glycogen is stored in both skeletal muscle and the liver. Muscle glycogen is important for fueling intense anaerobic or aerobic exercise. Liver glycogen is degraded into glucose, which is then transported to the blood to help maintain blood glucose levels during aerobic endurance exercise and between meals. This section explains how glycogen is synthesized.

In the synthesis of glycogen, intracellular glucose undergoes several modifications to generate uridine diphosphate (UDP)-glucose (48). This reaction takes place in three steps:

1. Intracellular glucose is **phosphorylated** (a phosphate group is added to it) by hexokinase as it enters the cell to generate glucose-6-phosphate.
2. Glucose-6-phosphate is then converted to glucose-1-phosphate (by phosphoglucomutase).
3. UDP-glucose is synthesized from glucose-1-phosphate and uridine triphosphate in a reaction catalyzed by UDP-glucose pyrophosphorylase.

The UDP-glucose that is formed is added to the growing glycogen molecule. This reaction is catalyzed by the enzyme glycogen synthase, which can add glucose residues only if the polysaccharide chain already contains more than four residues. Glycogen is not simply a long string of repeated glucose compounds; it is a highly branched polymer. Branching is important because it increases the solubility of glycogen. Branching also facilitates rapid glycogen synthesis and degradation (essential for providing glucose that can enter glycolysis for energy production during high-intensity exercise).

Glycogen Breakdown

The degradation of glycogen during exercise indicates that the body needs **ATP** to fuel skeletal muscle contraction. ATP is a high-energy phosphate compound synthesized and used by cells to release energy for cellular work. The goal of glycogen breakdown is to release glucose (specifically, glucose-1-phosphate) compounds so that they can enter the glycolytic pathway, which yields quick ATP production.

In the complex process of glycogen breakdown, individual glucose compounds are cleaved from glycogen to form glucose-1-phosphate (catalyzed by the enzyme glycogen phosphorylase). Phosphorylase catalyzes the sequential

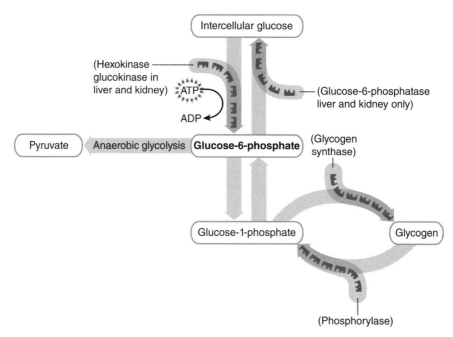

FIGURE 3.3 Central role of intercellular glucose-6-phosphate in glycolysis, glycogen storage, and glycogenolysis in skeletal muscle, liver, and kidney.

removal of glycosyl residues from the nonreducing end of the glycogen molecule. The glucose-1-phosphate formed in the phosphorolytic cleavage of glycogen is converted into glucose-6-phosphate by phosphoglucomutase. In skeletal muscle, the glycogen-liberated glucose-6-phosphate joins glucose-6-phosphate, derived from glucose that enters the cell from the blood, for metabolic fuel processing by the glycolytic enzymes. The liver, and to a limited extent the kidney, either can process the glycogen-liberated glucose-6-phosphate through glycolysis or can dephosphorylate the glycogen-liberated glucose-6-phosphate and release the glucose into the blood. In cellular glucose metabolism (i.e., glycogen synthesis and glycogen breakdown), the intermediate glucose-6-phosphate plays a central role in the various conversions between glucose storage and glucose oxidation (figure 3.3).

Glycolysis

During exercise, intense training, and sport performance, ATP is needed quickly for energy production. One of the fastest processes by which ATP can be generated is glycolysis. In general, glycolysis is the breakdown of carbohydrate (i.e., glucose) to produce ATP. Glycolysis occurs in the cytoplasm of cells including the muscle fiber. The key physiological outcome of glycolysis is relatively quick ATP production to be used for muscle contraction. As can be seen in figure 3.4, glycolysis is a series of 10 enzymatically controlled chemical reactions that starts with one six-carbon glucose and ends with two three-carbon pyruvate molecules.

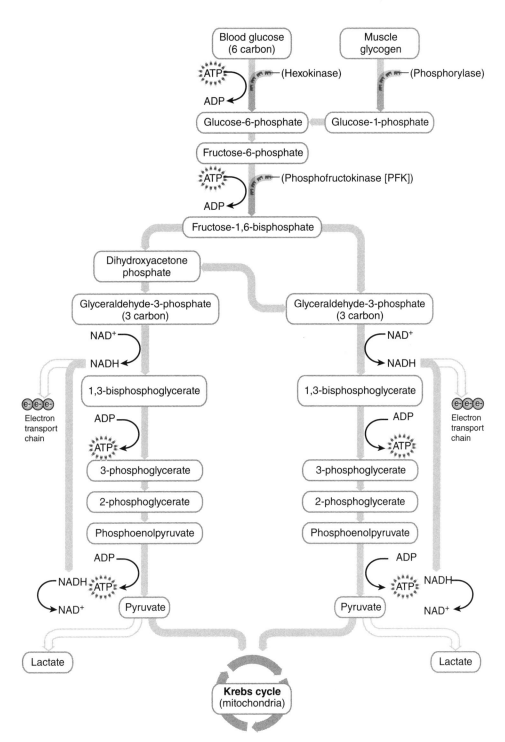

FIGURE 3.4   Glycolysis from blood glucose or glycogen uses ATP and requires the coenzyme NAD. The products of glycolysis include ATP, water, pyruvate or lactic acid, and NADH.

Reprinted by permission from NSCA, "Bioenergetics of Exercise and Training," by T.J. Herda and J.T. Cramer, in *Essentials of Strength Training and Conditioning*, 4th ed., edited by G.G. Haff and N.T. Triplett (Champaign, IL: Human Kinetics, 2016), 47.

The pyruvate that is produced at the end of glycolysis has two possible fates: It can be converted to lactate, or it can enter the **mitochondria (**the part of a cell responsible for the production of ATP with oxygen; it contains the enzymes for the Krebs cycle, electron transport chain, and the fatty acid cycle). The next section describes the production of lactic acid. Before pyruvate enters the mitochondria, it is converted to acetyl-CoA and then enters what is known as the Krebs cycle. The Krebs cycle further metabolizes the pyruvate–acetyl-CoA compounds in a series of enzyme-catalyzed chemical reactions. Ultimately, these reactions in the Krebs cycle generate NADH and $FADH_2$ compounds; these carry electrons that are taken up by the electron transport chain in the mitochondria. The electron transport chain facilitates the production of more ATP to fuel physiological processes including skeletal muscle contraction, but this ATP production occurs at a slower rate as compared with glycolytic ATP production. An important point to understand is that glycolysis produces ATP at a fast rate, which is needed during high-intensity training or exercise. Glycolysis produces significant amounts of pyruvate that can further be oxidized to produce ATP. The role of glucose in rapid ATP and pyruvate production makes it easy to appreciate the importance of having adequate carbohydrate in the diet to fuel intense exercise during training or competition.

Lactic Acid Production and Clearance

As already noted, the glycolysis end product is pyruvate. Pyruvate can be converted to acetyl-CoA and enter the Krebs cycle in the mitochondria, or it can be converted to lactic acid. Once produced inside the cell, lactic acid rapidly ionizes by releasing a hydrogen ion, contributing to a decline in **sarcoplasmic** (i.e., cytoplasmic) pH. The remaining ionized molecule is lactate. Reductions in cellular pH have deleterious effects on numerous metabolic and contractile processes. Therefore, the hydrogen ions must be buffered immediately inside the cell or expelled from the cell for extracellular buffering. At rest and during low-intensity exercise, a small amount of lactic acid is constantly produced; most of the associated hydrogen ions are easily buffered inside the cell, and some are transported outside of the cell where it is quickly rendered harmless. The plasma hemoglobin protein plays the most prominent extracellular buffering role; plasma bicarbonate also provides effective extracellular chemical buffering. The muscle pain or burning sensation that occurs during sustained, high-intensity muscle contraction is primarily due to irritation of free nerve endings outside the muscle cells by the lower pH. The remaining three-carbon lactate molecule can be used as a potential fuel source for nonexercising muscle, for the heart, and even for the exercising muscle itself (74). During moderate- to high-intensity exercise corresponding to the **lactate threshold** (a level of oxygen consumption at which blood lactate concentration increases rapidly and systematically), excess lactate is transported out of the cell. As the exercise intensity increases, blood levels of lactate rise in an exponential fashion. The free hydrogen ions resulting from the pronounced lactic acid production during higher-intensity exercise has detrimental effects on muscle performance. The formation of this metabolic by-product, however, helps facilitate accelerated anaerobic ATP production from carbohydrate for a short time.

Fatigue, as defined by an inability to maintain a desired power output or exercise intensity during short-term, high-intensity anaerobic exercise, is in part due to the release of the hydrogen ions associated with lactic acid in working muscles (leading to a drop in pH). Sustained, higher-intensity contractions can rapidly deplete exercising muscle glycogen. The decreasing intercellular glycogen and the limited rate of blood glucose availability quickly precipitate muscle fatigue as the anaerobic system's ability to sustain rapid ATP resynthesis is compromised. Muscle contractions may continue but at a lower intensity as aerobic ATP is contributing more to the total muscle exercise ATP needs.

Although lactate accumulation is correlated to fatigue, no nutritional practices can help to decrease lactate production during intense exercise. Rather, proper conditioning enables an athlete to work at higher intensity with greater reliance on aerobic metabolic pathways including enhanced use of lactate as a fuel, resulting in lower blood lactate levels. Broadly speaking, athletes must include optimal amounts of carbohydrate in the diet to enable them to perform high-intensity training, which will result in adaptations that promote energy production from oxidative (i.e., fat) sources of energy.

Carbohydrate availability in the body controls its use for energy. The concentration of blood glucose provides feedback regulation of the glucose output of the liver; an increase in blood glucose inhibits hepatic glucose release during exercise. Carbohydrate availability may also limit fat metabolism by decreasing both fatty acid mobilization and oxidation in the cell (68). Intuitively, this makes metabolic sense as the fatty acid oxidation is far too slow to contribute significantly to the ATP requirements and would act only to congest the mitochondrial NADH and acetyl-CoA concentrations, necessitating further lactic acid production to sustain anaerobic glycolysis.

Carbohydrate and Performance

The role of carbohydrate in exercise has been a topic of interest for nearly 100 years. In 1925, Gordon and colleagues demonstrated that the ingestion of a glucose candy during a marathon allowed runners to complete their task in "better condition" (26, 49). Our exploration of the role of carbohydrate in performance accelerated with the reintroduction of muscle biopsies in the 1960s, which enhanced the understanding of muscle glycogen and carbohydrate loading during the following two decades. The ergogenic effects of carbohydrate ingestion during prolonged exercise was demonstrated through an acceleration in the number of studies in the 1980s (18). Our knowledge of the potential ergogenic effects of carbohydrate in anaerobically based activities grew during the early 2000s (28, 29). The benefit of multiple forms of carbohydrate was seen in 2004; multiple forms of carbohydrate demonstrated an increase in exogenous carbohydrate oxidations rates (39, 40). At the same time, the body's recognition of carbohydrate in the mouth and its subsequent potential to enhance exercise performance was also demonstrated (10). The following sections provide more detail and discuss these seminal studies and others that built our current understanding of the role of carbohydrate for athletes.

Effect of Exercise on Carbohydrate Stores

At rest and during exercise, the liver produces glucose to maintain a blood glucose concentration of approximately 100 mg/dl (5.5 mmol/L) (43). Blood glucose may account for 30% of the total energy fuel required by exercising muscles; the remaining carbohydrate fuel is derived from stored muscle glycogen (17). In prolonged, intense exercise, blood glucose concentration eventually falls below normal levels because of liver glycogen depletion while active skeletal muscle continues to use the available blood glucose.

Liver glycogen declines overnight to maintain acceptable blood glucose. Additionally, the relatively small amount of stored liver glycogen can be rapidly reduced with aerobic exercise; a 2-hour bout of intense aerobic exercise may almost entirely deplete glycogen in the liver as well as in working muscle (18, 67). Depletion is of particular concern during exercise after a prolonged period without food, for example, early in the morning or after an exercise warm-up period. The result is that the athlete would begin a training session or competition with suboptimal liver glycogen levels.

Skeletal muscle glycogen is a readily available energy source for the working muscle. The amount of carbohydrate stored is influenced by both diet and training status (2). The rate at which glycogen is used depends largely on exercise intensity (figure 3.5). As the exercise intensity increases to high levels (i.e., above anaerobic threshold or >70-80% $\dot{V}O_2$max), the muscle energy requirements cannot be matched by accelerated mitochondrial oxidation of carbohydrate and fat. Muscle glycogen becomes the most important energy substrate, because anaerobic ATP production is required to match the rapid ATP use by the contractile machinery. Exercise-mediated depletion of muscle glycogen to less than 30 mmol/kg muscle will result in increased reliance on the relatively slower process of blood glucose uptake as a carbohydrate fuel source.

A decline in exercising muscle glycogen levels late in exercise results in an increased reliance on blood glucose as the carbohydrate source of the exercising muscles. Without ingestion of carbohydrate, hypoglycemia (<45 mg/dl; 2.5 mmol/L) can quickly ensue after liver and working muscle glycogen depletion (64). Hypoglycemia ultimately impairs exercise performance and can contribute to central nervous system fatigue associated with prolonged exercise.

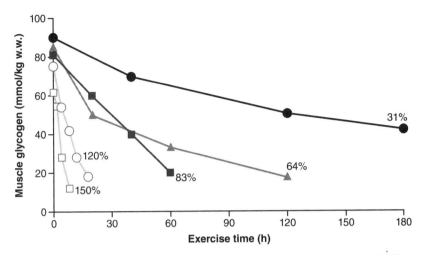

FIGURE 3.5   The effects of exercise intensity (shown as a percentage of $\dot{V}O_2$max) on muscle glycogen

Reprinted by permission from A.E. Jeukendrup and M. Gleeson, *Sport Nutrition,* 3rd ed. (Champaign, IL: Human Kinetics, 2019), 138.

Fatigue during prolonged aerobic exercise is caused primarily by depleted carbohydrate stores in the exercising muscle (60). Fatigue occurs despite sufficient oxygen supply to the muscle and almost unlimited stored energy available from fat. Aerobic endurance athletes commonly refer to this type of fatigue as "hitting the wall." Symptoms of significantly reduced blood glucose include weakness, dizziness, and decreased motivation. The decline in muscle glycogen results in perception of fatigue, and further decline and depletion necessitate termination of exercise or a significant reduction in exercise intensity (1, 6). Thus, it should not be surprising that optimal aerobic endurance performance is directly related to the initial muscle glycogen stores (1, 34).

Note that regardless of muscle glycogen content, fatigue during bouts of high-intensity exercise could likely result from the accompanying reductions in pH in and around the working muscle fibers. Thus, the importance of muscle carbohydrate stores with respect to exercise performance is more relevant during prolonged (i.e., >2 minutes) and intermittent high-intensity exercise bouts (e.g., drills and wind sprints).

High-intensity intermittent exercise includes numerous activities performed in various types of exercise training sessions and in team sport competitions. In the short rest period between intermittent bouts, the muscle has time to clear or buffer some of the hydrogen ions associated with metabolism (or do both), alleviating the potential detrimental effects of this by-product. Additionally, the performance of very high-intensity, short-duration (i.e., <10 seconds) exercise depends primarily on the provision of ATP through the phosphagen system. During repetitions of these exercise bursts, however, muscle glycogen plays an important role in maintaining the muscle ATP content over the course of a workout session consisting of many sets of high-intensity repetitions with short recovery periods.

Muscle Glycogen Optimization

Fatigue during exercise and sport is related to initial glycogen content. Therefore, beginning an exercise or training session with optimal muscle glycogen levels and rapidly replenishing glycogen after exercise before a subsequent performance is critically important for optimal performance. A carefully designed nutrition plan is important to ensure abundant muscle glycogen stores. Carbohydrate is an important fuel source for both aerobic and anaerobic exercise, because the rate of carbohydrate use and thus glycogen depletion is directly related to the intensity of the exercise (see figure 3.5). During lower-intensity, aerobic exercise, fatigue related to glycogen depletion occurs later in the exercise session, whereas fatigue related to glycogen depletion associated with higher-intensity, anaerobic exercise can develop much earlier (25).

Because of the cumulative glycogen use in muscle during a workout or competition, it has been suggested that consumption of higher levels of carbohydrate in the diet would improve muscle performance in these activities (4, 6, 12, 54, 61, 62, 69). Carbohydrate ingestion rates should reflect the duration and intensity of exercise training that an athlete undertakes each week. Most athletes can meet their carbohydrate needs though the ingestion of 5 to 10 g carbohydrate per kilogram body weight per day. Athletes who participate in light, low-intensity activity may suffice with 3 to 5 g carbohydrate per kilogram body weight per day, and athletes who participate in moderate-high intensity exercise for 4 to 5 hours per day may need up to 12 g carbohydrate per kilogram body weight per day (71).

Additionally, after prolonged exercise, replenishment of muscle glycogen to within a normal range is essential for maximizing the recovery process (31). The postexercise recovery period should be considered the initial preparation for an upcoming exercise challenge (37). Following exercise, athletes should ingest carbohydrate to take advantage of the up regulation of carbohydrate transport into the muscle cell.

Aerobic Endurance Exercise Effects

Optimizing preexercise muscle glycogen stores (i.e., >150 mmol/kg muscle) increases time to exhaustion by as much as 20% and increases aerobic endurance performance by reducing the time taken to complete a given workload (33). In general terms, focusing on grams of carbohydrate per kilogram body weight per day, an aerobic endurance athlete's carbohydrate consumption should account for approximately 55% to 65% of the total caloric intake (56). The generally recommended carbohydrate intake for this type of training is not drastically different from the typical American intake (~45% of total calories) (73). Keep in mind, however, that despite similar percentages, the absolute amount of recommended carbohydrate (in grams) will vary tremendously depending on the total dietary caloric intake.

Anaerobic Exercise and Resistance Training Effects

Despite the importance of carbohydrate in anaerobic activities, the general carbohydrate recommendations for these athletes are slightly less than those for an athlete performing aerobic endurance exercise. Therefore, the optimization of preexercise muscle glycogen levels and rapid replenishment of glycogen in previously exercised muscle are just as important during anaerobic training and competition. Because preexercise muscle glycogen levels are similar in aerobic and anaerobic athletes, daily carbohydrate consumption should account for 55% to 65% of caloric intake for anaerobic athletes as well. Specifically, anaerobic athletes who train or compete regularly should ingest 5 to 6 g carbohydrate per kilogram body weight per day.

Strength performance, as well as training to improve muscular strength, muscular endurance, and muscular power, consists of repetitive bouts of high-intensity work with relatively short rest intervals. Therefore, carbohydrate is the primary fuel source over the course of a resistance exercise session. As with anaerobic exercise, the intensity of the bout dictates the level of fast-twitch muscle fiber recruitment, which in large part determines the performance capabilities of a muscle or muscle group in resistance exercise. During high-intensity (i.e., >60% 1RM resistance exercise, more glycolytic fast-twitch fibers are heavily recruited, and they quickly fatigue as glycogen content is used. Not surprisingly, the recruitment of fast-twitch type IIx fibers (formerly referred to as type IIb) increases during eccentric and high-speed contractions (57, 69). Several studies, however, have demonstrated that the faster-twitch fiber types are recruited at moderate- (i.e., 60% 1RM) (70) and even lower-intensity (i.e., 20-40% 1RM) (25, 61) muscle contractions.

In Preparation for the Next Session or Day

Because many athletes perform intense training several times a week, adequate carbohydrate intake is necessary to prevent a gradual depletion of glycogen in trained muscle over time. Further, the amount of glycogen used in training sessions appears to be related to the combination of the total amount of work accomplished and the duration of the training bout. The translocation of glucose transporters to the surface of the muscle cell membrane during exercise aids in the uptake of glucose into the muscle. These transporters remain at the cell membrane for a short period following exercise and aid in the replenishment of muscle glycogen levels when carbohydrate is ingested shortly after exercise cessation.

Effect of Low-Carbohydrate Diets on Performance

A reduction in dietary carbohydrate intake is a common weight management technique in both recreational and competitive athletes. Research
has demonstrated the potential enhancement of fat use of athletes training
in a low-carbohydrate state (3). Most research demonstrates a decrement
in performance in most athletes following low-carbohydrate diets. A large
study conducted in race walkers who were consuming a low-carbohydrate
diet found a reduction in exercise economy, which resulted in an increase
in oxygen requirement at the same walking speeds (9). Although low-
carbohydrate diets may be an option for weight management, adequate
carbohydrate intakes are critical for people who desire performance optimization.

Carbohydrate Ingestion During Exercise

In addition to the benefits of optimizing muscle glycogen levels through diet,
the ergogenic effect of carbohydrate ingestion during exercise was clearly
demonstrated when blood samples and physical condition was recorded
in runners following the 1924 and 1925 Boston Marathons. Researchers
found that the ingestion of candies containing glucose during the 1925 race
improved the physical condition and performance in many of the runners.
The added benefit of carbohydrate intake during exercise is evident because
most of the runners reported consuming high-carbohydrate diets preceding
the race in both 1924 and 1925 (26, 49).

A concern about carbohydrate ingestion developed because of a study
reporting that carbohydrate ingestion before exercise could lead to an elevation in insulin that resulted in a drop in blood glucose, causing decrements in
performance (23). This concern that carbohydrate should be avoided around
the exercise occasion was coupled with an emphasis on maximizing muscle
glycogen levels several hours before exercise. Follow-up studies, however,
have shown that although an upregulation in insulin may occur, any effects
are not long lasting during exercise and a warm-up may further reduce any
possible negative effects (19, 53, 78).

Aerobic Endurance Exercise

The ingestion of carbohydrate during aerobic endurance exercise has been
shown to aid in the maintenance of blood glucose and sustained exercise.
One influential study found that cyclists were able to ride for 4 hours until
fatiguing with carbohydrate ingestion as opposed to fatiguing after 3 hours
without carbohydrate (18). This was one of the preliminary studies that led
to a large body of work focused on understanding ways to optimize carbohydrate type, dosage, and timing. The associated performance benefits have
been shown across a wide range of carbohydrate intakes (66, 67). A series

of studies investigating the use of exogenous carbohydrate demonstrated that the inclusion of multiple forms (glucose, fructose) of carbohydrate led to increased exogenous carbohydrate oxidation (39, 40). As carbohydrate is ingested it must be emptied by the stomach and absorbed by the intestine.

In a series of studies that investigated the effect of carbohydrate in exercise sessions lasting approximately 1 hour, the infusion of glucose directly into blood did not enhance performance whereas the ingestion of carbohydrate was found to enhance exercise performance (10, 11). These findings led to a number of studies demonstrating an ergogenic effect of rinsing the mouth with carbohydrate in aerobic endurance exercise sessions that would not typically be considered substantially detrimental to muscle glycogen stores. Functional magnetic resonance scans demonstrated activation of reward regions in the brain when carbohydrate was rinsed in the mouth as opposed to an artificial sweetener. This finding has led to the hypothesis that oral receptors in the mouth may recognize carbohydrate as opposed to strictly recognizing sweetness (13).

The combination of these findings has resulted in a recommendation to ingest a 6% to 8% carbohydrate solution at a rate of 30 to 60 g/h during exercise sessions lasting 1 to 2.5 hours. For exercise sessions shorter than 60 minutes, athletes are not likely to experience significant benefits from carbohydrate beyond mouth rinsing. When exercise sessions exceed 2.5 hours, athletes will likely benefit from carbohydrate intakes up to 90 g/h (71). As with all variables associated with sport, carbohydrate intake should be practiced before using it in competition to identify the methods and dosages that work with each athlete.

Anaerobic Exercise and Resistance Training

Despite the lack of consensus about ingestion of a high-carbohydrate diet or ingestion of carbohydrate before weightlifting performance, skeletal muscle carbohydrate sources facilitate overall resistance exercise performance by acting as the primary fuel source during this type of exercise. Having sufficient skeletal muscle carbohydrate is especially imperative over the course of an entire weight training session in which many individual muscles or muscle groups are worked to the point of fatigue (including possible glycogen depletion), which results in an associated prolonged postexercise period of energy-consuming muscle recovery. Therefore, the overall training regimen outcome (e.g., increased strength, power) would likely be affected negatively when carbohydrate ingestion is not optimal. Several studies have demonstrated ergogenic effects of carbohydrate ingestion on resistance training performance (30, 45, 75, 76). These ergogenic effects, however, are not as consistently observed with resistance training as compared with aerobic endurance activities (22, 28, 46).

Influence of Carbohydrate on Training Stress

Although much of the role of carbohydrate in exercise is to serve as a fuel source during moderate- to high-intensity exercise, carbohydrate levels in the body also influence longer-term responses to that exercise session. The ingestion of carbohydrate influences adaptation to exercise through metabolic and hormonal variations. Two hormones that have been found to be influenced by carbohydrate ingestion around exercise are cortisol and insulin. Reduced carbohydrate intake around aerobic exercise has also be shown to upregulate key signaling pathways in the development of mitochondria (5, 32).

Cortisol is a marker of stress that has been shown to rise in response to exercise. Although this rise is expected, cortisol has been shown to have a negative effect on protein synthesis. Acute elevations in cortisol in response to stressors such as exercise aid in the maintenance of blood glucose. Chronic elevations of cortisol are associated with several undesirable responses that can negatively affect health (20, 47). Carbohydrate ingestion during exercise has been shown to reduce cortisol levels in both aerobic endurance and resistance exercise (27, 35, 55, 58). Reductions in cortisol have been suggested to reduce the catabolic environment associated with exercise (65).

In addition to reducing the catabolic environment with cortisol, carbohydrate ingestion may enhance the anabolic environment by elevating insulin levels. Carbohydrate ingestion (particularly high-glycemic types) dramatically increases endogenous insulin secretion. Elevations in insulin is beneficial for athletes because of its role in both muscle development along with glycogen synthesis (7, 72).

Two of the effects of insulin release—increasing protein synthesis and decreasing protein breakdown—may improve the chronic anabolic adaptations of resistance exercise, particularly if insulin is elevated surrounding the period of each resistance exercise bout with carbohydrate consumption. Associated with this is the recommendation to ingest liquid carbohydrate before, during, and after exercise to promote faster recovery and gains in lean muscle mass (29). Chapter 10 expands on this concept of nutrient timing and the effect that carbohydrate ingestion has on endogenous insulin secretion, as well as the exercise performance improvements observed with such practices.

Professional Applications

Athletes can make informed decisions about the use of carbohydrate based on knowledge from multiple perspectives, including what types of carbohydrate can be ingested; how this ingested carbohydrate is regulated and used in the body; and how carbohydrate intake influences aerobic, anaerobic, and resistance training. One decision has to do with the choice of food that can best restore skeletal muscle glycogen that has been depleted by intense or long-duration exercise.

For example, if a soccer athlete is competing in several matches in a single day (as in tournament play), glycogen must be restored as soon as possible (within several hours) so that depleted glycogen levels do not induce fatigue for later matches. In this case, the soccer athlete should choose high-glycemic carbohydrate foods, because these have been shown to result in rapid restoration of skeletal muscle glycogen. For an athlete whose primary mode of training is resistance exercise, low-glycemic carbohydrate sources would be recommended for resistance training as part of everyday eating habits, whereas higher-glycemic foods would be recommended for the immediate postexercise period for optimal muscle glycogen repletion and insulin response (15).

The physiological processes of glycogen synthesis, glycogen breakdown, and glycolysis are all ways in which the body deals with ingested carbohydrate. These processes allow quick ATP production (glycogen breakdown and glycolysis) during intense exercise and the storing of glycogen (glycogen synthesis) in the skeletal muscle and liver for future training and conditioning.

To prevent suboptimal carbohydrate stores, an aerobic endurance athlete, such as a long-distance runner, should consume approximately 55% to 65% of total caloric intake in the form of carbohydrate (56). Although this recommendation provides a general range of carbohydrate ingestion as compared with protein and fat, the absolute amount of recommended carbohydrate (in grams) will vary tremendously depending on the total dietary caloric intake and physical activity level. As a general guide, athletes training or competing on a regular basis should ingest 5 to 7 g carbohydrate per kilogram body weight per day and consider increasing up to 10 g carbohydrate per kilogram body weight per day. Athletes participating in very high levels of training (moderate to high intensities for more than 4 hours/d) may need 12 g carbohydrate per kilogram body weight per day (71).

An anaerobic athlete, by comparison, would likely not need more than 5 to 7 g carbohydrate per kilogram body weight per day. Although an anaerobic athlete consistently trains at high intensity, the relative duration of such intensity is lower than that of an aerobic endurance athlete.

An athlete engaged in a resistance training program will, on a day-to-day basis, require more total energy than a nonactive, healthy counterpart of the same age. By obtaining 55% to 65% of total calories from carbohydrate, a resistance or power-training athlete can ensure having near-optimal energy. Athletes on a 3,500 kcal/day diet in which 65% of caloric intake is composed of carbohydrate should aim to consume approximately 570 g of carbohydrate daily (~8 g per kilogram body weight per day for a 70 kg [154 lb] person). In contrast, a nonactive adult consuming 2,500 kcal/day consisting of 55% carbohydrate would require considerably fewer grams of carbohydrate (i.e., 340 g) daily (~5 g per kilogram body weight per day for a 70 kg [154 lb] person).

The general carbohydrate prescriptions, based on an athlete's type and extent of energy expenditure, are merely rough guidelines to illustrate the need to be mindful of the percent of carbohydrate per daily caloric intake in an athlete's nutritional program. Specific carbohydrate intake strategies to optimize performance are recommended in chapter 8.

Summary Points

- Carbohydrate provides a vital source of energy production during anaerobic and aerobic exercise.

- Reductions of the body's carbohydrate sources during exercise decrease exercise performance and promote fatigue.

- Daily consumption of adequate carbohydrate (e.g., 55%-65% total calories) is critical for optimal athletic performance in most sports.

- Dietary carbohydrate is a vital component of exercise preparation, performance, and recovery. Thus, the carbohydrate requirement for athletes increases because of the repetitive nature of their training.

- During periods of intense physical training, most athletes can meet their carbohydrate needs with 5 to 10 g carbohydrate per kilogram body weight per day.

- Performance will likely improve with carbohydrate ingestion during moderate- to high-intensity activities lasting longer than 60 minutes.

- An athlete can take advantage of both high- and lower-glycemic food for optimal performance. Ingesting foods with a high glycemic index during prolonged exercise or immediately after exercise is a vital strategy that athletes are encouraged to use for peak performance and recovery.

- When people ingest lower-GI carbohydrate, they can prevent dramatic fluctuations in blood glucose while maintaining a prolonged, lower-level exposure of the previously exercised muscle to blood glucose. Thus, athletes benefit by ingesting low-glycemic foods as part of their normal diet between training sessions.

- By planning carbohydrate feeding schedules, athletes can ensure optimal muscle carbohydrate stores when beginning an exercise bout or training session, carbohydrate provision during exercise, and rapid replenishment of glycogen after exercise and before a subsequent performance.

Chapter 4

Protein

David Barr, CSCS, PPSC*M, CISSN, TSAC-F, RSCC

The fundamental unit of protein is the amino acid. These nitrogen-containing compounds have a particular structure with an amine group, a carboxyl group, and a side chain (figure 4.1). Amino acids can be joined together by peptide bonds, and 2 to 49 joined amino acids are known as peptides. A peptide chain that grows beyond 49 amino acids is known as a protein. Protein consumed in the diet is digested by stomach acid and enzymes and absorbed from the small intestine into the blood as amino acids or short peptides. These amino acids are available to be used by the body directly, as in the case of some neurotransmitters, stored in the body in small amounts as free amino acids, or synthesized into new proteins.

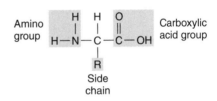

FIGURE 4.1 Amino acid structure.

The synthesis of new proteins from amino acids is appropriately known as protein synthesis and is the result of using DNA as the blueprint. Ultimately, DNA indicates the order (or sequence) in which amino acids are joined to create peptides or proteins. In its simplest description, DNA provides the blueprint for the creation of new peptide bonds (also known as amino acid sequences) and ultimately protein synthesis. Dietary protein provides the amino acids that serve as the raw material for protein synthesis, so that the body can create the specific proteins as needed (31).

Within the body, proteins are constantly being created and broken down. When these processes occur at an equal rate, protein balance is reached. For physiological adaptations to happen from training (for example, muscle hypertrophy), the rate of synthesis must be greater than that of breakdown. To accomplish this, both the training stress–stimulus and provision of dietary protein are needed. When resistance training happens in the absence of protein feeding, protein synthesis increases, as does the rate of breakdown. This process maintains protein balance so that no net synthesis will occur.

Amino Acids

The human body uses 21 amino acids to make peptides and proteins. These amino acids are known as **proteinogenic** amino acids. This group can be subdivided into **essential** and **nonessential amino acids** (**EAA** and **NEAA**, respectively). The former must be provided in the diet, whereas the latter can be synthesized by the body from the EAAs. A subgroup of NEAAs can be identified as **conditionally essential**, which means that they must be provided from the diet under conditions of exceptional stress or illness (10, 35). A list of the amino acids is provided in table 4.1.

A final group of amino acids are not directly incorporated during protein synthesis (i.e., they are nonproteinogenic) but are often used in different metabolic processes (such as L-DOPA or T_3 hormone), and many are sold as athletic supplements. Commonly encountered examples of these ingredients are listed in table 4.2.

TABLE 4.1 The 21 Proteinogenic Amino Acids

Essential (9)	Conditionally essential (7)	Nonessential (5)
Histidine (H)	Arginine (R)	Alanine (A)
Isoleucine (I)	Cysteine (C)	Aspartic acid (D)
Leucine (L)	Glutamine (Q)	Asparagine (N)
Lysine (K)	Glycine (G)	Glutamic acid (E)
Methionine (M)	Proline (P)	Selenocysteine (U)
Phenylalanine (F)	Serine (S)	
Threonine (T)	Tyrosine (Y)	
Tryptophan (W)		
Valine (V)		

TABLE 4.2 Examples of Common Nonproteinogenic Amino Acid Supplement Ingredients

Beta-alanine
Carnosine*
Citrulline
D-aspartic acid
Gamma-aminobutyric acid (GABA)
5-hydroxytryptophan (5-HTP)
Ornithine
Theanine

Note: Inclusion on this list is not meant to imply efficacy. The supplement ingredients carnitine and taurine have molecular structures similar to those of amino acids, and as a result they are commonly misidentified as such.

*Not to be confused with other supplement ingredients, creatine or carnitine.

Food Sources

In a reductive way, protein-containing foods can be thought of as sources of amino acids. By applying the understanding of EAAs and NEAAs, foods can be grouped into two categories: **complete** and **incomplete proteins**. The former is composed of animal protein and soy, and these sources contain all nine EAAs. Incomplete proteins are typically plant based and do not possess the full complement of EAAs. Vegan athletes can meet the body's EAA needs by consuming different protein sources that will collectively have all the EAAs. An example of this would be combining cereals and legumes in the diet. Cereals have high levels of sulfur-containing amino acids but are low in lysine. Legumes have the opposite amino acid profile (19). Incomplete protein sources that when combined provide all the EAAs are known as **complementary sources**.

Protein Quality

Another important concept related to the amino acid content of proteins is that of protein quality. One common measure of protein quality is the **protein digestibility-corrected amino acid score (PDCAAS)**. The PDCAAS is related to the quantity of specific amino acids it contains (also known as its amino acid profile), along with the digestibility of the protein source (18). As an example, a protein that is of higher quality would contain relatively high levels of the EAAs and be readily digestible. Whey is an example of this type of protein, and subsequently it has a high PDCAAS.

Recently, the **digestible indispensable amino acid score (DIAAS)** has been suggested as a more accurate measure of protein quality and ultimately as a replacement for the PDCAA. In contrast to the postdigestion and excretion fecal measurements on which the PDCAAS relies, the DIAAS used direct ileal (small intestine) absorption as its basis for quantifying absorption. As with the PDCAAS, a higher DIAAS score reflects greater protein quality, and this prospective transition is under evaluation (18). Although the exact scores are not practically relevant, the athlete can simply consider the fundamental concept of protein quality when choosing protein sources.

Protein Types

There are different types or sources of protein with different amounts and qualities of protein. Generally speaking, animal sources are higher in total protein and have higher quality protein (contain a greater amount of essential amino acids) when compared to other types of protein. The following sections provide an overview of the more popular protein sources that athletes may consider ingesting.

Collagen (Also Known as Gelatin)

As a protein supplement, collagen protein warrants a brief overview, but note that it may be consumed in an unconventional manner. Because of its incomplete amino acid profile, collagen is a poor source of amino acids compared with complete proteins. Instead, collagen ingestion is thought to facilitate the body's natural collagen synthesis by stimulating components of an immune reaction. This ability to alter immunity through food or supplement ingestion is known as **oral tolerance** (17). In doing so, collagen protein is hypothesized to promote joint health. The research in support of this concept is limited, and a thorough discussion of this concept is beyond the scope of this chapter. Briefly, one study found that healthy people who supplemented with 40 mg collagen for 120 days experienced improved knee range of motion and were able to exercise for longer before experiencing joint pain (17).

Dairy Proteins

Dairy is composed of two main types of protein, casein (80%) and whey (20%). Note that these classifications are practical and will be used throughout, but remain academically broad. Each type is composed of several different proteins such as α-lactalbumin and β-lactoglobulin for whey, and αS1-casein and β-casein within casein. Because their different digestive properties, whey and casein can have profoundly different biochemical effects that athletes can take advantage of (12).

Casein

The most predominant protein in milk, casein exhibits a high-quality amino acid profile (12). When this protein is ingested, stomach acid causes it to coagulate, which results in much slower digestion and subsequent absorption (28). The sustained release of amino acids into the blood make casein the ideal protein before periods of fasting, such as overnight. This concept is of such importance that it is isolated and explored later in the chapter.

Whey

Whey is the archetypal high-quality protein because it has high concentrations of the EAAs, is easily digestible, and is quickly absorbed (25). The unprocessed protein fraction extracted from dairy, known as native whey, still contains nonprotein elements such as lipids and lactose. Further refinement is required to minimize those elements, which results in the three most commonly available forms of whey supplements: whey protein concentrate (WPC), whey protein isolate (WPI), and whey protein hydrolysate (WPH). Whey protein concentrate is the least refined and quantitatively has a final postprocessing protein content below 90%. A more refined protein, WPI, has a protein content of 90% or greater, which could be important for athletes with lactose intolerance. Generalizing the final protein quantity of WPH is not possible because the degree of processing can vary wildly (12).

Although any protein can undergo the process of hydrolysis or predigestion, WPH is among the most common. Again, this classification is incredibly broad, because the numerous types of hydrolysis processes can yield different proteins and peptides, resulting in potentially different biochemical effects on the body (12). Although this area of research is intriguing, the variability makes it hard to make general conclusions about this broad class. The concept behind its application is that by creating new peptides through hydrolysis, the protein will be absorbed faster (because it does not have to undergo as much digestion), or novel peptides with their own nutraceutical effects will be created. The degree of hydrolysis (DH) is determined by several components of the reaction, including the enzymes used, the acidity, the temperature, and duration. Although it may seem intuitive that a protein that has undergone some predigestion and therefore has a higher DH may be absorbed more quickly (25), this is not always the case (9). This result occurs because of the heterogeneity of WPH reactions and subsequent difficulty in making subsequent generalizations.

Despite the variability between hydrolysates, some promising results exist. A study by Lockwood and colleagues (16) found that resistance-trained men experienced a relative 6% decrease in body fat mass after 8 weeks of training while consuming a WPH compared with consuming a carbohydrate placebo. More research is needed, using a greater homogeneity of WPH, before drawing firm conclusions about the benefits of this protein type. A meta-analysis exploring the results of studies that used WPC, WPI, and WPH has been completed (5). The analyses found that collectively, whey protein supplementation resulted in a decrease of fat mass. This effect was also significant in studies using WPC, although the authors acknowledge that an insufficient number of consistent studies exist to draw firm conclusions about any specific type of whey.

Insect Protein

As concerns for food availability grow with the increasing world population, finding sustainable protein sources becomes increasingly important. One potential candidate is protein derived from insects (36), as exemplified by the lesser mealworm (*Alphitobius diaperinus*), which has an amino acid profile similar to soy (40, 44). A study of untrained people found no difference between an insect protein-supplemented (0.8 g per kilogram per day) group and an isocaloric control after 8 weeks of resistance training. Although the results were not statistically significant, both groups added approximately 2.5 kg (5.5 lb) of lean muscle mass during that time (39). Given the importance of this prospective food source, athletes should be prepared to see far more research attempting to explore this area.

Soy

Soy, an unusual plant-based protein that has the full complement of EAAs, is of high overall quality (12). Soy is therefore ideal for vegan athletes and those with allergies to dairy or lactose intolerance. Soy also contains compounds known as phytoestrogens, which may exhibit estrogen-like properties in the human body. This attribute could be problematic if it caused a subsequent decrease in levels of the anabolic hormone testosterone in males. To investigate this issue, a meta-analysis of the published research has shown that soy consumption has no negative hormonal effect on men (11). Although soy does not possess the overall quality of animal-based protein, a review of the literature has found no differences in strength or lean muscle mass when supplementing with soy or protein derived from animals (20).

Food Matrix

Although research often uses protein supplements for the sake of experimental control and practical convenience, the use of whole foods reflects a more common method of protein consumption. Research has identified that whole-food sources may have different anabolic effects than those of their isolated components. The theory is that elements within the whole-food matrix other than protein may contribute to their biochemical effect on the body. A study by Elliot and colleagues (8) found that whole-milk consumption elicited a greater whole-body protein synthesis response than skim milk, when matched for calories and protein content. Similarly, whole-egg consumption has been shown to increase MPS to a greater extent that the consumption of an identical dose of egg white (37). Although complex, the potential ubiquity and positive effect of this applied concept makes it an important area of future investigation.

Protein and Recovery–Adaptation

Coaches and athletes should understand the context behind optimal protein intake because of the numerous factors that come into play when establishing this parameter. Better understanding will aid in developing ideal athlete-specific plans. In contrast to thinking of nutrients as mere passive substrates, the **nutraceutical effect** identifies specific nutrient sources as direct effectors of biochemical change. Although the concept is not always fully appreciated, in practice athletes commonly use it. For example, athletes often supplement with omega-3 fats, but not with saturated fats. Both fats contain the requisite 9 kcal per gram, but each has a profoundly different effect on human biochemistry. Within the scope of this chapter, the most relevant nutraceutical effect is the direct stimulation of muscle protein synthesis (MPS) by dietary protein ingestion (29). This effect is caused largely by the EAAs, and more specifically by the branched chain amino acids (BCAAs; leucine, isoleucine, and valine), in particular, leucine (6).

To apply the research, a useful approach is to think of MPS as the recovery–adaptation response that athletes desire. Although it is often associated with muscle hypertrophy, the response should be thought of as specific to the training stimulus. For example, the MPS response for aerobic endurance athletes will affect not only muscle structural proteins but also the aerobic enzymes that are related to performance (recall that enzymes are proteins). Note that this effect regularly happens outside the exercise stimulus; it occurs any time that protein is consumed in a fasted or semifasted state. An important criterion for this effect seems to be a feeding-induced increase in blood amino acid levels, which signals the muscle to synthesize proteins (41). Note that this effect is transient, or short lived. It becomes refractory after 1 to 2 hours, such that maintenance or further increases in amino acids will not yield further increases in this MPS-stimulating effect (2).

Although the concept may seem unusual, this auto-storage feature is easy to recognize with the other macronutrients. For example, amino acid storage is not completely dissimilar to the way in which carbohydrate consumption can facilitate its own storage as glycogen. The nutraceutical effect of protein causes amino acids to be synthesized in muscle, a tissue that is, after all, the body's reservoir, or de facto storage form, of amino acids (24). Taking advantage of this effect may provide an opportunity for improved recovery adaptation from excise, which will be explored later in this chapter.

Protein Dose

The **daily recommended intake** (DRI) established nutrient recommendations with the intent of eliminating malnutrition-based disease (43). In this regard implementation has been largely successful, but the elimination of disease is not the goal of the athlete. Considering performance and adaptation-based goals, protein needs of the athlete are typically much higher than the DRI, which is set at 0.8 g/kg (0.36 g/lb) (42). Other guidelines are needed for the athlete to optimize performance and adaptation to exercise.

In other circumstances a person may need more protein than the current recommendations. For this reason, the **adjusted macronutrient distribution score** (AMDR) has been developed. This measure provides a range for nutrient intake as a percentage of total caloric intake, based on the needs of the individual (31). For protein, the AMDR is 10% to 35% of daily caloric intake (42). The wide range is designed to offer greater flexibility and develop more specific guidelines tailored to the needs of the individual. For example, an athlete who is consuming more total calories will likely need a smaller proportion of this intake to come from protein.

This nutrient is of such importance that some sport dietitians begin to calculate macronutrient distribution by first establishing protein intake and then establishing the needs of the other macronutrients (31). Consistent with the application of the AMDR, a wide range of daily proteins intake can be appropriate for different athletes. In contrast to more traditional methodologies that classify athletes based on aerobic endurance versus strength, and provide static suggestions, a more flexible approach allows greater athlete-centric specificity of nutritional recommendations (32). In this way, nutrition specificity is like training specificity for the athlete. Some important considerations for determining athlete-specific protein intake include

- training age (also known as experience),
- current periodization phase and goals,
- food choices and preferences, and
- total caloric intake.

More experienced athletes, for example, may need less protein than those who are unaccustomed to exercise. Intense peaking phases will likely necessitate greater protein intake than periods during the offseason. Because of the reduced quality of plant-based protein, vegan athletes may need to consume more protein than those with an omnivorous diet. Finally, periods of caloric restriction require the consumption of greater quantities of protein. This common occurrence has such a profound effect on protein metabolism that a more robust discussion is provided (32).

Protein Dose: Acute

The lay media have offered many recommendations for protein intake per meal, but finding a solid understanding of the rationale behind them is difficult. Fundamentally, the reader can apply the nutraceutical effect and understand that the commonly cited 20 g limit is based not on protein digestion or absorption, but on the maximal stimulation of MPS. More specifically, this 20 g dose is the minimum required to cause maximal stimulation of MPS. Doses beyond this point will not further stimulate protein synthesis, but will progressively increase ingested protein breakdown (23, 41). The 20 g ceiling has been found with both whole-egg protein consumption (23) and whey protein (41).

To add further precision to this application, a bodyweight-specific protein dose per meal has been suggested as 0.31 g/kg (0.14 g/lb) to produce maximal stimulation of MPS (24). This quantity falls in line with the 1.4 g/kg (0.64 g/lb) daily dose and the AMDR.

Another factor in considering single-meal dose is the absorption speed of the protein. Those that are absorbed more slowly or consumed within whole-food meals may not be limited to the 20 g quantity, because their goal is to sustain training-induced MPS rather than cause a rapid pulse in blood amino acid levels (38). For this reason, daily protein intake is helpful for establishing per-meal protein quantity.

Protein Dose: Chronic

Chronic or daily protein dosing may be the most important consideration for optimizing the adaptive response from exercise (26). A protein dose of 1.4 to 1.7 g per kilogram body weight per day will be suitable for athletes most of the time (15). To provide some flexibility to account for atypical metabolic circumstances, such as calorie-restricted diets, a dose up to 2 g per kilogram body weight per day is suggested (32), which is consistent with the parameters of the AMDR (31).

Special Consideration: Calorie-Restricted Diet

During the period of a calorie-restricted diet, whole-body catabolism occurs. This action is often done intentionally to reduce body fat or overall body weight before a weigh-in. In this situation, the breakdown of all endogenous macronutrients occurs, including muscle protein. More specifically, the body oxidizes more amino acids for energy during periods of energy restriction. Without care, excessive protein loss can reduce lean muscle mass and impair performance (13). During this time, resistance training and increased dietary protein intake may help mitigate muscle protein loss (27). This effect has been shown in resistance-trained athletes undergoing 2 weeks of caloric restriction; more lean muscle mass was retained in those who consumed 2.3 g protein per kilogram body weight per day compared with those who ingested 1 g protein per kilogram body weight per day (21). Given the effect of caloric restriction on protein metabolism, intakes may be increased to meet athlete-specific needs in this situation.

Protein Timing and Frequency

The importance of nutrient timing was initially established with a carbohydrate-based postworkout window of opportunity. It is with this lens that the protein literature was initially viewed. A more robust body of research and better appreciation of the nutraceutical effect have contributed to a more recent higher fidelity understanding; there is no restrictive anabolic window for protein intake after exercise (7, 14). Although resistance training increases MPS and the magnitude and duration of the nutraceutical effect, this effect lasts for at least 24 hours (4). Rather than suggesting that protein timing is unimportant, the implication is that the opportunity window is much larger than anticipated, which provides more opportunity for optimization.

Although there is not a distinct effect in the postworkout period like that for carbohydrate, resistance exercise enhances the existing nutraceutical stimulation of MPS (22, 41). This elevation in MPS lasts for at least 24 hours (4) which may provide multiple opportunities for enhanced nutraceutical MPS to facilitate recovery–adaptation. It has been theorized that athletes could take advantage of this nutraceutical effect for maximal daily stimulation of MPS by employing multiple rapidly absorbed protein drinks throughout the day (3). This pattern would transiently elevate blood amino acids to induce the nutraceutical effect and then allow them to wane to minimize refractory period. Repeated consumption in this pulsatile manner could optimize MPS. In direct support of this concept, research has shown that pulse feeding with 4 meals of 20 g whey protein (about every 3 hours) after resistance training yields a greater total MPS response than consuming an equivalent amount of whey in two 40 g doses or more frequent 10 g doses (1). Although the ingested dose of 80 g over 12 hours is inadequate for the needs of athletes, this research provides an early step toward establishing optimization protocols.

Timing: Before Sleep

An often-ignored time for protein feeding occurs shortly before a prolonged sleep-induced fast. Note that the colloquial idea that "sleep is the most ana-bolic time" is not merely incorrect; it is directly opposite reality. The implica-tions are clear after considering that during the overnight fasted hours, neither the amino acid supply nor caloric energy is available to support muscle protein synthesis. As a result, the body cannibalizes its muscle tissue to harvest amino acids for ongoing necessary functions (34). Therefore, under fasted circumstances, sleep often becomes the most catabolic time for athletes. Subsequently, the topic warrants analysis. Note that it is not the act of sleep-ing, but rather the fasting that results in a catabolic metabolic environment (33). Eliminating this fast and preserving muscle protein each night could have an additive effect on an athlete's posttraining recovery–adaptation response.

In support of this theory, 40 g of casein supplementation before sleep was found to improve whole-body protein synthesis overnight compared with a noncaloric placebo (28). The results of this study show that protein ingested before sleep is digested and absorbed without any impairment from sleep itself. The overnight research has been followed up by a more robust, 12 weeks of casein supplementation before sleep (27.5 g protein, 15 g carbo-hydrate, 0.1 g fat) study. The athletes consuming the protein supplement experienced increased muscle strength and cross-sectional area compared with those in the placebo group (30).

Although casein is the commonly studied protein for overnight fasting, it may be cost-prohibitive or contraindicated because of lactose intolerance. Other protein sources may be used to acquire 40 g before sleep, such as the following (34):

- Seven cooked whole eggs
- 5 cups (1,025 ml) of low-fat milk
- 5 cups (1,176 ml) of low-fat yogurt
- Two chicken breasts (176 g [6.2 oz])

Professional Applications

Among the roles that protein and amino acids play in the body, the effect of MPS is often one of focus because it is the most highly sought after recovery–adaptation response to exercise. If athletes can use dietary protein to optimize this response, they may have a competitive advantage over those who do not. To this end, four general elements of protein intake have been addressed.

Quality

This concept is based on the quantity of EAAs within the protein as well as how easily they are absorbed. Higher-quality proteins contain amino acids that are more readily available to be used by the body for protein synthesis. These are often exemplified by soy and animal-derived proteins.

Dosing

The quantity of protein ingested per meal is described as an acute dose. The nutraceutical theory states that nutrient sources can directly induce biochemical change, rather than serve as passive substrate. Combining these ideas, it has been shown that quickly absorbed proteins can maximally stimulate MPS when consumed in a dose of approximately 20 g. Consistent with the idea of athlete specificity, this could be further refined to 0.31 g/kg body weight (0.14 g/lb). Proteins ingested along with whole-food meals are more common and are typically digested and absorbed more slowly than isolated supplements. The estimation of a daily protein dose is thus far more practical. With that idea in mind, protein intakes for athletes are approximately 1.4 to 1.7 g protein per kilogram body weight per day. Exceptional metabolic circumstances such as caloric restriction can increase the protein needs of the athlete beyond this but remain within the AMDR. Although a wide range for suggested protein intake may seem too general to be applicable, it provides the flexibility necessary to ensure athlete specificity. This variability can occur not only between individuals but also with the training and competition cycle for each athlete.

Timing

Initial consideration of protein timing was relative to an exercise bout. A short-lived metabolic window of opportunity does not seem to exist for protein as it does for carbohydrate ingestion; athletes can optimize their recovery–adaptation response over a much longer period. Another shift in protein timing has been toward the catabolic nature of the overnight fast, once thought to be a time of exceptional postexercise recovery. Research has shown this idea to be diametrically opposed with reality. The consumption of a slow protein like casein before sleep has been shown to improve performance outcomes induced by training.

Frequency

Taking advantage of the prolonged postexercise increase in MPS may be achieved using a combination of the other key elements. The strategic use of a rapidly absorbed protein at a dose of 30 g in a pulsatile manner after training may result in the greatest net stimulation of MPS.

Summary Points

- Flexibility of protein recommendations allows greater dietary specificity for each athlete.
- Factors affecting daily protein requirements include training age, periodization phase and goals, food choices, and caloric intake.
- Protein ingestion can directly stimulate muscle protein synthesis, which is known as a nutraceutical effect.
- Under most circumstances hard-training athletes can benefit from consuming 1.4 to 1.7 g protein per kilogram body weight per day.
- An overnight fast causes muscle breakdown, but this effect can be mitigated or reversed by consuming protein before sleep.

Chapter 5

Fat

Lonnie Lowery, PhD, RD, LD, FISSN

Unsurprisingly, new trends in dietary fat consumption, as well as new peer-reviewed literature on dietary fat and its metabolism, have emerged since the original 2011 printing of this chapter. Unfortunately, public interest in reduced-carbohydrate, higher-fat, and even more extreme ketogenic diets has arguably outpaced advances in the literature (12). As noted in the section Ketogenic Diets and Exercise, interest in increased fat "burning" (oxidation) and loss of body fat on **very low-carbohydrate ketogenic diets** (VLCKD) continue to receive attention in the scientific literature. Somewhat to the contrary, earlier findings of elevated perceived exertion coupled with inconsistent or decreased athletic performance also continue to be corroborated, although it is increasingly clear that this depends in part on the specific exercise test employed. The latter is affected by performance time frames, ranging from seconds to minutes, and the energy systems (phosphagen versus fast glycolysis versus oxidative) on which they rely. Other developments, or relative lack thereof, include the application of "medium-chain triglycerides" (actually, shorter fatty acids in free form or as part of a triacylglycerol), structured lipids, uncommon long-chain fatty acids that have previously received less attention, and ketone body supplements.

As a default fuel source for humans, fat (triacylglycerol) is abundant in the body. A relatively lean athlete with 15% body fat carries approximately 10,000 g of stored triacylglycerol in adipose tissue, providing 90,000 kcal of energy, enough energy to complete multiple marathons and many more resistance exercise sessions. Further, approximately 300 g (2,700 kcal) of triacylglycerol is present in intramuscular lipid droplets.

We thank Rachel Hawk and Hayley Maher for their support in this chapter.

Fat, however, is much more than fuel. A complex variety of fats exists, varying by their **fatty acid** makeup and placement on the **glycerol** backbone. Fatty acids are the major component of fats used by the body for energy and tissue development. Glycerol is a three-carbon substance that serves as the central structural component of triglycerides. These variations can exert pharmaceutical-like effects as they influence biological systems. Many (but not all) of these pharmaceutical-like effects occur because the dietary fats that an athlete ingests are incorporated into cell membranes, affecting biochemical processes and the physical nature of the cell. The results can include anti-inflammatory, antidepressive, anticatabolic, and other effects that are of interest to hard-training athletes (51). A large body of literature exists on the various fatty acid types and their physiology, but specific application to athletes is still in the early stages. The section Dietary Fat and Performance provides details on the relationship between fats and athletic performance.

Fat Digestion and Absorption

Of course, to take advantage of fat as a fuel source, or a "nutraceutical," an athlete must digest (break down) and absorb it into the body. Fat digestion begins in the mouth with an enzyme called lingual lipase; the fat is further broken down by gastric and pancreatic lipases. Bile, which is produced in the liver and stored and secreted on demand by the gallbladder, then mixes with and emulsifies the partially digested fat in the proximal small intestine. Then, almost strangely, these broken-up fatty acids and glycerol molecules are recombined in the intestinal cells as they are packaged into chylomicrons and sent into the lymphatic circulation. Ultimately, the absorbed packages of fat enter the blood and have their contents extracted by an enzyme lying in the capillary beds of tissues, lipoprotein lipase. Only then can the constituent fatty acids be transported into a fat cell or working muscle cell. Once in muscles, they can enter the mitochondrial "furnace" as a fuel (figure 5.1). During nonfed periods, the scenario changes somewhat. It is mostly at this time that the "free" fatty acids are derived from adipose cell storage, under the influence of adrenaline and the enzyme hormone-sensitive lipase. The mobilized free fatty acids can circulate to working muscles escorted by the albumin protein.

Types of Fat

Fat contains only three atoms (carbon, hydrogen, and oxygen), but the ways in which these atoms are bonded to each other and their numbers give fats various classifications and biological functions. The following discussion deals with these differences. An understanding of the differences enables the athlete to choose the types of fat that will optimize health and performance.

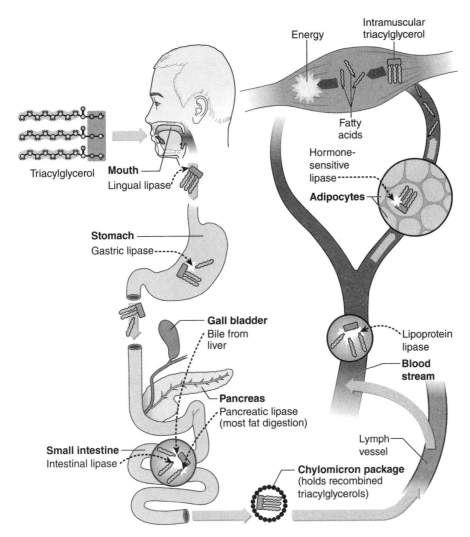

FIGURE 5.1 The steps in dietary fat digestion, absorption, transport, and usage.

Chemical Differences in the Types of Fat

Fats can be categorized into two major types, saturated and unsaturated, but making distinctions far deeper than this is important. A look at figure 5.2 will aid in the understanding of these differences. Nutrition scientists have increasingly appreciated why these many differences affect an athlete's physiology. Indeed, researchers have manipulated different types of fat to enhance exercise performance, impart healthy weight gain, induce body fat loss, and control inflammatory conditions as well as emotional states. So, what are these differences?

- Degrees of saturation: The number of carbon–carbon double bonds.
- Carbon–carbon double-bond position: The placement of the double bonds counted from either end of the fatty acid chain.

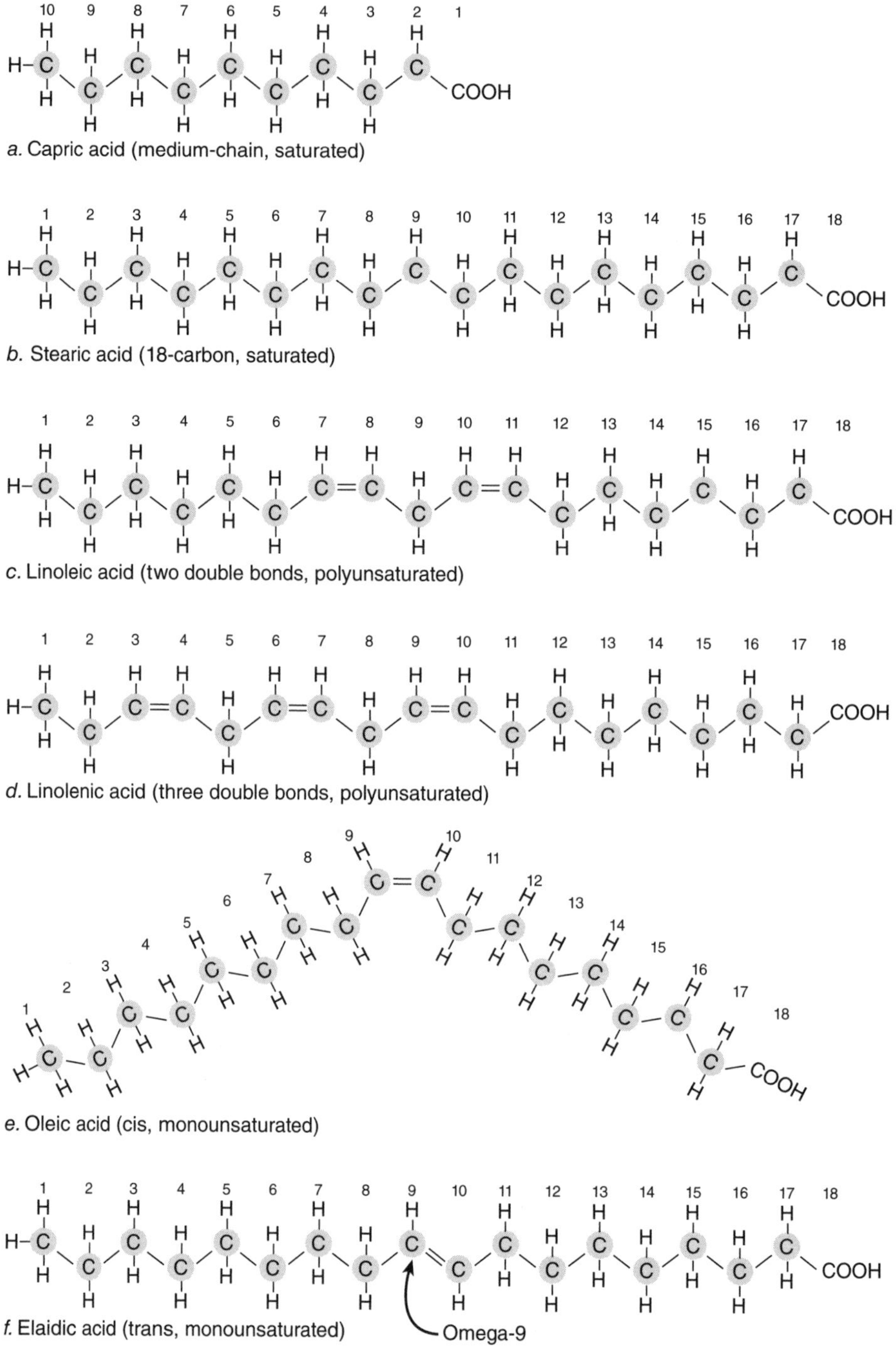

FIGURE 5.2 Six different triacylglycerol molecules show variation in the number of double bonds, placement of double bonds, and chain length. Also, the shape of the molecule varies in cis versus trans fatty acids, as seen in the elaidic acid and oleic acid examples.

- Chain length: The length of the carbon chain that makes up the fatty acids.
- Fatty acid placement. Differences in where the fatty acid chains are attached (or omitted) from the glycerol backbone of the fat molecule. Food chemists can manipulate these configurations to produce potential ergogenic effects.

Degrees of Saturation

Fatty acids are the business end of a fat (triacylglycerol) molecule. Fatty acid chains have most of the calories and the most pharmaceutical-like effects. It is from their degree of unsaturation (the number of carbon–carbon double bonds) that fatty acids, and thus their parent triacylglycerol molecule, get the designation *saturated*, *monounsaturated,* or *polyunsaturated*. That is, a fatty acid can contain zero, one, or multiple carbon–carbon double bonds, respectively (refer to figure 5.2). The more carbon–carbon double bonds on a fatty acid, the less saturated it is with hydrogen atoms.

Saturated fatty acids, the fatty acid chains with zero double bonds (refer to the capric and stearic acid chains in figure 5.2*a* and *b*), have been condemned for negatively affecting **low-density lipoprotein** (LDL) cholesterol receptors on the liver and thus increasing serum LDL cholesterol (and therefore heart disease risk). Educational materials since the early 1970s have included this observation, but more recent research suggests that differences exist even among the saturated fatty acids. For example, *stearic acid*, an 18-carbon fatty acid (figure 5.2*b*), does not appear to be as atherogenic as other saturated fatty acids (57). Further, recent research suggests a helpful role for higher serum cholesterol concentrations among strength athletes, as discussed later in this chapter.

Monounsaturated fatty acids have enjoyed a much more positive reception among dietitians. For example, *oleic acid* (figure 5.2*e*), which olive oil is so rich in, has been related to enhanced longevity and reduced morbidity. This beneficial effect is apparent from observations that the Mediterranean diet is rich in olive oil and that populations consuming this diet tend to live longer than others. Controlled research indicates that oils rich in this monounsaturated fat improve blood pressure and glucose metabolism compared with diets higher in carbohydrates or polyunsaturates (64, 70, 88). Canola oil is also rich in oleic acid, offering a cheaper and slightly more versatile alternative. Tree nuts, peanuts, and nut butters are also excellent sources of oleic acid.

Polyunsaturated fats (i.e., polyunsaturated fatty acids, from which the parent fat molecule gets its designation) have two or more carbon–carbon double bonds. Most notably, these include *linoleic acid* (two double bonds, figure 5.2*c*), which is heavily consumed in Western cultures; *linolenic acid* (three double bonds, figure 5.2*d*), which is underconsumed in Western cultures; and the fish oil fatty acids *eicosapentaenoic acid* (EPA, five double bonds) and *docosahexaenoic acid* (DHA, six double bonds), which are also underconsumed in Western cultures. These latter fatty acids, because of their large number of double bonds, are sometimes called *highly unsaturated fatty acids* (HUFA). A balance of the various polyunsaturates is important, because these fatty acids can have opposing effects in the body. That is, a diet too rich in linoleic acid increases low-grade inflammatory states that have been linked to cardiovascular disease, diabetes, and other chronic diseases prevalent in Western cultures (7, 15, 44, 77). Also, high-intensity exercise leads to an inflammatory state that can improve or worsen depending on the amounts of linolenic and linoleic acids ingested. Specifically, ingestion of EPA and DHA, which have anti-inflammatory properties, can counteract the low-grade inflammation brought on by high-intensity exercise (for more information on EPA and DHA, see the section Essential Fatty Acids on page 83). The inclusion of more fish oil–derived fatty acids moderates this effect. Unfortunately, little information currently exists about whether linoleic acid–based inflammation worsens athletic conditions such as bursitis and tendinitis.

Carbon–Carbon Double-Bond Position

No discussion of **polyunsaturated fatty acids** (PUFA) would be complete without an explanation of the position of the carbon–carbon double bonds. This is where the categories *omega-3* and *omega-6* become meaningful (monounsaturates are in the *omega-9* category, which tends to get less attention). *Omega* refers to the position of the first carbon–carbon double bond, counting from the methyl end (figure 5.2). This is important in relation to several nutraceutical effects. For example, fish oils contain omega-3 fatty acids and are anti-inflammatory, whereas most vegetable oils contain predominantly omega-6 fatty acids, which are proinflammatory. Typically, two "regular" carbon–carbon single bonds separate the rarer carbon–carbon double bonds on PUFA molecules. These double bonds can also be designated by counting from the "delta," or carboxyl, end (the end attaching to a glycerol when a full fat molecule is formed). Thus, linolenic acid, which is underconsumed from sources such as flax meal or walnuts, is fully described by counting from both ends of its chain. It is an omega-3, "delta" 9,12 polyunsaturated fatty acid. A popular supplemental fat is *conjugated linoleic acid* (CLA) found in beef and dairy. It has double bonds closer to each other than is typical; for example, one version of CLA is an omega-7, delta 9,11 fatty acid. The section Fat Supplements for Athletes discusses this supplemental fat in more detail.

Another positional difference relating to carbon–carbon double bonds does not concern the numerical position on the fatty acid chain. Instead, it concerns the localized type of a given double bond. This is the *cis* versus *trans* descriptor. Most "natural" fatty acids exhibit the cis configuration. In these fats, the carbon–carbon double bond is missing hydrogen atoms on the same side of the fatty acid chain. The resulting "hairpin" shape is evident in the oleic acid example in figure 5.2*e*. Conversely, trans-configured fatty acids (or **trans fat**), created by food producers have the missing hydrogen atoms on the opposite sides of the chain, giving them a straight shape much like the one exhibited by elaidic acid (figure 5.2*f*). These trans fatty acids are processed fats that are used in baked goods like doughnuts, breads, crackers, potato chips, cookies, and many other processed foods like margarine and salad dressings. Food scientists create these trans fats by **hydrogenation**—a process used in the food industry in which hydrogen gas is bubbled through oil at a high temperature to create trans fatty acids, which increases shelf life or spreadability (or both) of the original oil. Hydrogenated oils also impart certain beneficial "mouth feel" characteristics on finished food products. Indeed, the deleterious effects of manufactured trans fats, such as those in some pastries, crackers, fried chicken, and french fries, are much like those attributed to saturated fats (e.g., cardiovascular disease), both metabolically and physically. For example, a triacylglycerol with three very straight fatty acids attached to its glycerol backbone would pack more tightly with its fellows into a cell membrane compared with a triacylglycerol with "bent" fatty acids.

Chain Length

On a deeper level than degree of unsaturation, the physical fact of chain length is also important. Fatty acid chains range widely from 4 to 22 carbons in length but are more typically 16 to 22 carbons long. Examples of (rarer) short-chain fatty acids (less than 6 carbons long) are those made by bacteria in the gut as they act on dietary fiber or those present in cow's butter. Examples of (also rare) medium-chain fatty acids (6-12 carbons long) are capric acid and lauric acid derived from tropical oils that are sold as sport supplements. Long-chain fatty acids (i.e., 16-22 carbons long) are most common and include all of the mono- and polyunsaturated fats previously discussed, including linoleic acid (omega-6, cis type, 18 carbons), linolenic acid (omega-3, cis type, 18 carbons), oleic acid (omega-9, cis type, 18 carbons), elaidic acid (omega-9, trans type, 18 carbons), EPA (omega-3, cis type, 20 carbons), and DHA (omega-3, cis type, 22 carbons). See table 5.1 for types of dietary fat. Fatty acid chains that are classified as medium-chain fatty acids (6-12 carbons long) have been studied in terms of improving aerobic endurance performance. The theoretical rationale of ingesting these **medium-chain triglycerides** (MCT) is that they may spare muscle glycogen and improve aerobic endurance performance. Unfortunately, most studies investigating this aspect of MCT ingestion have not supported improvements in aerobic endurance performance. But as noted in the section Medium-Chain Fatty Acids, athletes may gain other benefits by ingesting these types of fat.

TABLE 5.1 Types of Dietary Fat

Type and examples	Number of carbon atoms: number of c–c double bonds	Dietary sources	Recommended intakes[a]
SATURATED FATTY ACIDS			
Butyric acid	4:0	Cow's butter	—
Various medium-chain types (e.g., capric and lauric acids)	6-12:0	Tropical oils, dietary and medical supplements	<30 g per serving to prevent intestinal distress
Palmitic acid	16:0	Animal fat, palm oil	Saturated fat <33% of fat intake; <10% of caloric intake
Stearic acid	18:0	Animal fat, cocoa butter	Saturated fat <33% of fat intake; <10% of caloric intake
MONOUNSATURATED FATTY ACIDS			
(cis, n-9) oleic acid	18:1	Olive, canola, peanut oils	>33% of fat intake; ~15% caloric intake
(trans, n-9) elaidic acid	18:1	Partially hydrogenated oils: some margarines, pastries, crackers, fried chicken, French fries	Minimize
POLYUNSATURATED FATTY ACIDS			
(all cis, n-6) linoleic acid[b]	18:2	Most vegetable oils: snack foods, bottled oils including corn, cottonseed, safflower, and so on	Adequate Intake: 17 g daily men, 12 g daily women
(cis + trans, n-7 or n-6) conjugated linoleic acids[c]	18:2	Beef and dairy, dietary supplements	3.0-7.5 g research dose; typical intakes <250 mg daily
(all cis, n-3) linolenic acid[b]	18:3	Walnuts, flax products, canola oil, and soybean oil (some)	Adequate Intake: 1.6 g daily men, 1.1 g daily women
(all cis) gamma-linolenic acid	18:3	Primrose, borage and black currant oils, dietary supplements; produced in body from other fatty acids	~500 mg daily research dose
(all cis, n-3) eicosapentaenoic acid (EPA)	20:5	Salmon, sardines, herring, dietary supplements	160 mg Daily Value (extrapolated); dose–response effects (more = larger effect); limit total EPA and DHA to <3.0 g daily
(all cis, n-3) docosahexaenoic acid (DHA)	22:6	Salmon, sardines, herring, dietary supplements	160 mg Daily Value (extrapolated); dose–response effects (more = larger effect); limit total EPA and DHA to <3.0 g daily
UNCOMMON TRIACYLGLYCEROLS (TWO OR THREE FATTY ACIDS AND GLYCEROL)			
Structured triacylglycerols	–	Research and medical formulas	10 g (oral) research dose
Diacylglycerol	–	Enova oil	14 g per tablespoon serving

[a]Method of recommendations may vary: % of total kilocalories or % of total fat intake, grams or milligrams; recommendations based on USDA suggestions, Daily Values, Adequate Intakes, intervention and observational studies, and computational estimates by author.

[b]Essential fatty acid.

[c]Conjugated linoleic acid is multiple fatty acids, commonly cis-9, trans-11 or trans-10, or cis-12 versions.

Data from U.S. Department of Health and Human Services and U.S. Department of Agriculture (2017).

Fatty Acid Placement

Fatty acid placement is a final difference, and one that can be manipulated; food chemists can specifically arrange or omit fatty acids from the glycerol backbone of a triacylglycerol molecule. The result can be what is known as a *structured triacylglycerol* (careful arrangement of different fatty acids on the glycerol molecule) or alternatively a *diacylglycerol* (omitting the middle, or sn-2, fatty acid). These manipulations are perhaps the cutting edge of fat technology for athletes and are discussed in the section Dietary Fat and Performance later in the chapter.

Essential Fatty Acids

The potent and varied physiological effects of the many fatty acids are perhaps best exemplified by the fact that humans must consume certain ones to prevent deficiency symptoms. The two nutritionally essential fatty acids are **linoleic acid** (omega-6) and **linolenic acid** (omega-3). The omega-6 linoleic acid is an 18-carbon fatty acid with two double bonds, and, in most Western diets, is overconsumed relative to the omega-3 linolenic acid. Linolenic acid is also an 18-carbon fatty acid, but it has three double bonds and is underconsumed in most Western diets.

Consumption of these fatty acids is necessary because humans lack the enzymes delta-12 and delta-15 desaturase. These cellular enzymes would add carbon–carbon double bonds (points of unsaturation) at the 12 and 15 positions in fatty acid synthesis as the chain is built. Again, note that linolenic acid is an (essential) omega-3 fatty acid with double bonds at the 9, 12, and 15 positions, counting from the delta (carboxyl) end. Without the provision of such double bonds and thus these fatty acids, vertebrates (e.g., humans) exhibit symptoms such as retarded growth, dermatitis, kidney lesions, and even death. This is partly because consumed linoleic acid and linolenic acid are built into longer physiologically important fatty acids that become part of cell membranes and form eicosanoids. Eicosanoids, derived from the essential fatty acids, influence many bodily systems and play key roles in inflammation and immunity.

An interesting additional example is the omega-3 fatty acid docosahexaenoic acid (DHA). As another fatty acid with effects on cell membranes, eicosanoid production (e.g., prostaglandins), and gene interactions, DHA also produces valuable physiological effects (5). In fact, some have argued for the formal recognition of DHA as an essential fat because these effects are more than merely helpful. Animal, epidemiological, and human intervention studies suggest that DHA improves neurological and visual function in developing infants (36, 39, 98). Docosahexaenoic acid is a major component of cerebral gray matter. Provision of DHA as part of a fish oil supplement improves mood and may benefit psychological depression (49, 85).

The benefits of DHA extend beyond the brain and eyes. Supplementation with n-3 fatty acids including DHA lessens the inflammatory component of several chronic diseases, some more than others (10, 15). A fish oil supplement containing 1.1 g EPA and 0.7 g/day DHA has been shown to reduce the cortisol response to stress (19). Supplementing DHA with EPA reduces total serum triacylglycerol concentrations, blood pressure, platelet aggregation, and inflammation and decreases arrhythmic cardiac death (8, 73). Indeed, research suggests that some of the effects of (essential, omega-3) linolenic acid are more potently exhibited by DHA (8, 15, 22, 84). For these reasons, DHA is arguably a third essential fatty acid (61).

Note, though, that more research is necessary to elucidate whether DHA, EPA, or some combination is best for cardiovascular and other benefits (8). This breakdown could be of particular relevance to male athletes, whose higher testosterone concentrations depress tissue levels of DHA (17). Regarding dose, Arterburn and colleagues (5) reported that a large dose (2 g) of DHA daily maximizes plasma concentrations in one month. Table 5.1 shows recommended daily intakes of individual fatty acids. Note also that DHA can be converted in the body to EPA, but the reverse does not occur (5). Many natural sources and dietary supplements include a mixture of DHA and EPA (mixed omega-3), and some recommend a combined dose of less than 3 g daily (60).

Discussions of essential fatty acids are, however, insufficient to emphasize the impact of dietary fat on health. In the context of the "balanced diet" concept, it is helpful to realize that Western society does not encourage a balanced intake regarding dietary fat. According to the Institute of Medicine (IOM), intakes of omega-6 to omega-3 fatty acids should approximate a 7-to-1 ratio (41). Some researchers and dietitians suggest an even lower ratio. These recommendations, based on physiological, paleonutritional, and other evidence, are very different from the nearly 17-to-1 ratio that Westerners consume (77). To state this differently, Western populations such as Americans, Britons, and Australians vastly overconsume omega-6 fat while vastly underconsuming omega-3 fat (77, 52, 58). Because of the competition of these types of fat with respect to incorporation into cell membranes, prostaglandin production, cytokine concentrations, gene interactions, and other effects, this is a prescription for inflammation, thrombosis, and other physiological aberrations. Also connected to the concept of balance are the well-known health benefits of the Mediterranean diet with its emphasis on olive oil. This rich source of omega-9 fatty acids (oleic acid) is part of the reason that the Mediterranean diet is considered healthy (65). Although considered more neutral relative to inflammation, rather than anti-inflammatory in itself, oleic acid can nonetheless alter the ratio of (inflammatory) omega-6 fats to omega-3 fats if it replaces some of the omega-6 fat in the diet.

Scientific research on essential fatty acids and athletic performance is in its infancy. Although the health benefits of essential fatty acid ingestion for athletes are clear, performance studies are lacking. A recent study, however, examined the effects of omega-3 supplementation on young wrestlers' (approximately 18 years old) pulmonary function during intensive wrestling training. Wrestlers consumed capsules containing 1,000 mg/day of omega-3 (180 mg EPA and 120 mg DHA) while participating in wrestling training three times a week for 12 weeks. The authors reported that at the end of the 12-week study, wrestlers ingesting the omega-3 supplement significantly improved their pulmonary function as compared with a placebo group undergoing the same training and pulmonary testing. With the popularity and attention that essential fatty acids are attaining, more research on essential fatty acids and exercise performance is likely.

Cholesterol

Cholesterol is not classified as a dietary fat, but it is an important lipid. Cholesterol is a complex fatty substance that has many important functions in the body. It can be made in the body or supplied through foods of animal origin. Although it may hold negative connotations for most Americans, dietary cholesterol is actually a controversial substance. First, interpretations of its deleterious effects have differed between the United States and Canada. Canadian authorities have deemphasized its effect on actual serum cholesterol concentrations and cardiovascular risk (55) and still do not consider the once-common U.S. recommendation to restrict dietary cholesterol to less than 300 mg per day important enough for inclusion in Canada's dietary guidelines. This is not to say that Canadians view circulating cholesterol as without effect on cardiovascular risk; instead, the view is that dietary cholesterol has a relatively minor influence on blood levels of cholesterol and probably cardiovascular disease. The United States Dietary Guidelines have recently followed suit, removing recommendations to limit dietary cholesterol (89).

Second, dietary cholesterol may play as yet unrecognized roles in strength athletes. In a sense, dietary cholesterol may be emerging as advantageous. Early work by Riechman and colleagues (74) suggests correlations between dietary cholesterol intake and lean muscle mass and strength gains among older resistance trainers (60-69 years). Although not causal, the relationship with lean muscle mass gain was significant ($R^2 = 0.27$), suggesting that more than a quarter of the variance in observed lean muscle mass gain during resistance training was attributable to dietary cholesterol. This finding lends some credence to historical, less scientific suggestions from coaches that strength athletes should consume large amounts of whole eggs and beef. More research is necessary in younger persons. Because this cholesterol research is in its early stages, it is not clear how best to reconcile any potential benefits with the controversial potential adverse effects on vascular health.

Dietary Fat and Performance

Certain examples suggest how the effects of fat differ between athletes and sedentary healthy persons or patients in clinical settings. For instance, physical training can favorably change the tissue ratios of fatty acids in the body (2, 35). This beneficial, nondietary shift toward greater omega-3 content is not seen in nonexercisers. In addition, consumption of the lower-fat diet often pursued by athletes favorably changes tissue ratios of fatty acids (69). This change occurs at least in part because of a lower presence of (and thus less competition from) omega-6 fatty acids. Many athletes do not realize they can reduce (improve) their tissue ratios of omega-6 to omega-3 by simply consuming less overall dietary fat.

Extreme diets, however, can become problematic. As one example, the "benefits" of very low-fat, high-fiber diets suggested by some researchers induce changes that athletes may want to avoid. For instance, reduced testosterone concentrations (10, 29, 72) from such intakes may be beneficial to a patient with risk of androgen-dependent prostate cancer but may not be beneficial to an athlete who needs the additional 10% to 15% circulating testosterone. Most athletes are aware that testosterone is advantageous for athletic recovery and muscular growth.

Another popular and sometimes extreme dietary recommendation, decreased calorie intake, may also be problematic for athletes. With the often large calorie expenditures of training or the caloric demands of adding lean muscle mass, athletes do not benefit by restricting the very energy that drives progress. All things considered, fat content of the diet can range from 20% to 40% of total calories with no effect on strength performance (91).

Fat as Exercise Fuel

The longer-term effects of dietary fat on an athlete are not the only consideration; more acute issues are important as well. Regarding dietary fat as fuel during exercise, two major phenomena are the metabolic crossover effect (table 5.2) and the duration effect, or "fat shift" (table 5.3). The former involves a crossover from fat oxidation at rest and at lower intensities toward carbohydrate usage at high intensities. That is, an inverse relationship exists between direct fat "burning" (measured by respiratory exchange ratio) and exercise intensity (measured by heart rate or $\dot{V}O_2max$) (9, 45, 75). Biochemical control and the immediacy of need for energy are reasons for this crossover. Even highly trained aerobic endurance athletes, with their enhanced capacity to oxidize fat, eventually cross over to carbohydrate use, albeit at higher intensities than less aerobically fit persons.

The duration effect, however, involves the opposite relationship. Exercise duration is positively correlated with fat use (51). During prolonged, low-intensity exercise (longer than 30 minutes), the use of carbohydrate to fuel the activity gradually shifts toward an increasing reliance on fat as

TABLE 5.2 Fat Versus Carbohydrate Oxidation During Fasted Exercise of Different Intensities

Exercise intensity[a]	RER[b]	Fuel type	Biochemistry[c]
Low (<25% $\dot{V}O_2$max)	0.70	Fat	$C_{16}H_{32}O_2 + 23\,O_2 \rightarrow$ $16\,CO_2 + 16\,H_2O$
Moderate (50% $\dot{V}O_2$max)	0.85	Fat and carbohydrate (increasingly carbohydrate)	Mix of palmitate and glucose usage
High (100%)	1.00	Carbohydrate	$C_6H_{12}O_6 + 6\,O_2 \rightarrow$ $6\,CO_2 + 6\,H_2O$

[a]Low-intensity exercise can be prolonged (several hours) and moderate-intensity exercise somewhat less (perhaps 1-4 h), whereas high-intensity exercise is measured in just minutes.

[b]Respiratory exchange ratio (RER) assessed on a metabolic cart (volume of CO_2 produced / volume of O_2 consumed each minute) is often used interchangeably with respiratory quotient (RQ), which is technically a cellular respiration term. RER measures validate the biochemistry at the far right in the table.

[c]Note that, as with RER measurements, the CO_2 produced / O_2 consumed for palmitate "burning" = 16 / 23 = 0.70, which rises with intensity toward glucose use where 6 / 6 = 1.00.

TABLE 5.3 Fat Mobilization During Fasted Exercise of Different Durations

Exercise duration	Serum glycerol*
Prolonged, >60 min	Higher
Moderate, 30 to 60 min	Moderate
Brief, <30 min	Lower

*Serum glycerol concentrations (fat breakdown and mobilization) are high during prolonged fasting (i.e., even at rest) as well as during low- to moderate-intensity prolonged exercise; in general, greater fat mobilization during exercise relates to greater fat oxidation.

the fuel. The greater reliance on fat can be demonstrated by measurement of glycerol levels in the blood. Recall that a triglyceride molecule consists of a glycerol molecule and three fatty acids. If fat is going to be used to fuel activity, the triglyceride molecule needs to be broken down (chemists use the term *hydrolysis* to refer to this reaction) into a free glycerol molecule and three free fatty acids. The glycerol and fatty acids are said to be "free" because they are not bound to each other as they were in the triglyceride form. As exercise duration increases, an associated increase of blood glycerol levels occurs (table 5.3), indicating that triglycerides have been broken down and that the fatty acids are being used to fuel the low-intensity exercise.

Two points about exercise for body fat loss are worth reiterating here. First, not all bodily fat is stored in adipose cells. A significant percentage comes from the roughly 300 g of stored intramuscular triacylglycerol. Research has clarified that these muscle lipid droplets are a portion of the oxidized fat seen with use of metabolic cart systems. Second, the crossover and the duration phenomena do not necessarily suggest that body fat reduction is achieved directly only during fasted, low- to moderate-intensity prolonged exercise. Indeed, repeat bouts of high-intensity exercise stimulate mitochondrial bio-genesis that would enhance fat usage throughout an athlete's day. Further, high-intensity training reduces glycogen stores that would subsequently be refilled by ingested carbohydrate, a nutrient that may otherwise be converted and stored as body fat (these are key reasons that many power athletes are so lean). The choice of exercise intensity and duration, then, is partly determined by the athlete's need for aerobic conditioning versus the need for rest and prevention of (sympathetic type) overtraining.

Fat Loading

To augment and support the adaptations of physical training, athletes have increasingly sought to manipulate dietary fat through both food manipulation and dietary supplement administration. Food manipulations center on the fact that eating more fat—even "fat loading"—can increase muscle concentrations of stored triacylglycerol and increase the activity of "fat-burning" enzymes. Raising the roughly 300 g of stored intramuscular triacylglycerol would appear advantageous regarding simple fuel supply. A look inside a muscle cell reveals lipid droplets immediately adjacent to the mitochondrial furnaces that drive aerobic endurance performance, leading to interest in increasing these readily accessible depots of fuel. This point is especially true given that aerobic endurance athletes have increased capacity to store these fat droplets compared with nonexercisers (90) (note that cellular fat accumulation is part of the mechanism behind diabetes but in athletes is not deleterious). Eating more dietary fat, however, is not intended simply to increase the content of a person's intramuscular fuel tank. By adapting to a higher-fat diet, an athlete becomes better at using stored fat (25, 100). One strategy, then, is to devise a preevent dietary regimen that allows for 1 to 2 weeks of increased lipid storage and (fat oxidative) enzyme enhancement.

Unfortunately, the primary finding of fat-loading studies appears to be an increased (rather than decreased) rate of perceived exertion (RPE), with inconsistent or decreased overall performance. Although some studies have suggested a prolonged time to exhaustion after a fat load (which is good), the increased sense of effort coupled with no enhancement of aerobic power (25, 30, 81) has led many researchers and coaches to abandon or modify the fat-loading strategy. Simply having more intramuscular fat or even enhanced fat oxidation does not appear to equate to better performance in most sports. This conclusion has prompted researchers to try fat-loading regimens followed by ample pre- and midexercise carbohydrate consumption. Despite showing marked and seemingly favorable changes in fuel metabolism, however, these investigations remain equivocal regarding actual performance (71). A potential mechanism for these inconsistent findings may be reduced or delayed activity of the pyruvate dehydrogenase (PDH) reaction that links glycolysis and the citric acid cycle (80). Having increased carbohydrate stores after a fat-then-carbohydrate load would be less useful if the glycogen is not efficiently accessed.

Ketogenic Diets and Exercise

Related to fat loading, but more chronic and perhaps more extreme in nature, is the concept of ketogenic diets. As stated by Ma and Suzuki (53),

> A ketogenic diet involves using fat, a high-density substrate, as the main source in daily calorie intake while restricting carbohydrate intake. . . . In this way, the liver is forced to produce and release ketone bodies into the circulation. . . . This phenomenon is called nutritional ketosis (p. 1).

Very low-carbohydrate ketogenic diets (VLCKD), approximating 50 g or less of daily carbohydrate, continue to be popular with athletes and weight-conscious people (56, 92). Efficacy and relative agreement in the peer-reviewed literature, however, depends on species type (62) and desired outcomes. For example, enhanced fat oxidation or reduced body fatness on ad libitum higher-fat VLCD is repeatedly reported (11, 33, 56, 92). The reduced fat mass in athletes who can comply with VLCKD may be a reason for the popularity of these diets. Even in those in a hyperenergetic state, Vargas and colleagues (92) found reduced fat mass among ketotic subjects during 8 weeks of resistance training compared with nonketotic controls. Exercise performance results, however, vary more widely, depending on athlete type and methodology (12, 13, 28, 33, 42, 56). Investigation of VLCKD has even been done on hypertrophy during hyperenergetic mesocycles, but without enhancement (92). At present, fat loss, as opposed to exercise performance or lean muscle mass gains, appears to be the primary beneficial outcome of VLCKD.

The metabolic mechanisms underlying greater loss of body fatness compared with higher-carbohydrate diets involve both increased free fatty acid mobilization from adipose tissue and elevated fatty acid oxidation (13, 33, 56, 80). Moderately reduced circulating glucose and insulin (62) and several intracellular and enzymatic changes in fat and muscle tissue (12, 42, 76) underlie these elevated lipolytic and oxidative effects. As noted elsewhere in this chapter, the elevated presence of ketone bodies such as beta-hydroxybutyrate indicates that fatty acid mobilization outweighs their oxidation; it is thus used as a confirmation that a very low-carbohydrate diet is indeed putting intervention groups in nutritional ketosis (13, 56, 62, 82). Whether the metabolic and fat loss benefits coincide with reduced lean muscle mass, however, appears more equivocal (28, 53, 92). A 2019 review (53) stated, "A [ketogenic diet] may induce muscle loss and excess oxidative stress. To prevent oxidative damage, oxidative state and muscle mass may need to be occasionally monitored." When lean muscle mass is reportedly lost, however, it may not be enough to be ergolytic. Green and colleagues (28) concluded that when it did occur, "lean mass losses were not reflected in lifting performances" (p. 3373).

Attempts at actual performance enhancements often cite similar metabolic changes to those invoked during body composition discussions, including a shift in endocrine status and adaptation toward using fat as a fuel (42, 53, 62). Not providing the primary fuel source during intense crossed-over exercise, however, high-fat-low-carbohydrate diets are often reported to hamper power output and perceived exertion (33, 42, 53). Even for aerobic endurance athletes operating at lower power levels, VLCKD have been related to poorer exercise economy (more oxygen required per unit of performance output) (13). Again, however, the type of exercise testing matters: Work done at Ohio State University suggests that *brief* power performance tests (that would rely more on the phosphagen system as opposed to fast glycolysis) may benefit (56).

When examining VLCKD, it is important to distinguish between the period necessary to achieve ketosis (about 3-4 days) (82) and the longer period for "fat adaptation." Researchers and athletes have both posited that a long enough period of fat adaptation may lead to improved performance of intense exercise, but these hypotheses have been met with inconsistent data as noted earlier. The period of metabolic adaptation toward reaching elevated serum ketone bodies was summarized by Burke (12) to be 2 to 3 weeks—a scenario that could affect compliance. Whether such compliance can be improved with specialized ketogenic meals that mimic carbohydrates remains to be established (62).

Fat Supplements for Athletes

Although they are relatively rare in the Western food supply, specialty fat supplements are of interest because of two biological facts. First, cell membranes generally incorporate the newly ingested fat, a rather profound phenomenon. For example, in relatively large amounts, EPA and DHA can displace the more inflammatory arachidonic acid (all-cis, n-6, 20:4) in cell membranes, altering the cellular prostaglandin cascade (7). Using the analogy of a water balloon to depict a cell, this means that the "rubber" of the balloon changes—not simply its contents, as would be true with carbohydrate ingestion. Further, the cell membrane can remain altered for long periods. Some studies using fish oils report washout periods of 10 to 18 weeks (23, 46). Second, cell contents and operations change when uncommon types of fat are provided as fuel. For example, medium-chain triacylglycerol supplements (which are distinguished by the length of the fatty acids rather than their unsaturation) can be more readily absorbed and "burned" (oxidized) in cells, as discussed next.

Fish Oils

Probably the most pervasive type of special lipid supplementation is fish oils. These supply both EPA and DHA at roughly 50% of the total contents of the (gel) capsule; EPA is usually predominant. More concentrated products, sometimes called extra-strength fish oils, contain more of the active ingredients EPA and DHA and may alter the ratio toward more or less DHA. For this reason, fish oil enthusiasts justifiably look for the total dose of EPA and DHA in a product rather than simply dosing by total grams of gross fish oil. Fatty foods, on the other hand, provide a sometimes broad mix of fatty acids and tend toward only one predominant type or another.

Typically, claims about sport supplements purported to confer multiple beneficial effects are exaggerated or deliberately misleading, but the myriad effects of consuming EPA–DHA supplements are more evidence based, making them popular. Fish oils offer benefits beyond the long washout periods (which could be negative as well as positive). The simple fact that omega-3 fat is underconsumed in most Western cultures creates a state of relative deficiency or imbalance. This relative deficiency is what underlies the various physiological effects noted earlier in the chapter. For example, Archer and colleagues (4) reported that the U.S. population, particularly in the Midwest, eats too little fatty fish to garner cardioprotective effects. Therefore, supplementation is of interest. Other factors that add to the interest in fish oil supplements include the low level of concern about heavy metal contamination (mercury) in comparison with some seafood (51) and a recommendation from the American Heart Association that supplementation may be necessary in select populations (8). As a rule, dietitians recognize that correcting a deficiency induces more reliable and potentially broader positive effects than does hypersupplementation of a nutrient that is adequately consumed.

Reviews addressing how EPA and DHA may benefit athletes are rare and include an element of speculation because of a dearth of population-specific research. But some research has been conducted on healthy persons and those with athletic injuries or issues. A review by Lowery (51) suggested that the anti-inflammatory and antidepressive (mood-elevating) effects of these omega-3 fatty acids may benefit athletes who train hard or who are overtrained. A later study by Simopoulos (78) also indicated that the anti-inflammatory effects were beneficial for athletes, suggesting 1 to 2 g of daily EPA plus DHA.

Conditions such as tendinitis, bursitis, osteoarthritis, and even overtraining syndrome (e.g., depression) are examples of athlete-specific maladies that may be improved through omega-3 supplementation. The protective effect against cartilage breakdown, for example, in arthritic conditions (18), may be beneficial to an athlete's career longevity, as may the bone-protective effects (24), although more sport-specific research is needed. Benefits to exercise-related bronchoconstriction have also been reported (59). Further, emerging research may suggest a role for omega-3 fat in reduction of body fat. This research has a sound basis because of the known inflammatory nature of obesity, particularly visceral obesity (e.g., cytokines) (6), and the corrective anti-inflammatory characteristics of fish oils. Such work is in the early stages, however, and has not yet provided the critical mass of evidence needed to call for recommendations related to body composition. Finally, research on the relation between omega-3 fat and muscle recovery and soreness from exercise is mixed and appears dose and age related (16, 47, 66).

Conjugated Linoleic Acid

Perhaps the next most popular fatty acid supplement among athletes, which is a group of positional **isomers**, is *conjugated linoleic acid* (CLA). Isomers are compounds that have identical molecular formulas but differ in the nature or sequence of bonding of their atoms. Since before the First International Conference on CLA in 2001, however, researchers realized that humans are "hyporesponders" compared with animals such as mice. In a sense this characteristic is unfortunate because of the dramatic anticatabolic and body fat–reducing qualities exhibited by CLA in these animals (63, 64). A second generation of animal research has since ascribed individual qualities to the cis-9, trans-11 isomer (growth enhancing) versus the trans-10, cis-12 isomer (antilipogenic, lipolytic, or both) (63). Any consistent benefits to humans and to athletes, however, have yet to be elucidated. Reasons for the relative inefficacy in human studies could include different dosing methods (often 3 g daily in human research versus 0.5% to 1.0% of food weight or total calories in animal studies), study duration, and species differences. The faster metabolic rates and growth curves of rodents compared with humans appear to be confounders.

Human intakes of CLA from foods such as dairy and meats have been reported to be 151 mg daily for women and 212 mg daily for men; almost all of this is the cis-9, trans-11 type (87). Limited human research suggests increases in strength or lean muscle mass, or both, with supplementation (50, 87), and other data suggest a small reduction in body fat (71). Strength and body composition protocols in human studies have not been standardized, however, and thus no clear benefits have been substantiated. Since publication of the few positive findings on body composition, concerns have emerged over potentially hampered insulin sensitivity and fatty liver (1, 97) and unimpressive effects regarding body weight and fat reduction in pigs and humans (97). Thus, human studies remain rare compared with animal research, which is continuing. Although one meta-analysis has indicated a modest and variable body fat–reducing effect in humans that approximates 1 kg (2.2 lb) of loss over 12 weeks (99), at the present time CLA isomers do not appear to be as advantageous to humans as other fatty acid supplements.

Medium-Chain Fatty Acids

As mentioned earlier, another important aspect of fatty acid selection in sport nutrition is fatty acid length. Short, medium, and long fatty acids exert different physiological effects. For example, although EPA and DHA are discussed in the section Carbon–Carbon Double-Bond, their length also matters. They are longer than more common fatty acids and thus are distinguished by their chain length, not simply the presence of the omega-3 double bond. About half as long as EPA and DHA are the medium-chain fatty acids capric acid (10 carbons, figure 5.2*a*) and lauric acid (12 carbons), typically derived from coconut oil and palm kernel oil. The relative shortness of the fatty acid chains in medium-chain triglycerides (MCT) makes them behave differently in the body.

Compared with common 16- and 18-carbon fatty acids, MCT are water soluble enough to be absorbed directly into the blood, without need for the lymphatic vessels as is typical (see figure 5.1). Once in the bloodstream and after reaching tissues such as liver or skeletal muscle, MCT can also be taken into the mitochondrial furnaces of cells without the usual need for carnitine transferase enzymes. Thus, great interest was generated in the 1980s in testing MCT as an immediate performance fuel. Unfortunately, this research, using approximately 25 to 30 g MCT preexercise and sometimes along with carbohydrate, revealed no benefit regarding improved performance or glycogen sparing during exercise (37, 95, 100). Speculation then was that larger amounts may be needed to offer a benefit, but gastrointestinal distress was already a problem with many subjects. Research has been done with large 71 to 85 g doses of MCT, but symptoms such as cramping and diarrhea were again problematic (14, 43).

Interest in the ergogenic effects of MCT, however logical, may have taken the focus away from other potential benefits to athletes. A good deal of sport nutrition involves weight gain and body recompositioning. This may be an avenue of future interest for MCT. Medium-chain triglycerides are a calorie source that is biochemically less likely to be stored as body fat because of rapid transport to the liver (for beta-oxidation of the fatty acids and ketone formation) and increased thermogenesis compared with long-chain triacylglycerol (3). Indeed, new research suggests reduced body fat over a period of MCT ingestion (3, 86). Researchers have explained that additional fat and calories benefit commonly underfed athletes (38, 51, 93, 94), and MCT or similar nutrients may be an advantageous way to provide them.

One recent public trend in MCT use among athletes has been "keto-coffee" and similar products. By adding specific fats (coconut oil being 60% MCT) (40) to coffee, athletes can obtain MCT and necessary calories in doses that do not cause gastrointestinal distress and do not increase carbohydrate intake or risk loss of a ketotic state. Lay Internet sources (21) have accurately acknowledged that little to no peer-reviewed data exist to support performance or body composition claims from fat-added coffees, and the unblinded consumer perception would likely be skewed by the fact that coffee itself is uniquely ergogenic in preexercise settings (27, 31, 68, 79).

Structured Triglycerides

Medium-chain fatty acids are again garnering attention, in part because of the renewed (actually ongoing) research on structured triglycerides. Structured triglycerides are a special triacylglycerol molecule formed through a chemical process known as esterification. During this process, specifically chosen fatty acids are placed onto a glycerol backbone. Early research suggested body fat–reducing qualities and a lack of intestinal distress surrounding structured triacylglycerols that contain a mix of medium-chain and long-chain fatty acids (3, 86). Further, a structured triacylglycerol with a targeted fatty acid at the middle, or sn-2 position, may better deliver that fatty acid into the body. Structured triacylglycerols confer enhanced nitrogen retention and less liver stress than simple physical mixtures of various types of fat in clinical situations (48, 67). Nonetheless, barriers, such as technology or cost, continue to prevent widespread use in sport nutrition.

Apart from structured triglycerides (also known as structured triacylglycerols), the other major adjustment of whole fat molecules is the use of diacylglycerols. These molecules were introduced in Japan in 1999 as cooking oil and were once widely available in the United States (26). In diacylglycerols, the glycerol backbone of the source triacylglycerol has the middle (sn-2) fatty acid removed. These oils are oxidized more readily (rather than stored in the body) when they replace typical oils (26). The mechanism involves a lack of 2-monoacylglycerol during digestion, which affects absorption and metabolism. Controversy regarding absolute safety has removed direct-to-consumer sale of diacylglycerol cooking oil; whether they see renewed market presence in the future is uncertain.

Ketone Salts and Esters

Supplementation with ketone products related to beta-hydroxybutyrate—as opposed to generating them endogenously through very low-carbohydrate intake—creates a novel scenario whereby physiologic ketosis may be achieved in a carbohydrate-replete state (32). The simultaneous and ongoing presence of elevated blood glucose, insulin, *and* ketone bodies is not something normally encountered by the human body, making outcomes uncertain. For example, glucose and ketone bodies have similar Michaelis-Menten constants (Km) for transport into the brain (62), so their competition in this all-inclusive condition is a curious one. As of 2018, however, just six studies were published on exogenous ketone body ingestion (83). Contrasting results from these existing studies using different ketone compounds, performance tests, dosages, and analytic techniques highlight that further research is required. In any case, this technological development opens a heretofore unheard-of metabolic state that warrants investigation.

Professional Applications

How much fat is recommended in an athlete's diet? Unfortunately, no firm standards exist for optimal lipid intake. The acceptable macronutrient distribution range for fat is 20% to 35% of energy intake (41). When fat intake is at 30% of total calories, *Dietary Guidelines for Americans* (89) recommends that the proportion of energy from fatty acids be 10% saturated, 10% polyunsaturated, and 10% monounsaturated and that sources of essential fatty acids be included. In general, athletes report an average fat intake of 35% of total calories (34). The area in which most athletes need to plan is fat source distribution. A fat intake with an equal balance of saturated, polyunsaturated, and monounsaturated fats is not likely to occur by chance. Saturated fats are abundant in the typical American diet and are found in animal fat such as beef and dark meat in poultry. Monounsaturated fats are found in vegetable oils, such as olive oil and canola oil, and in peanut butter. Polyunsaturated fats are found in most vegetable oils, nuts, cheese to some extent, and fish. When considering polyunsaturates it is always important to remember the sometimes-divergent biological effects of omega-3 versus omega-6 subtypes. Athletes need to make sure that they are selecting a variety of foods to obtain the recommended balance between the types of fat.

Although the research is limited, it appears that fat intake can vary as a percentage of total calories and not affect exercise performance. When fat intake was 20% of total calories as compared with 40% of total calories, no effect on exercise training or strength exercise performance occurred in moderately trained males (91). In relation to aerobic exercise, researchers from Switzerland (96) compared the effects of a diet containing 53% fat and a diet containing only 17% fat in 11 male duathletes (a duathlon consists of running and cycling). After subjects ingested the high-fat or low-fat diet for 5 weeks, no difference was seen in the time it took to run a half marathon or in the total work output during a 20-minute all-out time trial on a cycle ergometer. Further, recent data suggest that more extreme very low-carbohydrate, high-fat ketogenic diets may induce loss of lean muscle mass, but of a magnitude that does not affect power performance in brief tests (56).

From these studies it appears that the percentage of total calories derived from fat does not have a large effect on exercise or athletic performance. Nevertheless, athletes need to be careful not to go to extremes by eating too much or too little dietary fat. Consuming too much fat can lead to the overconsumption of total calories, which leads to weight gain in the form of body fat. Because fat tissue does not contribute to movement, it acts as dead weight and decreases relative force production. Athletes in sports in which greater physical size is beneficial may be more prone to this problem. For example, American football linemen are more likely to consume excess calories and be classified as overweight or obese than athletes who play other positions (54).

On the other hand, if fat intake is too low, performance can decline. Athletes who participate in gymnastics, figure skating, and weight-class events (e.g., wrestling) are more likely to consume too little dietary fat. Horvath and

(continued)

Professional Applications *(continued)*

coworkers assessed the aerobic endurance performance of male and female aerobic endurance athletes after they ingested isocaloric diets with varying fat content (38). The athletes consumed isocaloric diets consisting of either 16% fat, 31% fat, or 44% fat for 4 weeks before running at 80% $\dot{V}O_2$max until voluntary exhaustion. The authors reported that the 31% fat diet resulted in a significant improvement in aerobic endurance performance in comparison with the 16% fat diet. No difference was seen, however, in aerobic endurance performance between the 31% fat and the 44% fat diet groups.

The recommendation is that athletes consume a habitual diet of approximately 30% fat. Of this 30%, 10% should be saturated, 10% polyunsaturated, and 10% monounsaturated. Following these fat intake suggestions avoids the extreme practices of consuming too little or too much dietary fat.

Summary Points

- Classification of fat includes degrees of saturation (the number of carbon–carbon double bonds); carbon–carbon double-bond position (the placement of the double bonds counted from either end of the fatty acid chain); chain length (the length of the carbon chain that makes up the fatty acids); and fatty acid placement (differences in where the fatty acid chains are attached or omitted from the glycerol backbone of the fat molecule). An understanding of these differences enables athletes to choose the proper types of fat to optimize health and performance.
- Fat is the primary fuel at rest and during low-intensity exercise.
- Fat comes in a wide variety of types, some of which are essential, including linolenic acid from flax and walnuts (omega-3, polyunsaturated), EPA and DHA from fish oil (omega-3, polyunsaturated), and oleic acid from olive and canola oils (omega-9, monounsaturated).
- Fat confers nutraceutical benefits, including helping to maintain sex hormones, potentially enhancing mood, reducing inflammation, and assisting in body fat control.
- Athletes should consume a habitual diet of approximately 30% fat. Of this 30%, 10% should be saturated, 10% polyunsaturated, and 10% monounsaturated.
- Diets that are too low in fat are associated with reduced testosterone concentrations and exercise performance.
- Consuming too much fat can lead to the overconsumption of total calories, which leads to weight gain in the form of body fat.
- Fat supplements (conjugated linoleic acid, medium-chain fatty acids, structured triglycerides, and ketone body products) have not consistently demonstrated improvements in exercise performance.

Chapter 6

Fluids

Jennifer Bunn, PhD

Water is the most important nutrient for the human body. It composes approximately 60% of a person's body weight and can fluctuate between 45% and 75% (14). The amount of water in a person's body depends on factors such as age, gender, body composition, and overall body size. Water is stored in different locations in the body including fat, bone, muscle, and blood plasma (14). Typically, blood is 90% water, skeletal muscle is 75% water, bone is 25% water, and adipose tissue is 5% water. **Euhydration**, the state in which the amount of water is adequate to meet the body's physiological demands, should be the daily goal for any active person. **Hyperhydration**, an excess amount of water, and **hypohydration** (sometimes referred to as dehydration), an insufficient amount of water, are two extremes of fluid intake that can be dangerous. All hydration states are temporary and are subject to change based on fluid and electrolyte balance as dictated by hormones, thermoregulation, excretion, and ingestion.

Total body water is separated into two compartments in the body: intracellular fluid (ICF), which stores about 65% of the total body water, and extracellular fluid (ECF), which contains the remaining 35% of total body water. ECF is further separated into the fluid in the interstitial space between cells, intravascular water within the blood, and fluid in other locations, such as cerebrospinal fluid. Despite barriers that separate the compartments, water moves quite easily between the ICF and ECF. The ECF acts as a passageway for water to enter the ICF space (63).

The ICF and ECF are composed of similar substances but in very different concentrations as shown in figure 6.1. In the ECF, the major **cation** (positively charged ion) is sodium, and the major **anions** (negatively charged ions) are chloride and bicarbonate. Other substances found in the ECF include potassium and protein. The composition in the ICF is quite different. Potassium is the major cation, and phosphate and protein are the major anions. Sodium is

The author would like to acknowledge the significant contributions of Bob Seebohar to this chapter.

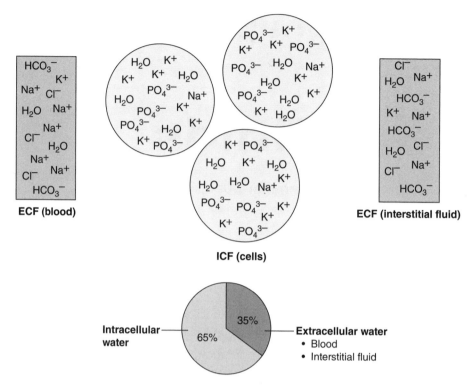

FIGURE 6.1   When the body is in fluid balance, most of the water (H_2O), potassium (K^+), and phosphate (PO_4^{3-}) will be in the intracellular fluid (ICF) and most of the sodium (Na^+), chloride (Cl^-), and bicarbonate (HCO_3^-) will be in the extracellular fluid (ECF). Although the types of compounds in these two spaces are different, the total concentration of solutes (osmolarity) is the same. If the total concentration of solutes changes in either space, the body moves water from one space to the other to maintain balance.

Adapted by permission from M. Dunford, *Fundamentals of Sport and Exercise Nutrition* (Champaign, IL: Human Kinetics, 2010), 114; Adapted by permission from M. Dunford, *Exercise Nutrition,* version 2.0 (Champaign, IL: Human Kinetics, 2009), 33.

present but in much smaller concentrations. These different compositions between the ECF and ICF are important for the transport of fluid and **electrolytes** across cell membranes. Electrolytes are the ionized components in a cell or fluid. There is constant pressure for sodium to "leak" into cells and for potassium to "leak" out of cells, and these concentrations are regulated by sodium–potassium pumps on the cell membranes (63). The body also aims to have water and electrolyte balance between the ECF and ICF, so water can also move between the two fluid compartments to help achieve that balance.

Although the composition of these two spaces differs, the **osmolarity**, or total concentration of solutes in a solution, is the same. If the concentration in either compartment changes, a shift occurs. For example, during heavy sweating, water is lost and plasma volume changes, resulting in a higher concentration of sodium in the plasma. To balance the concentrations between

ECF and ICF, water moves out of the cells and the cells shrink in volume. The body is efficient at maintaining **homeostasis** (a state of equilibrium and balance), and thus the opposite also holds true: If the sodium concentration in the ECF is low, then the osmolarity is less than in the ICF and the body moves water into the cells (63).

When a solution (or beverage) contains a total solute concentration that is equal to the solute concentration of human blood, the solution is considered **isotonic**. Fluids are absorbed best in the human body when they are isotonic. A **hypotonic beverage** is a solution whose osmolarity is less than that of the body and is emptied from the stomach more quickly. Water is a hypotonic beverage that helps with rapid hydration and with water loss but does not replenish any minerals or provide carbohydrate. If an athlete consumes a balanced diet that includes electrolytes and participates in exercise for less than 1 hour at a time, then water may be the only "sport drink" needed for hydration. A **hypertonic beverage** is a solution with higher osmolarity than that of the normal body and is emptied from the stomach more slowly. This slow emptying could cause gastrointestinal distress such as discomfort, cramping, and nausea. Milk, coffee, and fruit juices are examples of hypertonic beverages. These drinks appear to serve the body best for replenishment of fluids and electrolytes during recovery from exercise. Most beverages advertised as sport drinks are **isotonic beverages**. Isotonic drinks also frequently have carbohydrate. The combination of water, carbohydrate, and electrolytes appears to be useful for maintaining performance during active bouts of 1 hour or longer (2).

Fluid Balance During Exercise

During exercise, an increase in core body temperature increases blood flow to the skin and sweat loss to cool the body. Evaporation, the primary method of heat loss during exercise, can be substantial in warmer environments (2). Individual characteristics such as body weight, genetic predisposition, and state of heat acclimatization influence sweat rate for any activity (72). Thus, people within the same sport and those in different sports and player positions have a large range of sweat and electrolyte losses. Sweat losses profoundly affect total body water, and therefore ECF and ICF. Water losses can be fully replaced to establish normal total body water, within 0.2% to 0.5% of body weight if adequate fluid and electrolytes are consumed over a period of 8 to 24 hours (9).

In addition to sweat rate, glycogen can also affect total body water. Greater stored glycogen can increase total body water because 3 to 4 g of water is bound to each gram of glycogen stored (51). This consideration is important for some athletes who compete in weight-class or acrobatic sports such as wrestling, weightlifting, boxing, gymnastics, taekwondo, and figure skating. Although keeping glycogen stores maxed out is important, eating a high-carbohydrate diet within the days before weigh-in for weight-class sports can alter an athlete's weight class for participation. Athletes in many aesthetic and weight-class sports must eat a diet tailored to their physique and weight needs, and glycogen content in relationship to total body water should be considered.

Dehydration

Normal hydration is vital not only for good athletic performance but also for cardiovascular and thermoregulatory functions (52). Dehydration from loss of iso-osmotic fluid, compared with the blood plasma, results in greater dehydration of the ECF. This type of dehydration, referred to as **extracellular dehydration**, typically results from the use of diuretics, not from exercise. In contrast, **intracellular dehydration** is the loss of hypo-osmotic fluid that creates an osmotic gradient, causing water to move from the ICF to the ECF (12). This type of dehydration results from normal urinary losses, low consumption of fluid during exercise, and consuming or losing only water during exercise. Intracellular dehydration can be assessed by monitoring urine color and urine specific gravity, and is referred to simply as dehydration throughout this chapter.

Dehydration greater than 2% of body weight is the threshold for impaired aerobic endurance performance (2), but the threshold may be higher for resistance training or anaerobic exercise performance (17). Physiologic functions are generally maintained until approximately 68 fluid ounces (2 L) of total body water is lost, which is 2% to 3% loss of body weight in a 155 to 176 lb (70-80 kg) person (2). The major cause of dehydration in athletes is sweat losses that are not compensated for through fluid intake, and thirst is the first physiological indicator of dehydration. Each athlete has a different sweat rate based on environmental conditions, clothing type, equipment worn, metabolic rate, and body surface area. Also, the onset of sweating is largely determined by an athlete's metabolic rate and core body temperature, which depends on exercise intensity and body weight (22). Following fluid loss from sweat, plasma volume decreases and plasma osmolality increases. This change in osmolality affects how heat is released from the body, causing increased heat storage (19). The change in plasma volume also causes the heart rate to increase, stroke volume to decrease, and perceived effort to increase (21). The risk of dehydration and subsequently heat illness is greater in hot, humid environments and at altitude, subsequently increasing a person's risk of developing potentially life-threatening heatstroke. Athletes exercising at altitudes above 8,200 feet (2,300 m) are likely to experience fluid losses beyond those that result from exercise (36).

Given the factors that contribute to sweat losses, athletes in particular sports and particular positions within those sports are at greater risk for dehydration in comparison with their fellow athletes. American football players, wrestlers, as well as athletes who play hockey, basketball, tennis, and soccer all have increased risk for dehydration based on various factors not related to exercise (50). Risk of dehydration tends to be higher in athletes who have a large body surface area (22), wear a lot of protective equipment (49), engage in harmful weight-loss practices (38), and participate in sports that offer infrequent water breaks (50). Overall, the environment for competition, requirement for high-intensity efforts, fluid availability, hydration education, and frequency of drinking opportunities seem to dictate the risk of hypohydration.

Hyponatremia

Exercise-associated **hyponatremia**, a low concentration of sodium in the blood, is common in aerobic endurance athletes and was first described in the 1980s. Although the exact mechanism is unclear, factors associated with hyponatremia include

- overconsumption of hypotonic fluids,
- excessive loss of sodium through sweat, and
- extensive sweating with the ingestion of low-sodium fluids.

In general, symptomatic hyponatremia in events lasting less than 4 hours is attributable to drinking too much fluid and taking in little sodium before, during, and sometimes after the event (40). Most athletes who develop hyponatremia consume too much hypotonic fluids in excess of their losses, resulting in an increase in total body water and reduction in sodium blood concentration. The natural stimulus of exercise on **antidiuretic hormone** (ADH), or arginine vasopressin, can exacerbate this condition. ADH is released from the posterior pituitary gland and functions to preserve water in the blood and reduce fluid loss through urine. Hypo-osmolality attenuates the release of ADH, but this function may be suppressed in some athletes (27, 65, 67). Excessive sweat loss may also contribute to risk of hyponatremia if the loss is enough to cause a large loss of volume and stimulate ADH to be released (28). The signs and symptoms of **hyponatremia** include weight gain during exercise, disorientation, confusion, headache, nausea, vomiting, and muscle weakness. If left untreated, this condition can rapidly progress and cause seizures, brain swelling, coma, pulmonary edema, and cardiorespiratory arrest (45).

Women may be at higher risk for developing hyponatremia in longer aerobic endurance events, possibly because of several psychosocial and biological factors (2). Fluid intake recommendations for women have often been based on sweat loss data from men, which are obviously too high for most women and may have led to greater sodium dilution in the body because of smaller total body water stores (67). Although most documented exercise-associated hyponatremia cases are in women, a large study performed with marathon runners showed that this sex difference disappeared after adjusting for body mass index and race times (1).

Athletes who experience hyponatremia may not recognize the early signs and symptoms, which appear when blood sodium concentration reaches 130 mmol/L (67). These signs and symptoms include bloating, puffiness, nausea, vomiting, and headache (26). As the severity of hyponatremia increases and blood sodium concentration dips below 125 mmol/L, more serious signs and symptoms appear, including altered mental status (e.g., confusion, disorientation, and agitation), seizures, respiratory distress (due to pulmonary edema), and unresponsiveness. Exercise-associated hyponatremia has also been associated with cases of exercise-induced rhabdomyolysis (7). At the extreme, hyponatremia can be extremely dangerous and result in coma and death (26).

Athletes can easily become hyponatremic and dehydrated by choosing water alone or food and drink with little to no sodium. For people who have a high sweat rate and sweat sodium concentration, commercial sport drinks may not contain enough sodium to help with preventing hyponatremia. In general, the recommendation is to choose a sport drink containing a minimum of 20 mEq sodium (460 mg) per 34 fluid ounces (1 L).

No concrete recommendation has been offered about electrolyte intake before exercise, although many athletes consume salty foods and drinks beforehand to prevent hyponatremia. Consuming an adequate amount of salt daily, especially for salty sweaters, is recommended. In some cases, the use of salt tablets may be warranted during exercise as long as they are consumed with enough fluid to maintain fluid and electrolyte balance. Active people should limit fluid intake to what is needed to minimize dehydration and should consume sodium-rich foods and beverages during exercise longer than 2 hours to prevent excessive drinking and limit the risk of developing hyponatremia (67). Thirst is a practical physiological symptom to pay attention to, because it will result in some level of dehydration during the exercise activity but should not hinder performance (23).

Measuring Hydration Status

An athlete's hydration status should be assessed during training to ensure adequate hydration both during exercise and at rest. Ideally, the hydration testing method should be sensitive and accurate enough to detect total body water changes of 2% to 3% body weight. Testing hydration status in the field should be practical from a time, cost, and technical standpoint. **Urine specific gravity** (USG) is a quantifiable field test and is the preferred method for assessing hydration status before exercise in athletes. Urine specific gravity can be tested using a refractometer in a lab setting or a dipstick that can be taken almost anywhere. Testing with a dipstick is much cheaper than lab tests but also less accurate. Urine should be assessed using the first morning samples of the day, which reflect 24-hour concentrations (24). Assessing the osmolality of saliva has also been shown to measure ECF osmolality accurately and through noninvasive methods (47).

People can assess their own hydration status by examining the quantity of urine they produce, evaluating urine color, and estimating changes in body weight. Using one of these measures of hydration alone is not recommended because each has limitations. The color of urine is determined primarily by the amount of urochrome, a breakdown product of hemoglobin (42). When a large amount of urine is excreted, the urine is dilute and the solutes are less concentrated, giving urine a pale color. When a small amount of urine is excreted, the urine is more concentrated, giving urine a darker color (42). The urine color chart shows eight colors on a scale that reflects a linear relationship between the color of urine and its specific gravity and osmolarity (3). Note that certain dietary compounds can make urine appear darker, including B-complex vitamins, beta carotene, betacyanins, and some artificial food colors and medications (42). Athletes should pay attention to these factors if they are using urine color frequently to determine hydration status.

When an athlete is hydrated, the urine should be pale in color and plentiful, although athletes should keep in mind that it may appear darker and brighter if they have taken a multivitamin or B complex within an hour or so before urinating. In general, urine should be the same color as diluted lemonade. If it is darker and concentrated, the athlete is dehydrated. If urine is orange or brown, the athlete must see a physician immediately.

Body weight is another hydration status tool. For well-hydrated people who are in energy balance, body weight (measured in the morning after urinating) fluctuations should be plus or minus 1%. Keep in mind that morning body weight changes can be influenced by changes in bowel movements and eating habits. In women, hormonal fluctuations during the menstrual cycle may influence body weight. During the second half of menstruation, body weight increases slightly (39), and in the days before menstruation, women may have an increase in water retention and body weight gain (59).

Weighing before and after an exercise session can also be useful to help determine if athletes are meeting their fluid needs during training. The easiest approach is for athletes to weigh in the nude before a training session (preferably one at competition intensity) and then immediately after the workout. The difference in weight will provide a good estimate of fluid losses and the amount of fluid that should be ingested subsequently to maintain hydration status. After exercise, a person should consume 24 fluid ounces (710 ml) for every pound (0.45 kg) lost during exercise (41), and consumption should occur slowly to enhance retention and avoid urine production. For example, for someone who weighs 170 pounds (77 kg) before a session and 168 pounds (76 kg) afterward, the loss is 2 pounds (0.9 kg). This athlete should consume 48 fluid ounces (1,420 ml) of fluid to achieve euhydration. Testing the first urine of the morning for color, assessing USG, and noting changes in body weight should provide enough information to detect any changes in water balance (2).

Hydration and Performance

Athletes must pay close attention to fluid and electrolyte balance during aerobic endurance exercise because of the increased likelihood of becoming dehydrated, becoming overheated, or experiencing the consequences of altered electrolyte balance. Anaerobic events and sports other than running and cycling may have similar consequences. American football, soccer, hockey, tennis, and a variety of other sports also have increased risk for dehydration, heat illness, and low blood sodium levels.

Compared with the attention given to fluid balance in aerobic endurance athletes, significantly less attention has been paid to fluid balance during strength and power exercise. A plausible explanation is that athletes are more likely to become dehydrated during long bouts of aerobic exercise; the short duration of many strength and power events and the ready availability of fluids makes dehydration less of a concern.

Aerobic Endurance Exercise

Maintaining fluid and electrolyte balance is crucial for people who engage in aerobic endurance exercise. In fact, a fluid loss of 2% to 3% of body weight has been shown to reduce exercise performance in both hot and temperate environments (31, 42). Aerobic athletes should aim to be euhydrated before the start of the activity or performance, expect to have a mild net loss of body fluid during the exercise, and then replenish the loss of fluid, carbohydrate, and electrolytes after completion of the bout.

Before Exercise

People should begin exercise euhydrated and with normal electrolyte levels. Good hydration practices during the day, focusing on the consumption of fluids and foods with high water content such as fruits and vegetables, should be the main goal. If at least 8 to 12 hours have passed since the last exercise session and fluid consumption is sufficient, the person should be close to a euhydrated state. On the other hand, for someone who has lost a significant amount of fluid and has not replenished with fluids and electrolytes in the amounts needed to establish euhydration, an aggressive preexercise hydration protocol is in order (2).

Hydration should begin several hours before exercise to allow absorption and urine output. At least 4 hours before exercise, athletes should consume approximately 0.08 to 0.1 fluid ounces per pound (5-7 ml/kg) of body weight. They should consume more fluid at a slow rate—0.05 to 0.08 fluid ounces per pound (3 to 5 ml/kg) of body weight in addition to the aforementioned fluid recommendations—2 hours before exercise if the person is not urinating or if the urine is dark (2). Consuming sodium-rich foods at this time can help stimulate thirst and retain fluids. If sodium is consumed in a beverage, the recommended amount is 20 to 50 mEq/L (460-1,150 mg/L) of fluid (2).

A common practice for athletes before an event is to attempt to hyperhydrate with water. This practice is not advised because it increases the risk of urination during the event and could dilute the sodium levels in the body, thus increasing the risk of hyponatremia (40). For promotion of a euhydrated state before training or competition, fluid palatability is of utmost importance. Palatability or the lack of it will contribute to or detract from preexercise hydration strategies. The fluids should typically be lightly sweetened, should contain sodium, and should be cool in temperature. Beverages with carbohydrate and sodium have been shown to promote fluid retention up to 4 hours after ingestion while in a euhydrated state (43).

During Exercise

The goal of drinking during exercise is to prevent excessive dehydration (greater than 3% of body weight reduction from water loss) and excessive changes in electrolyte balance (2). Athletes may also choose to drink ad libitum, or according to their thirst preferences. This method of hydrating has been shown to result in 2% to 3% loss of body weight with no negative effect on performance (23). Other fluid guidelines suggest that athletes may follow an individualized fluid plan but should aim for 3 to 8 fluid ounces (90-240 ml) of a 6% to 8% carbohydrate–electrolyte beverage every 15 to 20 minutes during exercise lasting longer than 60 to 90 minutes (2, 69). Note, however, that a recent meta-analysis showed that drinking ad libitum during aerobic exercise caused greater weight loss of about 2% of body weight compared with programmed drinking in which athletes lost only 1% of their body weight during exercise (23). Further, ad libitum drinking improved performance over programmed drinking by approximately 1% (23). Evidence does not seem to support drinking as much as possible during exercise to attenuate all fluid losses, and research also suggests not to exceed ingestion of more than 27 fluid ounces per hour (800 ml/h) during exercise (48).

Consuming carbohydrate during exercise maintains blood glucose levels and reduces fatigue. A sport drink typically contains the following (31, 32):

- 20 to 30 mEq of sodium (460-690 mg) per liter
- 2 to 5 mEq of potassium (78-195 mg) per liter
- About 5% to 10% carbohydrate concentration

Energy bars, gels, and other foods, depending on a person's needs and preferences, can also supply this combination (10). Consuming beverages with sodium (20-30 mEq/L fluid) or snacks containing sodium will help stimulate thirst and retain water (53). Like sodium, a sport beverage with protein may increase fluid retention, but take caution because this item could result in some gastrointestinal distress (64). Athletes should train first with the beverage they intend to consume for any performance or race days.

After Exercise

After exercise, the goal is to fully replenish any fluid and electrolyte deficit from the exercise bout (2). Athletes should consume 150% of the lost weight to achieve normal hydration within 6 hours after exercise (42). Therefore, practically speaking, the recommendation is to ingest 24 fluid ounces (720 ml) of fluids for every pound (0.45 kg) of body weight lost during training. Although plain water is effective for rehydration, athletes should consider a sport drink or consume their water with foods that contain electrolytes such as sodium and chloride to replace electrolyte losses (14).

As a whole, alcoholic and caffeinated beverages have diuretic effects, but such effects are transient and therefore those beverages do contribute to daily hydration recommendations. But if rapid rehydration is the goal postexercise, the recommendation is to avoid alcoholic and caffeinated beverages in the first few hours after activity (14). The fluid chosen in the postexercise period should promote rapid rehydration.

Depending on the amount of time before the next exercise session, consuming sodium-rich foods and beverages with water after competition or a training session should suffice. Sodium is one of the key nutrients that athletes should consume in the postexercise period to return to a euhydrated state because it will help retain ingested fluids and stimulate thirst. Although sweat sodium losses differ among individuals, which can make individual sodium prescription difficult during this period, a little extra salt added to meals or snacks may be particularly useful for those with high sweat sodium losses (2).

Power and Sport Performance

Although a plethora of studies have led to recommendations for fluid consumption and measuring hydration status in aerobic endurance athletes, fewer studies have looked at the effects of fluid consumption on power output and sport performance. Collectively, these studies have yielded mixed results; some indicate that mild dehydration can affect certain aspects of performance, whereas others suggest that even severe dehydration has no effect. The varying results may be due, in part, to differences in methodology and measures obtained.

Regarding power, vertical jump height—a surrogate measure for vertical power—and jump squat height have shown no changes with dehydration in recreational or team sport athletes (25, 34, 50). But anaerobic power measured through 10-second cycling performance was affected in baseball players, who lost approximately 4% of their body weight from hypohydration (73). Sprint times in soccer and basketball were also slowed with dehydration of 2% to 4% loss of body weight, especially in the late stages of a game (50). Additionally, high-intensity running efforts were also affected at the same level of hypohydration (13, 15). Regarding sport-specific skills, results are conflicting. A review by Nuccio and colleagues concluded that shooting in basketball and bowling or throwing in cricket are both negatively affected at 2% to 4% hypohydration, but skills are not affected in soccer, field hockey, or tennis at this same level of dehydration (50).

Overall, evidence suggests that hypohydration appears to decrease strength by approximately 2%, power by approximately 3%, and high-intensity muscular endurance by approximately 10% (33). Many sports are multifaceted and require muscular endurance, strength, anaerobic power, and aerobic endurance, and therefore hypohydration will likely affect more than one component contributing to athletic performance in these sports. For example, athletes on a lightweight crew team who dehydrate to make weight may be able to participate, but their performance may be subpar at best. In addition, depending on the environmental conditions, athletes may be putting themselves at increased risk of heat illness. In addition to potentially hampering aerobic and muscular endurance and increasing the risk of heat illness, dehydration may increase an athlete's risk of developing rhabdomyolysis, a potentially serious injury to skeletal muscle that results in leakage of large quantities of intracellular contents to plasma (4, 5).

Resistance Training

Resistance exercise is associated with unique metabolic demands. Little research, however, has evaluated the effect of dehydration on resistance training, and there is no consensus on whether dehydration decreases muscle performance. Hypohydration of 1% to 3% has been shown to cause a marked reduction in isometric leg extension strength (25), and hypohydration of 2.5% to 5% reduced back squat performance (34). This high level of dehydration may also affect the endocrine and metabolic internal environments before and after the training bout. Specifically, catabolic hormones, cortisol, epinephrine, and norepinephrine increased, which altered the postexercise anabolic response (35). These data suggest that a dehydrated state enhances the stress of a resistance exercise session and may interfere with training adaptations. A dehydrated state, however, does not appear to affect markers of muscle damage—myoglobin and creatine kinase. Although the finding was not statistically significant, the authors noted that the more dehydrated the participants were, the less total work they performed (72).

In summary, resistance-trained athletes should be encouraged to emphasize good hydration techniques throughout the day to remain as hydrated as possible before, during, and after training. Data are insufficient to support a scientifically based hydration protocol, so a prudent approach to hydration is likely safe.

Age-Related Fluid Needs

The two population groups that may be of concern with hydration are children and the elderly. Because these two groups are more likely to experience hydration-related issues and, in the case of elderly persons, alterations in electrolyte balance, sport nutritionists must be aware of the issue in these populations and educate parents and coaches.

Children

Fluid needs for children are more challenging and problematic than for adults because few empirical studies formulate guidelines and recommendations. The research available indicates that concerns with children exist because of differences in heat production (18) and sweat rate (20, 30). Boys tend to sweat less than their adult male counterparts (30), but this physiological difference does not hold true for girls and women (56), unless training in the heat (20). Despite these concerns, the evidence indicates that dehydration, thermoregulation, and risk of heat illness are not collectively different from that of an adult (44, 60). The detriment of dehydration on performance, however, does appear to differ between adults and children. Dehydration of 2% of body weight in adults seems to decrease work capacity and decrease performance, whereas a mere 1% dehydration has the same effects in boys (70). More research should be conducted in this area to confirm these results and evaluate the effects in girls.

Ad libitum drinking appears to offset dehydration in children better than in adults, replenishing 66% to 100% of the sweat-related fluid deficits in children (20, 29, 61). General fluid recommendations for children during exercise include drinking 0.2 fluid ounces per pound per hour (13 ml · kg^{-1} · hr^{-1}) (62). This recommendation is slightly lower than the guidelines provided by the American Academy of Pediatrics (AAP), suggesting that consuming 3 to 8 fluid ounces (100-250 ml) every 20 minutes is appropriate for children (11). The recommendations from the AAP are geared for 9- to 12-year-olds and may indicate too much fluid for younger, smaller children. If a fluid deficit exists after exercise, it should be replenished by drinking 16 fluid ounces (480 ml) per pound (0.45 kg) of body weight lost (62). This fluid should be fully replaced during recovery and before the next bout of exercise. Studies in children are equivocal regarding the use of fluid palatability, glucose, and sodium to encourage more ad libitum drinking; therefore, choosing water or a sport drink that a child will drink is a sufficient choice (71). The addition of carbohydrate to a beverage, however, does appear to improve performance in efforts longer than 60 minutes in children, as it does in adults (55).

Elderly Persons

Fluid and electrolyte imbalances are common in older adults because aging is associated with certain physiological changes in renal adaptation, blood flow responses, sweat rates, thirst sensation, altered sensitivity to ADH, and fluid and electrolyte status that all affect thermoregulation (46, 58, 66). Age-related changes include decreased renal functioning, which can cause kidney water excretion to be higher than in younger adults (57). Additionally, aging leads to structural changes in the blood vessels that decrease blood flow to the skin to dissipate heat. In fact, older adults can have between 25% and 40% less skin blood flow at a given thermic load than younger adults (37). Finally, elderly people may have lower sweat rates and may begin sweating later in an exercise session in comparison with younger adults (6). These three changes can predispose older individuals to fluid imbalances, especially when an exercise stimulus is introduced. Additional renal changes due to biological aging include:

- a decline in glomerular filtration rate (GFR) (a measure of kidney function indicating the rate at which blood is being filtered by the kidneys),
- reduced urinary concentrating ability (68),
- less efficient sodium-conserving ability (54), and
- decreased ability to excrete a large amount of water (57).

These changes reduce fluid and electrolyte homeostasis, which can predispose people who are elderly to **hypovolemia** (an abnormal decrease in blood volume) and dehydration (57, 58). Elderly persons are also at risk for **hypernatremia**, an increase in plasma sodium concentrations greater than 145 mEq/L. This state can result from excessive loss of water and electrolytes caused by polyuria (excessive urine production), diarrhea, excessive sweating, or inadequate water intake. For many elderly people, however, the age-related decrease in thirst may be the primary cause (16). Overall, when fluid choices are palatable and no illness is present, elderly persons seem to have no problem maintaining fluid balance during sedentary conditions.

During exercise, older athletes can experience similar alterations in fluid balance as their younger counterparts with risks related to both hyponatremia and dehydration. The effects of biological aging on the kidneys can result in slowed excretion of water and electrolytes (57), which may then increase the risk of hyponatremia (66). With dehydration, older athletes experience similar detriments to performance as younger adults do with a loss of 2% of their body weight. But this level of dehydration also has a negative effect on short-term memory and psychomotor and visual motor skills (66). Thus, older athletes should evaluate their sweat and urination rates when making decisions about fluid intake.

No published data exist on which to base an exact fluid replacement strategy for elderly people. Fluid replacement guidelines for younger athletes can be used to establish a hydration plan for masters athletes with a few exceptions related to individualized renal function (58). Rehydration after exercise periods tends to be longer for older adults, in comparison with younger adults, after they have experienced dehydration (16). Consumption of fluids should begin early in an exercise session to prevent the onset of dehydration (8).

Professional Applications

Careful monitoring of hydration status and electrolyte balance is crucial not only for athletic performance but also for prevention of heat illness, heatstroke, and hyponatremia. Therefore, sport nutritionists must not only help athletes monitor their hydration and electrolyte status but also teach them how to do this for themselves and to be aware of the signs of dehydration, overheating, and hyponatremia.

Athletes can do two simple things to assess their hydration status. First, they should pay attention to the frequency of urination, urine color, and quantity. Urine should be pale yellow and plentiful (though consuming B vitamins in the form of a B complex, multivitamin, or functional food can make urine brighter and darker). Athletes should also get into the habit of weighing themselves before and after each training session. If they lose more than 2% of their body weight from before to after a session, they need to do a better job hydrating before and during training. For each pound (0.45 kg) lost, they should consume 24 fluid ounces (720 ml). Optimal replenishment should be done by consuming water and eating foods that replenish electrolytes, but sport drinks may be used for convenience.

Every year, people die from hyponatremia. Although the marathoner who takes a long time to finish (>4 hours) and consumes too much fluid is more likely to suffer from hyponatremia than a basketball player, sport nutritionists should be aware of the potential for hyponatremia in a wide range of athletes. Athletes who participate in sports that allow frequent water breaks may also be susceptible to hyponatremia if they overconsume fluids. Drinking according to thirst, rather than following programmed drinking, can prevent incidences of hyponatremia.

Dehydration can hamper most kinds of athletic performance, from aerobic endurance exercise to sports requiring explosive power movements. Two groups that need to be closely monitored and educated regarding dehydration and heat illness are children and the elderly. The following are some general hydration recommendations for athletes, which should be adapted as necessary to meet the unique needs of the sport and the individual:

- At least 4 hours before exercise, athletes need to drink approximately 0.08 to 0.1 fluid ounces per pound (5 to 7 ml/kg) of body weight and an additional 0.05 to 0.08 fluid ounces per pound (3 to 5 ml/kg) of body weight 2 hours beforehand if they are not urinating or if the urine is dark (2). The athlete is aiming to be euhydrated before training or performance.

- The fluid consumed before exercise should contain 20 to 30 mEq (460-690 mg) of sodium/L of fluid (2).

- Athletes may consume 3 to 8 fluid ounces (90-240 ml) of a 5% to 10% carbohydrate–electrolyte beverage every 15 to 20 minutes during exercise lasting longer than 60 to 90 minutes (2, 32). Athletes who drink according to thirst, however, consume on average 27 fluid ounces per hour (800 ml/h) with no negative affect on performance and reduction of body weight of only 1% (23).

- Athletes should choose a sport drink that contains 20 to 30 mEq of sodium/L (460-690 mg), 2 to 5 mEq of potassium/L (78-195 mg), and about 6% to 8% carbohydrate concentration for use during exercise (31, 32). Most sport drinks on the market meet these descriptions.
- Athletes should consume 24 fluid ounces (720 ml) for every pound (0.45 kg) of body weight lost after training. Plain water should be used after exercise only when it is combined with foods that contain sodium (14).

Summary Points

- Fluids are of utmost importance to maintaining good health and performance for anyone participating in sport. Many variables affect hydration needs and status; thus, proper timing and implementation of hydration and rehydration strategies throughout the training year are important to fine-tune individual fluid prescriptions.

- Normal hydration is essential for athletic performance and normal cardiovascular and thermoregulatory functions. Dehydration greater than 2% to 3% of body weight can impair athletic performance. Dehydration also increases the risk of heat illness. Drinking ad libitum is an effective strategy to mitigate fluid and electrolyte losses during exercise, and full replenishment should occur after the bout is complete.

- There is no conclusive evidence of significant performance decrements in resistance training when it is performed in a hypohydrated state. Hypohydration can reduce power output by 3% and high-intensity muscular endurance by up to 10% (33). Multifaceted sports requiring muscular endurance, strength, anaerobic power, and aerobic endurance may therefore be affected by hypohydration. All athletes should be encouraged to observe good hydration techniques throughout the day to remain as hydrated as possible before and after a training session.

- Factors associated with hyponatremia include overdrinking hypotonic fluids, excessive loss of sodium through sweat, and extensive sweating. In general, hyponatremia in events lasting less than 4 hours can be attributed to drinking too much fluid and taking in too little sodium before, during, and sometimes after the event (40).

- Athletes should limit fluid intake to only what is needed to minimize dehydration and should consume sodium-rich foods and beverages during exercise longer than 2 hours to prevent excessive drinking and hyponatremia (67).

- Drinking according to thirst appears to offset dehydration in children, replenishing 66% to 100% of the sweat-related fluid deficits (20, 29, 61). Fluid recommendations for children during exercise include drinking 0.2 fluid ounces per pound per hour (13 ml · kg^{-1} · hr^{-1}) (62).

- No current data provide the basis for an exact fluid replacement strategy for elderly persons; fluid replacement guidelines for younger athletes can be used to establish a hydration plan for masters athletes (58).

Chapter 7

Vitamins and Minerals

Henry C. Lukaski, PhD, FSLAN

The field of sport and performance nutrition began in the early 1900s with a focus on macronutrients (protein, fat, and carbohydrate) to support training, performance, and recovery of athletes. Subsequent public health awareness of the synergy between diet and physical activity in promoting wellness stimulated interest in the roles that **micronutrients** (vitamins, minerals, or other substances that are essential for growth or metabolism) play in the physiological processes to attain health, optimal function, and peak physical performance. Evidence of increased activity of micronutrient-dependent and energy-producing metabolic pathways, biochemical adaptations in tissues, and elevated rates of turnover and losses has built interest in the interaction of micronutrient nutrition and physical activity (167). The food content of vitamins and minerals is small (micrograms [mcg] to milligrams [mg]) compared with that of protein, carbohydrate, and fat (up to hundreds of grams [g]). Micronutrients, however, exert potent biological effects as components of proteins. In this capacity, micronutrients enable the complex reactions that are required to use the potential energy in macronutrients to fuel the biological processes inherent in physical training and recovery (106, 175).

The Dietary Reference Intakes (DRIs) are recommendations for intake to prevent nutritional inadequacy that could lead to deficiency and impair health and function (73-79, 120). The Recommended Dietary Allowance (RDA) is a value that meets the needs of approximately 98% of healthy people, whereas the Adequate Intake (AI) is the value that is set sufficiently high to prevent inadequacy. An RDA is calculated from data derived from rigorous scientific studies; the AI is derived from less complete research information. An important point is that physical activity was considered a factor in the DRI for only one-third of the nutrients (tables 7.1 and 7.2).

TABLE 7.1 Exercise-Related Functions and Recommended Dietary Allowances (RDAs) of Micronutrients for Individuals (19-50 Years)

Nutrient	Function	RDA Males	RDA Females	Physical activity considered	Activity effect on requirement
VITAMINS					
Thiamin (B$_1$), mg	Reactions in energy production pathways	1.2	1.1	Yes	Limited evidence[a]
Riboflavin (B$_2$), mg	Electron transfer in oxidative production	1.3	1.1	No	Small effect[b]
Niacin, NE[c]	Electron transfer in oxidative energy production	16	14	No	—
Pyridoxine (B$_6$), mg	Amino acid and glycogen breakdown	1.3	1.3	Yes	Small effect[d]
Cyanocobalamin (B$_{12}$), mcg	Folate recycling and hemoglobin synthesis	2.4	2.4	No	—
Folate, mcg DFE[e]	Cell regeneration and hemoglobin synthesis	400	400	No	—
Ascorbic acid (vitamin C), mg	Antioxidant	90	75	Yes	No demonstrated effect[f]
Retinol (vitamin A), mcg RAE[g]	Antioxidant	900	700	No	—
Tocopherol (vitamin E), mg	Antioxidant	15	15	Yes	—
MINERALS					
Iron, mg	Aerobic energy production	8	18	Yes	Increased need[h]
Magnesium, mg	Aerobic energy production	400	310	Yes	Limited effect[i]
Zinc, mg	Energy metabolism and gas exchange	11	8	No	Limited effect[j]
Copper, mcg	Iron metabolism, aerobic energy production, and antioxidant	900	900	No	—
Phosphorus, mg	Energy metabolism	700	700	No	—
Selenium, mcg	Antioxidant	55	55	No	—
Iodine, mcg	Energy metabolism	150	150	No	—
Molybdenum, mcg	Unknown	45	45	No	—

[a]Limited evidence of increased need with prolonged exercise.

[b]Increased performance with B$_2$ supplementation of low-status subjects; otherwise inconsistent results.

[c]NE = niacin equivalents.

[d]Based on decreases in B$_6$ status in athletes and not requirement per se.

[e]DFE = dietary folate equivalents (1 mcg folate from food or 0.6 mcg folic acid from fortified foods or supplements).

[f]Based on physical activity and vitamin C status.

[g]RAE = retinol activity equivalents (1 mcg retinol = 12 mcg beta-carotene) (74).

[h]Increase intake for regular heavy, intense exercise (30%-70%); beneficial effects in iron-deficient, nonanemic women.

[i]Limited evidence of an effect of magnesium depletion on some measures of performance.

[j]Limited evidence of an effect of low zinc status on some measures of performance.

TABLE 7.2   Exercise-Related Functions and Adequate Intakes (AIs) of Micronutrients for Individuals (19-50 Years)

| Nutrient | Function | AI | | Physical activity considered | Activity effect on requirement |
		Males	Females		
VITAMINS					
Vitamin D, mcg	Calcium absorption and use	5	5	No	—
Vitamin K, mcg	Clotting and bone formation	120	90	No	—
Biotin, mcg	Gluconeogenesis	30	30	No	—
Pantothenic acid, mg	Glycogen synthesis	5	5	No	—
Choline, mg	Acetylcholine, creatine, and lecithin formation	550	425	Yes	Possible effects*
MINERALS					
Calcium, mg	Bone formation	1,000	1,000	Yes	Insufficient evidence
Fluoride, mg	Unknown	4	3	No	—
Chromium, mcg	Facilitate insulin	35	25	No	—
Manganese, mg	Antioxidant	2.3	1.8	No	—
Sodium, g	Fluid regulation, nerve conduction, and muscle contraction	1.5	1.5	Yes	—
Potassium, g	Fluid regulation, glucose transport, glycogen storage, and ATP production	4.7	4.7	No	—
Chloride, g	Fluid regulation, nerve conduction, and muscle contraction	2.3	2.3	Yes	—

*Strenuous exercise decreased plasma choline concentrations; supplements slightly increased performance.

This chapter provides an overview of the biological roles of vitamins and minerals in support of physiological function during exercise, and it highlights the effects of reduced micronutrient status on measures of physical performance. The chapter also identifies the points at which micronutrients can affect metabolism during physical activity and outlines the effects of reduced and, in a few cases, excess intakes of micronutrients on physical activity.

Micronutrient Requirements for Athletes

Micronutrients include vitamins, which are **organic compounds** (made mostly of carbon atoms), and minerals, which are inorganic elements that exist as solids; they cannot be produced by the body and thus must be consumed in food and beverages. Micronutrients form bioactive compounds, generally proteins. They are not direct sources of energy but facilitate energy production and use from carbohydrate, fat, and protein; transport oxygen and carbon dioxide; regulate fluid balance; and protect against oxidative damage. As shown in figure 7.1, many of the B vitamins (thiamin, riboflavin, niacin, B_6, and pantothenic acid) and some minerals (iron, magnesium, copper, and zinc) are needed for the metabolism of carbohydrate into energy for muscle work. Iron, copper, B_6, B_{12}, and folate are required for red blood cell (RBC) formation and oxygen (O_2) transport to muscle cells. Zinc is essential for removal of carbon dioxide (CO_2) from working muscle and recycling of lactate to glucose. In the adrenal gland, vitamin C is necessary to produce epinephrine, which acts to release free fatty acids (FFA) from adipose tissue. Niacin may block the release of FFA during exercise. Vitamins C and E, beta-carotene, and some minerals (zinc, copper, and manganese) neutralize reactive oxygen (ROS) and reactive nitrogen species (RNS) and prevent free radical damage in muscle and other tissues.

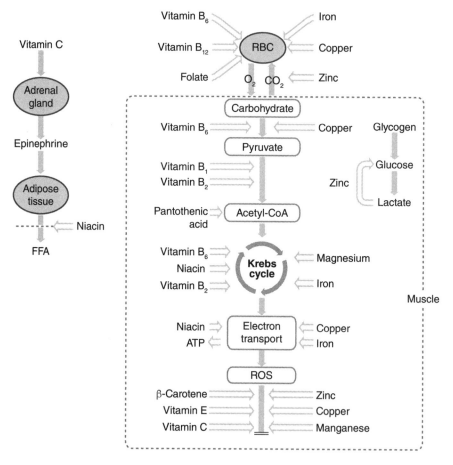

FIGURE 7.1 Summary of the roles of vitamins and minerals related to physical performance.

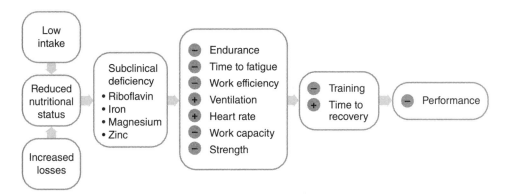

FIGURE 7.2   Outline of the effects of reduced micronutrient nutrition on aspects of physical performance.

Evaluation of micronutrient needs for optimal physical performance requires concurrent assessment of nutrient intake and biochemical measures of nutritional status (63, 96, 109). Only a limited number of investigations have met these criteria. Sole reliance on self-reported food intake to characterize nutritional status is problematic because of underreporting of food intake (111). Assessment of the adequacy of micronutrient intakes relies on the appropriate DRI (RDA or AI) (77). Low micronutrient intakes generally result in subclinical deficiencies characterized by decreased biochemical indicators of nutritional status and impaired physiological function. Figure 7.2 presents an overview of how a subclinical deficiency of several minerals (zinc, iron, riboflavin, and magnesium) leads to reductions in exercise performance and markers of performance. Overt or clinical deficiency is rare without excess loss, decreased absorption, or prolonged periods of deprivation (73-76, 79, 102).

Vitamins and Performance

Thirteen vitamins are required for life. They are described as water or fat soluble. Adequate Intake of B vitamins (water-soluble vitamins) is important to ensure optimum energy production and the building and repair of muscle tissue (184). The B-complex vitamins have several major functions directly related to exercise—energy production during exercise and the production of red blood cells, as well as involvement in protein synthesis and in tissue repair and maintenance including the central nervous system. Despite these important roles for vitamins, few studies on vitamin intakes have directly determined an ergogenic value for athletes. Some vitamins, however, may help athletes tolerate training to a greater degree by reducing oxidative damage, helping to maintain a healthy immune system during heavy training, or both. The following sections provide more detail on the specific roles that the vitamins play in an athlete's diet and performance outcomes.

Water-Soluble Vitamins

Nine vitamins are **water soluble** (eight B vitamins and vitamin C). Their solubility in water limits their storage in the body for extended periods. Excessive intake of water-soluble vitamins in supplement form results in excretion of the excess in urine.

Thiamin

Thiamin is the common term for vitamin B_1. The biologically active form of B_1 is thiamin pyrophosphate, which acts as a **coenzyme** in the metabolism of carbohydrate and protein to produce energy (74). A coenzyme is any small molecule necessary for the functioning of an enzyme. It converts pyruvate to acetyl coenzyme A and α-ketoglutarate to succinyl coenzyme A in the Krebs cycle for oxidative energy production, particularly during exercise (figure 7.1 on page 116). It also participates in the decarboxylation (removal of a CO_2 group) of branched-chain amino acids that contributes to energy production in muscle. Thiamin is widely distributed in foods, including whole grains and enriched cereals and breads, beans, green leafy vegetables, pork, sunflower seeds, and oranges.

The RDA for thiamin is 1.2 and 1.1 mg/day for men and women, respectively, and is also related to energy intake, 0.5 mg/1,000 kcal per day (74). According to the research, female gymnasts and wrestlers consume less than RDA levels of vitamin B_1 (39, 101, 152). Thus, athletes who consume low-energy diets to meet weight standards appear to be at risk for low thiamin status. Evidence of an adverse effect of low thiamin intake is lacking. In a classic study it was reported that neither muscle strength nor running performance was adversely affected in young men fed diets with variable thiamin content (0.23, 0.33, 0.53, and 0.63 mg/1,000 kcal per day) (85). Men fed 0.5 and 5 mg thiamin showed no change in aerobic endurance capacity despite impaired biochemical markers of thiamin status (decreased erythrocyte transketolase activity and increased thiamin pyrophosphate activity) (183). Other studies failed to show a benefit of supplemental thiamin on muscle strength or exercise performance despite improvements in thiamin nutritional status (36, 50, 178).

Riboflavin

Riboflavin is the common term for vitamin B_2. Riboflavin functions in the mitochondrial electron transport system as the coenzymes flavin mononucleotide (FMN) and flavin adenine dinucleotide (FAD). These enzymes participate in the transfer of electrons from breakdown of carbohydrate and fat to formation of adenosine triphosphate (ATP). Riboflavin is also necessary for the conversion of vitamin B_6 to its active form (74). Food sources of riboflavin include milk and dairy products, eggs, whole grains and cereals, lean meats, broccoli, yogurt, whey protein, and almonds.

The RDA for riboflavin intake is 1.3 and 1.1 mg/day for men and women, respectively, or 0.6 mg/1,000 kcal (74). Athletes generally have adequate riboflavin intakes, except for female gymnasts (12, 39, 90, 101). Physical training increases riboflavin needs of adults. During training, athletes experience decreased riboflavin status (50, 83). Metabolic studies of women fed 0.2 compared with 0.6 mg riboflavin daily for 12 weeks, with and without weight loss, showed reduced riboflavin status (decreased erythrocyte glutathione reductase activity) (9, 10). Although gains in peak oxygen uptake after training did not differ with adequate riboflavin intake, the study was not designed to detect performance differences (9, 10). Nineteen percent of adolescent athletes participating in physical training had low riboflavin status at entry; status improved with riboflavin supplementation (2 mg/day, six days a week, for two months), as did physical fitness (164). This finding is consistent with a previous observation of improved aerobic endurance performance after supplementation with multiple B vitamins (170).

Niacin

Niacin is the common term for vitamin B_3. This B vitamin exists as nicotinic acid and nicotinamide, which is metabolized to form nicotinamide adenine nucleotide (NAD) and nicotinamide adenine dinucleotide phosphate (NADP) that serve as coenzymes. The NAD is an electron carrier in the breakdown of carbohydrate, fat, protein, and glycogen to produce ATP; NADP is a hydrogen donor in the pentose phosphate shunt (74). Foods with high protein content are good sources of niacin. Lean meats, fish, poultry, whole-grain products, beans, peanuts, and enriched foods provide ample niacin.

The RDAs for niacin are 14 and 16 mg/day for women and men, respectively (74). Although niacin is an essential nutrient for energy metabolism, there is no evidence of any beneficial effect with supplementation at doses exceeding the RDA (65). Doses of niacin exceeding 50 mg (compared with the RDA of 14 to 16 mg) administered acutely before exercise blocked fat mobilization and decreased aerobic endurance performance (52, 119, 133).

Vitamin B_6

Vitamin B_6 is also commonly referred to as pyridoxine. This term includes all biologically active forms of the vitamin; pyridoxine, pyridoxal, and pyridoxamine are the forms commonly found in foods. Pyridoxal phosphate is a cofactor for enzymes that transform amino acids. It also serves as a cofactor for glycogen phosphorylase that regulates gluconeogenesis and glycogenolysis during exercise (74). The highest levels of B_6 are found in high-protein foods (meats, poultry, fish, wheat germ, whole-grain products, and eggs). Other sources are bananas, soybeans, raw carrots, broccoli, spinach, and avocados.

The RDAs for vitamin B_6 are 1.3 mg/day for men and women, respectively, from 19 to 50 years of age, and then increase to 1.7 to 1.5 mg/day for men and women, respectively, from 51 to 70 years of age (74). Approximately one-third of female and 10% of male athletes fail to meet the RDA (98, 112). Low energy intakes and poor food choices contribute to decreased vitamin B_6 intakes. Surveys of physically active men and women show that 5% to 60% of athletes have decreased B_6 status (50). Aerobic endurance performance did not change in physically active men fed diets containing 2.3 or 22 mg B_6 for nine days (173). Based on increased urinary loss of B_6, however, data suggest that 1.5 to 2.3 mg of B_6 is needed to maintain adequate B_6 status of adults participating in aerobic endurance training (50, 112).

Folate

Another name for folate is vitamin B_9. This B vitamin acts as a coenzyme for many enzymes facilitating one carbon transfer that is critical for DNA synthesis and amino acid metabolism. It also acts in cell repair and growth, including red blood cell formation (74). Dietary sources of folate include green leafy vegetables, fortified cereals, grains, nuts, legumes, liver, and brewer's yeast. Ready-to-eat cereals, bread, and other grain products are good sources of folate.

The RDA for folate is 400 mcg of Dietary Folate Equivalents (DFEs) daily. One DFE corresponds to 1 mcg of food folate, 0.6 mcg of folic acid in fortified foods, or 0.5 mcg of folic acid supplement (74). Active men have adequate folate intakes, but women tend to consume 130 to 364 mcg/day (44, 84, 184). Among female aerobic endurance athletes, 8% to 33% have low plasma folate concentrations (8, 113). Plasma folate concentrations were not different between recreational aerobic endurance athletes (median of 8.6 ng/ml) and gender-matched controls (8.3 ng/ml) (66). Folate supplementation of folate-deficient, but not anemic, athletes did not improve physical performance. Female marathoners with low plasma folate (<4.5 ng/ml) supplemented with folate (5 mg/day for 10 weeks) increased hematological parameters but did not improve treadmill performance, cardiorespiratory function, or metabolic response during exercise as compared with placebo-treated, folate-depleted controls (113).

Vitamin B_{12}

Vitamin B_{12} is also known as cobalamin. Cobalamin is a general term for the group of cobalt-containing compounds called corrinoids. It functions as a coenzyme for the transfer of methyl groups in the formation of DNA, particularly with folate in the formation of hemoglobin (74). Vitamin B_{12} is found only in foods from animal sources such as meats, poultry, fish, eggs, cheese, and milk.

The adult RDA is 2.4 mcg/day; the average omnivore diet contains 5 to 15 mcg (74). Intakes of B_{12} were low in female aerobic endurance athletes (82) but adequate in other groups of male and female athletes (162, 187). Avoidance of animal-based foods increases the risk for low B_{12} intakes. Evidence of improved performance with B_{12} supplementation is lacking. Early studies clearly established that performance does not improve with

B_{12} supplementation. Adolescent males supplemented daily with 50 mcg of B_{12} for seven weeks did not improve running performance or work capacity (116). In addition, other supplementation trials with young men undergoing various regimens (injection of 1 mg, three times a week for six weeks (168) or 0.5 mcg/day for six weeks (141) failed to show any beneficial effect on strength or aerobic endurance.

Other B Vitamins

Pantothenic acid is a component of coenzyme A that is the major substrate for energy production in the Krebs cycle (figure 7.1 on page 116). It is also involved in gluconeogenesis (74). Biotin is a coenzyme involved in amino acid metabolism and a coenzyme for gluconeogenesis (74). Pantothenic acid is found in animal and plant products including meats, eggs, legumes, and whole grains. Sources of biotin include egg yolks, liver, legumes, dark green leafy vegetables, nuts, and soybeans.

The RDAs for pantothenic acid and biotin are 5 mg and 30 mcg, respectively (74). Data on the usual intakes of these B vitamins and biochemical indicators of status are lacking. Supplementation of pantothenic acid (1.8 g/day for seven days) had no beneficial effects on metabolic responses during a 50 km (31.1 mi) time trial or performance (178). Data on the effects of biotin supplementation on performance measures are not available.

Choline functions as a neurotransmitter (acetylcholine), a methyl donor in the formation of creatine, and a lipid transporter (phosphatidylcholine or lecithin). Although exercise affects plasma choline levels differently (e.g., dependent on intensity and duration), initial evidence suggests that supplemental choline administered regularly during prolonged exercise can improve performance (33). More studies are needed to determine if this improvement in performance is consistent and can be repeated.

Vitamin B Complex

Knowledge that B vitamins cumulatively affect energy metabolism has led to research on the effects of supplementation with multiple vitamins on physical performance. Combined restriction of dietary thiamin, riboflavin, and B_6 significantly decreased peak aerobic capacity (~12%), decreased peak power (~10%), and hastened onset of blood lactate accumulation (7%) in trained male cyclists (170). Although no single B vitamin was identified with any performance impairment, this finding emphasizes the importance of the B vitamins for optimal performance.

Vitamin C

Vitamin C is also referred to as ascorbic acid. This vitamin has various biological functions that could affect physical performance. Although it does not directly influence enzyme actions, vitamin C is needed to synthesize catecholamines and carnitine, which transport fatty acids into mitochondria for energy production. It reduces inorganic iron for absorption in the intestine and serves as a potent **antioxidant** to regenerate vitamin E from its oxidized by-product (75). An antioxidant is a substance that prevents damage caused by free radicals. Free radicals are highly reactive chemicals that often contain oxygen. They are produced when molecules are split to give products that have unpaired electrons. This process is called oxidation. Food sources of vitamin C include fruits and vegetables (especially citrus fruits and green leafy vegetables), such as broccoli, potatoes, tomatoes, and strawberries.

The RDA for ascorbic acid is 90 and 75 mg for men and women, respectively (75). Physiological stressors increase vitamin C needs. Although many athletes consume adequate amounts of vitamin C, 10% to 30% of male collegiate athletes and female aerobic endurance athletes consume less than the RDA (84). Up to 15% of athletes have plasma vitamin C concentrations indicative of deficiency (165). In a classic study, it was demonstrated that low vitamin C status impairs performance. Adolescents who consumed a diet low in vitamin C and then supplemented with vitamin C (100 mg/day for four months) improved work capacity by 48% compared with placebo-treated controls who consumed a diet low in vitamin C, whose work capacity increased by only 12% (99). Adults deficient in vitamin C who supplemented with vitamin C (500 mg/day for two weeks or RDA levels for eight weeks) significantly increased work efficiency and aerobic power during treadmill exercise (81, 169).

Fat-Soluble Vitamins

Vitamins A, D, E, and K are associated with sources of dietary fat and stored in adipose tissue (75, 76, 79). These **fat-soluble** vitamins are capable of being dissolved in fat and have no direct role in energy production (tables 7.1 and 7.2 on pages 114 and 115). No evidence currently links vitamin K to physical performance.

Vitamin A

The physiologically active form of vitamin A is retinol, which can be formed from beta-carotene, a provitamin. Vitamin A protects epithelial cells from damage, plays an important role in vision, and helps maintain immune function (76). Its role in exercise is as an antioxidant. Dietary sources of vitamin A include liver, butter, cheese, eggs, and fortified dairy products. Beta-carotene, the precursor of retinol, is found in yellow-orange vegetables and fruits, as well as dark green leafy vegetables.

Different chemical forms of vitamin A (retinol, beta-carotene, and other carotenoids) contribute to meeting the RDA, which is expressed as retinol equivalents (REs). The RDA is 900 RE or 4,500 IU for men, and 700 RE or 3,500 IU for women (76). Athletes generally report vitamin A intakes in excess of the RDA. Distance runners (135), professional ballet dancers (29), and female (180) and male collegiate athletes (61, 121) have satisfactory intakes of vitamin A. Some studies that have investigated adolescents and young adults (wrestlers [161], ballerinas [11], and gymnasts [100]) reported that these athletes tend to consume only 30% to 40% of the RDA for vitamin A, which is attributable to avoidance of dietary fat. Conversely, other studies have reported that vitamin A intakes were adequate in adolescent gymnasts and ballet dancers (46, 158). Surveys of international athletes show no evidence of low plasma retinol values but do indicate variable ranges (160). The effects of vitamin A supplementation on physical performance are not intensively studied. An early study reported no change in running performance of men maintained on a diet low in vitamin A for six months followed by a six-week repletion phase (176).

Vitamin E

Vitamin E is sometimes referred to as α-tocopherol, though α-tocopherol is just one of the eight isomers within the vitamin E family. The generic term, vitamin E, refers to naturally occurring compounds termed tocopherols and tocotrienols, of which α-tocopherol is considered the most biologically active. Vitamin E serves as an antioxidant in cell membranes and protects against oxidative stress (75). Major sources of dietary vitamin E include vegetables, nuts, whole grains, wheat germ, and peanut butter.

The RDA for vitamin E is 15 mg of α-tocopherol for adults (75). Surveys of athletes reveal adequate vitamin E intake (diet and supplements) (39). When only dietary sources were considered, however, 53% of college athletes (61), 50% of adolescent gymnasts (100, 101), and 38% of ballerinas (11) consumed less than 70% of the RDA. The mean intake of vitamin E for athletes was 77% of the RDA as compared with only 60% of the RDA among sedentary controls, which suggests a similar, albeit reduced, vitamin E intake among physically active and sedentary people (61).

The effects of supplemental vitamin E on physical performance are unclear (126). Vitamin E supplementation did not affect performance during a 1-mile (1.6 km) run, bench step test, 400 m swim test, and motor fitness tests of male adolescents supplemented with 400 mg α-tocopherol daily for six weeks (149); work capacity and muscle strength of collegiate male swimmers given 1,200 IU vitamin E for 85 days (151); peak oxygen uptake in ice hockey players given 800 mg daily for 50 days (177); aerobic endurance and blood lactate response in competitive swimmers given 600 mg daily for six months (97); or motor fitness tests, cardiorespiratory function during ergocycle tests, and 400 m swim times in male and female trained swimmers given 400 mg daily for six weeks (150). Supplementation of elite cyclists with α-tocopherol (400 mg) for five months did not improve performance (145). In contrast, men who supplemented with α-tocopherol (400 mg for 10 weeks) at altitude had lower levels of lactate during exercise compared with the placebo group (154). It was postulated that a potential benefit of supplemental vitamin E, alone or in combination with vitamin C, could decrease production of oxidative stress. Performance effects of these combined antioxidants are inconclusive (1, 24, 51).

Vitamin D

Vitamin D is sometimes referred to as cholecalciferol. Current guidelines for assessment of vitamin D status recommend measurement of serum 25 hydroxyvitamin D [25(OH)D], which is the most abundant metabolite of vitamin D in the circulation (79). Classification of vitamin D status is based on its central role in calcium use and bone health. Serum 25(OH)D concentration guidelines are the following: Less than 30 nmol/L indicates increased risk for deficiency, 50 nmol/L indicates sufficient, 50 to 100 nmol/L is optimal, and greater than 150 nmol/L indicates excess or toxicity (79). Food sources of vitamin D are fortified dairy products, eggs, tuna, salmon, herring, oysters, shrimp, and mackerel. Further, skin exposure to sun is required to synthesize the biologically active form of vitamin D [1,25(OH)$_2$D]. The adequate daily intake of vitamin D is 600 IU (15 mcg) for adults, and intakes of 4,000 IU (100 mcg) are considered excessive (79). The Endocrine Society raised the cumulative intake (diet plus supplements) of vitamin D to 1,500 IU to account for the physiological role of vitamin D in nonosseous tissues (70).

Although the central role of vitamin D is calcium absorption and bone metabolism (79), the ubiquitous distribution of vitamin D receptors (VDR) in nucleated cells, specifically skeletal muscle, suggests a role for vitamin D in muscle strength and function (57, 58). Vitamin D supplementation (4,000 IU for four months) of deficient elderly women [25(OH)D <20 to 60 nmol/L] significantly increased type I and II muscle fiber volume and increased VDR expression in muscle fibers (23). Signs of extraosseous vitamin D deficiency include musculoskeletal pain and neuromuscular dysfunction (72, 136, 138). Older adults with low serum 25(OH)D (<40 nmol/L) have decreased lower body strength (13). Institutionalized and community-living elderly with vitamin D deficiency and supplemented with a range of therapeutic doses of vitamin D (1,000 IU/d to a single dose [bolus] of 150,000 IU once per month for 6 to 12 months) significantly increased lower body strength 16% to 25% and walking speed 17%, independent of physical training (117, 186). Systematic reviews of the independent effects of vitamin D supplementation (400 to 1,920 IU/d for 16 to 24 weeks) added to resistance exercise training (RET), and conversely RET plus vitamin D supplementation (400 to 2,000 IU/d for 12 to 24 weeks) of elderly reveal important observations (2). Vitamin D supplementation significantly enhanced the benefit of RET on increasing lower body muscle strength, and RET added to supplemental vitamin D significantly increased lower body muscle strength and functional measures of mobility. The greatest gains in strength occurred in people with low vitamin

D status before supplementation. No conclusions about dose (nutritional or therapeutic) and duration of vitamin D supplementation, however, can be made without more detailed clinical investigations.

Peak physical and athletic performance is seasonal and coincides with vitamin D status among athletes. Cannell and colleagues (22) observed peak performance when vitamin D levels were at their highest, declined as vitamin D levels decreased, and reached a low point when vitamin D levels were at their lowest. Overall, athletes who practice and compete indoors while avoiding sun exposure are at increased risk for decreased vitamin D levels at any time of the year (3, 22, 71, 94, 188).

Vitamin D deficiency is common among adult athletes worldwide; the prevalence is estimated to range from 26% to 90% (2, 22, 27, 45). Vitamin D deficiency results in atrophy of type II muscle fibers (23); therefore, it is associated with impaired muscle strength and power (57, 136). Vitamin D supplementation of athletes, however, yields inconsistent results on performance (94, 125, 126). Despite consistently low vitamin D status, moderating factors contribute to the equivocal outcomes and include variable dosages of vitamin D supplementation (600 to 5,000 IU daily) for inconsistent durations (eight days to four months), diverse ethnicity of athletes, genetic difference in VDR, uncontrolled exposure to sun and UV light, varying dietary intake of vitamin D, and a lack of standardization of physical performance assessment measures (45, 94). A consistent observation, however, is that athletes with low vitamin D status (<40 nmol/L) tend to respond positively to daily vitamin D supplementation (600 IU or 15 mg).

Vitamin D supplementation of male and female elite athletes improves vitamin D status. Athletes who were vitamin D adequate (>75 nmol/L), deficient [25(OH)D <50 nmol/L], and insufficient [25(OH)D 50 to <75 nmol/L] were assigned randomly and received an oral vitamin D supplement (440, 1,100 or 2,200 IU daily) for one year (3). After 3 months, the serum 25(OH)D levels of the deficient and insufficient significantly increased to greater than 75 nmol/L with the 2,200 IU/day supplement. Average estimated daily intake of vitamin D was 168 IU, which is substantially less than the recommended intake of 600 IU/day (42, 79).

Interest in vitamin D as an ergogenic aid for elite athletes prompted study of supranutritional doses of this nutrient (125). Vitamin D deficiency [plasma 25(OH)D < 50 nmol/L] was identified in approximately 60% of club athletes, who then received one of two therapeutic doses of vitamin D (20,000 or 40,000 IU per week) or placebo for 6- and 12-week periods (27). Plasma 25(OH)D reached sufficient levels (>75 nmol/L) in 6 weeks, and no gain in physical performance measures occurred at 12 weeks. Elite athletes with optimal serum 25(OH)D levels (mean: 86 nmol/L) received either 35,000 IU or 70,000 IU/week for 12 weeks. The average daily dose was 5,000 or 10,000 IU daily, which substantially exceeds the safe upper limit recommendations of cumulative intake (diet plus supplement), which range from 1,500 IU (70) from the Endocrine Society to 4,000 IU (41) and

8,000 IU (79) for bone health. Serum 25(OH)D concentrations increased significantly during the supplementation period, returned to basal levels in the moderately supplemented group six weeks after cessation of supplementation, but remained elevated in the athletes supplemented with the larger dose. Serum levels of 24,25(OH)D, a metabolite of 25(OH)D, increased significantly in both supplemented groups and decreased after supplementation only in the athletes consuming the moderate level of supplemental vitamin D. Elevated levels of 24,25(OH)D block VDR, impair the physiological action of 1,25(OH)$_2$D, and deleteriously affect skeletal muscle function. In both groups, parathyroid hormone concentration increased significantly—an indication of a negative effect of these elevated levels of vitamin D supplementation (79).

Accumulating evidence from long-term supplementation trials with therapeutic doses of vitamin D in elderly women reveal increased rates of falls. Elderly women supplemented with 500,000 IU/year (approximately 1,370 IU/day) had 15% more falls and 26% more fractures than the placebo-treated cohort (147). A study of graded vitamin D supplementation for 12 months revealed that fall rates were significantly lower (21% compared with 60% and 72%, respectively) on moderate (1,600 to 3,200 IU/day) compared with lower (400 to 800 IU/d) and higher (3,200 to 4,800 IU/d) doses (157). These findings emphasize the need for caution in use of megadoses of vitamin D supplements in maintenance of skeletal muscle function in athletes and elderly (53).

Emerging evidence suggests a beneficial role of supplemental vitamin D on recovery after intense physical activity. Untrained healthy adults with low vitamin D status [25(OH)D (~30 nmol/L)] underwent a single bout of intense exercise with one leg. Muscle weakness, defined as the difference between single-leg isometric force of the exercised and nonexercised leg, assessed immediately and up to three days after the exercise bout, was significantly and inversely related to serum 25(OH)D levels (6). Recreationally active men with low 25(OH)D concentrations received either a 4,000 IU vitamin D supplement or a placebo daily for 35 days randomly and performed one bout of isometric–concentric jumps. Supplemental vitamin D enhanced recovery of peak isometric force and attenuated the immediate and delayed (two- and three-day) increase in chemical biomarkers of muscle damage with no effect on self-reported muscle soreness (7). Owens and colleagues (124) reported a controlled study of men with low 25(OH)D (40 nmol/L) and supplemented with 4,000 IU vitamin D or placebo for six weeks and then exposed to damaging knee extensor exercise. They confirmed that supplemental vitamin D enhanced peak force recovery during the following seven days and identified in vitro improved muscle regeneration with elevated 1,25(OH)$_2$D using a muscle injury model with muscle biopsy samples from other men with low 25(OH)D levels. These observations provide new insight to a potential value of vitamin D supplementation in people with low vitamin D status.

Minerals and Performance

Minerals are inorganic elements that exist as solids (73, 75, 76, 120). Sodium, potassium, chloride, calcium, phosphorus, magnesium, and sulfur are designated as macrominerals because the recommended intakes exceed 100 mg/day and the body contains more than 5 g. Hormones control the levels of many of the macrominerals in the body. Iron, copper, chromium, selenium, and zinc are termed trace elements because recommended intakes are less than 100 mg/day. Precise mechanisms for absorption and excretion homeostatically regulate the trace element content of cells. Fluoride, boron, iodine, manganese, and molybdenum are ultratrace elements that have intakes less than 5 mg/day (tables 7.1 and 7.2, pages 114 and 115).

In contrast to the situation with vitamins, burgeoning data are available on the adverse effects of low intakes of some minerals on measures of physical performance. Research on the interactions among performance, intake, and status of copper, phosphorus, selenium, iodine, molybdenum, potassium, and chloride is lacking. Therefore, this section focuses on iron, magnesium, zinc, and chromium and emphasizes findings since the publication of the DRIs for minerals.

Macrominerals

Minerals fall into two categories: macrominerals and trace minerals. The total mineral content of the body is approximately 4% of body weight. Macrominerals are present in the body in larger amounts than trace minerals and include calcium, phosphorus, magnesium, sodium, chloride, and potassium.

Sodium, Potassium, and Chloride

These minerals exist as electrolytes principally in body fluids (120). Sodium is an extracellular cation that maintains body fluid and acid–base balance, as well as nerve function. Potassium is predominantly an intracellular cation and regulates water balance, impulse transmission from nerves to muscle, energy use in muscle cells, and production of ATP. Chloride is largely an extracellular anion that participates in fluid balance and nerve impulse transmission. Sodium is distributed widely in foods along with chloride. Potassium is found in fruits and vegetables, dairy products, meat, and fish.

Sodium, chloride, and potassium modulate fluid exchange within the body's fluid compartments, allowing a well-regulated exchange of nutrients and waste products between the cell and its external fluid environment. Individualized recommended sodium intakes may depend on sweat rate and sodium losses during exercise. For example, Division I collegiate football players differed in their sodium losses during a two-a-day training camp. Specifically, football players with a history of heat cramps lost about two times more sodium in their sweat when compared with football players without a history of heat cramps (163). For most people without a history of heat cramps, attainment of the recommended intake of sodium (1.5 g/day) is adequate to maintain sodium balance.

Calcium and Phosphorus

These minerals have key roles in the formation of bone; more than 90% is contained in bone (73, 79). Calcium is needed for nerve conduction and muscle contraction, as well as the synthesis and breakdown of glycogen. Phosphorus is present in every cell as a component of DNA, ATP, phosphocreatine, and 2,3 diphosphoglycerate (2,3 DPG), which regulates the release of oxygen to muscles during exercise. Dietary sources of calcium and phosphorus are milk, dairy products, broccoli, kale, turnip greens, nuts, and legumes.

The Adequate Intake for calcium for adults is 1,000 mg per day. The adult RDA for phosphorus is 700 mg for both men and women. Clinical studies using athletes and calcium supplementation are rare; when conducted, they supply the research participants with an amount of calcium or phosphorus well above the Adequate Intake or recommended dietary intake for these minerals.

One such study provided 35 mg calcium per kilogram body weight per day for a four-week period in conjunction with 90 minutes of aerobic endurance training per day, five days per week. The investigators assessed the total and free testosterone production in response to the calcium supplementation before and after an intense training routine. At the end of the four-week exercise training and calcium supplementation intervention, no significant differences were seen in either total or free testosterone in athletes who ingested the calcium supplement as compared with athletes assigned to an exercise-only group. Scientific data on phosphorus supplementation are more prevalent, but most of the published studies do not support improvements in aerobic endurance exercise performance (16, 92).

Magnesium

Bone contains almost 60% of the magnesium in the body. Only a small percentage of magnesium, which exists as a component of more than 300 enzymes, is in soft tissue (73). Magnesium regulates many physiological processes, including energy metabolism as a component of adenosine triphosphatase (ATPase) and 2,3 DPG, and gluconeogenesis. Food sources of magnesium include fruits, vegetables, nuts, seafood, and whole-grain and dairy products. Some bottled waters and hard water are practical sources of magnesium.

The RDA for men and women is 400 and 310 mg/day, respectively (73). Dietary surveys of athletes reveal that magnesium intakes equal or exceed the RDA for males but not female athletes, who consume 60% to 65% of the RDA (122). Regardless of gender, athletes participating in sports that have weight classifications, or in which the competition includes an aesthetic component, tended to consume inadequate amounts of dietary magnesium (<55% of the RDA) (67). Magnesium intakes of athletes assessed as they ate in a training center environment, however, exceeded the RDA (49).

Loss of magnesium from the body increases after heavy exercise. Intense anaerobic exercise caused 21% more urinary magnesium losses on the day of exercise, as compared with control or nonexercise conditions; values returned to nonexercise levels on the day after the exercise (31). The amount of urinary magnesium was related to the degree of exercise-induced anaerobiosis, indexed by postexercise oxygen consumption and plasma lactate concentration (32). Thus, magnesium needs increase when glycolytic metabolism is dominant.

Magnesium supplementation of competitive athletes can improve cellular function. Among competitive female athletes with plasma magnesium concentrations at the low end of the range of normal values, serum total creatine kinase decreased after training in the women supplemented daily with magnesium (360 mg/day for three weeks) compared with the athletes receiving placebo (59). Serum lactate concentration and oxygen uptake during an exhaustive rowing performance test decreased in elite female rowers with initial low serum magnesium and supplemented with magnesium (360 mg/day) for four weeks, as compared with the rowers receiving placebo (59). In response to a seven-week resistance training program, leg strength increased more in young men consuming supplemental magnesium (250 mg) in addition to the magnesium included in the diet (totaling 8 mg/kg body weight) compared with placebo (17).

Alterations in dietary magnesium affect magnesium nutrition and performance (105). Women given a controlled low magnesium intake compared with adequate magnesium intake (180 vs. 320 mg) had negative retention (intake minus losses) and decreased indicators of magnesium status (red blood cell and muscle magnesium concentrations). During submaximal exercise, heart rate increased (10 beats per minute) and work efficiency decreased (10%) with the low magnesium intake.

Trace Elements

By definition, trace elements are chemical components that naturally occur in soil, plants, and animals in minute concentrations. Although required in much smaller quantities than macrominerals, trace elements, also known as trace minerals, are necessary for optimal health and performance.

Iron

This metallic element is critical in the formation of compounds needed for oxygen transport and cellular use. Hemoglobin, the principal iron-containing compound, transports oxygen to cells. Cellular iron compounds include myoglobin, the cytochromes, and some enzymes in the Krebs cycle (aconitase, NADH dehydrogenase, and succinate dehydrogenase) that enable substrate use for energy production. Almost 30% of iron is stored in tissues, and 70% is involved in oxygen metabolism (76). Food sources of iron include heme protein (hemoglobin and myoglobin) found in animal flesh foods. Nonheme iron sources include dried fruits, vegetables, legumes, whole-grain products, and fortified cereals. Heme iron is better absorbed and used than nonheme iron (10%-35% vs. 2%-10%) (76). Diet composition has negligible effect on heme iron absorption, whereas many constituents of a meal significantly affect nonheme iron absorption (30). Meat protein and vitamin C both increase the absorption of nonheme iron; and tannins (found in tea, wine, and some foods), calcium, polyphenols, and phytates (found in whole grains) decrease the absorption of nonheme iron (30, 76).

The RDA for iron is 8 and 18 mg/day for men and women, respectively (76). Male athletes generally consume adequate amounts of iron, but female athletes participating in aerobic endurance sports or activities requiring low body weight (e.g., ballerinas and gymnasts) tend to consume less than the RDA for iron (64). Iron intakes of female athletes consuming supplements exceed the RDA (34). Low intake of iron is the principal cause of iron deficiency in women and is exacerbated by iron losses during menstruation.

Iron deficiency occurs in stages. Early tissue iron depletion, characterized by low serum ferritin (<12 mcg/L) and increased total iron-binding capacity (>400 mcg/dl), is prevalent in 15% to 20% of women, 20% to 37% of female athletes, in 20% to 25% of girls, and 25% to 47% of young female athletes. Although less than 12 mcg/L for serum ferritin is accepted as the clinical cutoff, a broader range to identify iron depletion, 20 and 35 mcg/L, is designated for premenopausal female athletes. Low serum ferritin signals increased iron absorption. Next, the iron content of red blood cells decreases; the number of transferrin receptors on cells increases, and then the number of these receptors increases in serum. Elevated soluble serum transferrin receptor (sTfR) concentrations (>8.5 mg/L) indicate a functional iron deficiency. The final stage of iron deficiency is preceded by stage 2 iron deficiency without anemia, or IDNA. The final stage of iron deficiency is **anemia** with decreased hemoglobin (<130 g/L for men and <120 g/L for women). Anemia is a decrease in the number of red blood cells, which reduces the amount of oxygen transport to the tissues. The prevalence of anemia is 5% in women, 5% to 12% in female athletes, and 6% for girls regardless of athletic participation (76). Estimates of IDNA range from 15% to 35% and 3% to 11% in female and male athletes, respectively (153).

Assessment of human iron status involves multiple blood biochemical measurements because infection and inflammation directly affect individual indicators (e.g., decrease serum iron and ferritin). Multiple biomarkers (erythrocyte protoporphyrin, red cell distribution width, mean corpuscular volume, transferrin saturation, and serum ferritin) are used to ascertain altered iron status (137). For athletes, however, the minimal assessment measurements include serum ferritin, hemoglobin, and transferrin (25).

Anemia reduces peak oxygen uptake, reduces work capacity and aerobic endurance, and raises plasma lactate; these impairments are corrected with iron supplementation (40, 54). Controversy exists, however, regarding the effects of IDNA on performance and metabolism (62, 128). Although supplementation trials of female athletes with IDNA showed increased serum ferritin and decreased lactate during exercise in laboratory tests without improvements in measurements of performance (103, 113, 148), other studies of adolescent female athletes and women during training with IDNA showed improved aerobic endurance performance or peak oxygen uptake (139, 146). One factor that could explain the inconsistency in findings is the confounding effect of inflammation that reduces circulating ferritin levels (115). Acute exercise increases expression of proinflammatory cytokines, notably interleukin 6 (IL-6), that boost synthesis and release of hepcidin from the liver (131). Elevated circulating hepcidin levels increase iron storage within intestinal mucosal cells and macrophages thus reducing iron available for physiological functions necessary to support the increased metabolic demands of physical activity (132).

Accumulating evidence supports beneficial effects of iron supplementation on performance of people with IDNA. During aerobic training, women with IDNA who were supplemented with iron (8 mg/day for six weeks) significantly decreased sTfR and increased ferritin without any change in hemoglobin. Although both groups improved cycling times, the iron-supplemented women improved 15 km cycle time trial and decreased plasma lactate more than the placebo-treated women (68). Also, women with IDNA (sTfR > 8.5 mg/L) supplemented with iron (8 mg/day for 10 weeks) and trained on cycle ergometers significantly reduced time to complete a simulated 15 km (9.3 mi) trial by exercising at a significantly higher work rate and using a lower percentage of aerobic capacity than women treated with placebo (18). Similarly, iron supplementation (10 mg/day for six weeks) compared with placebo reduced muscle fatigue during knee extensor exercise in women with IDNA (20). Iron supplementation (30 mg elemental iron for six weeks) significantly increased energetic efficiency of male and female athletes with IDNA (serum ferritin <12 mcg/L and sTfR >8.0 mg/L) randomly assigned to supplementation or placebo (69). The DRI panel summarized research findings showing that regular aerobic endurance training raised iron losses up to 3 mg/day (76). Thus, people who regularly engage in aerobic endurance training should increase iron intakes 30% to 70% to accommodate the increased iron loss.

Copper

Copper functions as a metalloenzyme needed for nonheme iron uptake and hemoglobin formation (ceruloplasmin), for energy production in the mitochondria (cytochrome c oxidase), and as an antioxidant (superoxide dismutase)

(76). Despite these possible opportunities to influence performance, clear evidence of impaired performance with inadequate copper intake is lacking. Copper is widely distributed in foods; appreciable amounts are found in nuts, beans, whole-grain products, shellfish, and organs. The RDA for copper is 900 mcg/day for adult males and females.

Zinc

Zinc is found in all tissues of the body as a component of more than 100 metalloenzymes. Zinc-containing enzymes regulate some aspects of energy metabolism, including oxygen–carbon dioxide transport (carbonic anhydrase) and lactic acid metabolism (lactate dehydrogenase), and control breakdown and synthesis of macronutrients, growth and development, immune function, and wound healing (76). Seafood, meats, lima beans, black-eyed peas, white beans, whole-grain products, and fortified cereals are sources of zinc. Diets high in protein provide substantial amounts of zinc. Zinc availability is reduced from diets high in fiber and phytic acid.

Physically active adults generally consume the RDA for zinc (11 and 8 mg/day for men and women, respectively) (102, 108). Female athletes in aerobic endurance sports and gymnastics have marginal intakes partially because of food restriction (152). Zinc status is an indicator of performance. Serum zinc levels were low, compared with the range of normal values, in 25% of male distance runners and were inversely correlated with training distances (37). Surveys of aerobic endurance athletes and runners revealed that the prevalence of low serum zinc was 20% to 25% compared with 13% for gender-matched controls (102, 155).

Accumulating evidence indicates that low zinc status affects physical performance. Zinc enhances in vitro muscle contraction (80, 142). Zinc supplementation, compared with placebo, in middle-aged women increased muscle strength and muscular endurance (93). Because these muscle functions rely on recruitment of fast-twitch glycolytic muscle fibers, zinc supplementation may enhance the activity of lactate dehydrogenase, a zinc-dependent enzyme. Male subjects fed diets with low, compared with adequate, zinc content (1 vs. 12 mg/day) had decreased serum zinc and zinc retention, as well as decreased upper and lower body muscle strength (171). Serum zinc concentrations of adolescent gymnasts were decreased compared with values in nonathletic age- and gender-matched controls; half of the athletes were characterized with subclinical zinc deficiency. Serum zinc was positively correlated with adductor muscle strength in the gymnasts (19). Elite male soccer players with low, compared with normal, serum zinc concentrations had decreased peak power output and increased blood lactate during cycle ergometer tests (87). The authors explained these findings with an observation that the supplemental zinc significantly decreased exercise-induced red blood cell deformity and thus improved blood flow to muscles during exercise (88). Men fed whole-food diets moderately low in zinc (3-4 mg/day) had increased ventilation rates with decreased oxygen uptake and decreased carbon dioxide output and respiratory exchange ratio during prolonged submaximal cycle ergometer exercise (107). The low-zinc diet resulted in decreased zinc status (serum zinc and zinc retention). The activity of carbonic anhydrase (a zinc-dependent enzyme) in red blood cells decreased with the low-zinc diet.

Selenium

Selenium exists as selenoproteins that exert biological actions including protection against oxidative damage to cells (glutathione peroxidase). Selenium acts with vitamin E as an antioxidant (75). Evidence supporting a role for selenium in performance is lacking. Selenium is linked with protein content of the diet. Foods high in selenium include seafood, meats, whole-grain products, liver, wheat bran, and some vegetables (broccoli and cauliflower). The RDA for selenium is 55 mcg/day for adult males and females.

Chromium

Emerging evidence suggests that chromium facilitates the action of insulin in cells of people with insulin resistance. Its role in promoting physical performance is controversial (104, 172). Whole grains, cheese, beans, mushrooms, oysters, wine, apples, pork, chicken, and brewer's yeast are sources of chromium.

Chromium is provisionally essential; Adequate Intakes are 35 and 25 mcg/day for men and women, respectively (76). Assessment of dietary chromium and chromium nutritional status is problematic (104), which limits evaluation of its importance in physical activity. Because of the putative role of chromium in regulating glucose metabolism and potentially anabolism (43), numerous studies have been conducted to determine the effect of supplemental trivalent chromium, generally as chromium picolinate, on strength gain and body composition change. Consistent results showing a beneficial effect of supplemental chromium on strength gain, muscle accretion, or glycogen synthesis after exercise in healthy men and women are lacking (110, 174).

Other Minerals

Boron, vanadium, cobalt, fluoride, iodine, manganese, and molybdenum have reported biological functions that theoretically would negatively affect performance when consumed in suboptimal amounts (73, 76). But no published research has presented evidence that restricted intakes of these minerals has negative effects on physical performance. Further, vanadium and manganese play roles in carbohydrate and lipid metabolism in animals, but dietary deficiencies in humans are rare.

Supplementation With Antioxidant Vitamins

Regular physical activity and exercise training offer pervasive health and performance benefits. But observations that exercise increases production of free radicals, ROS and RNS, that could cause muscle damage raised concerns about their biological significance (4, 15, 34) and prompted interest in use of supplements to decrease free radicals (55). Initial studies aimed to control excess exercise-induced free radicals and hypothesized a potential benefit of nutritional antioxidants to attenuate muscle damage, facilitate recovery, and enhance performance. Vitamins C and E were the supplemental nutritional antioxidants used because of their solubility in water and lipid, respectively. Research findings exposed paradoxical findings; they failed to support supplementation with nutritional antioxidants as beneficial and led to the propitious discovery of regulatory roles of free radicals as essential in the signaling processes of skeletal muscle adaptation to exercise (28, 134).

Adverse Effects of Vitamin C and E Supplementation

Supplementation with vitamins C and E of physically active adults consistently reveals evidence of increased exercise-induced free radical production. Usual measurements of oxidative stress included ROS and indicators of lipid peroxidation or damage and protein damage. Researchers supplemented athletes with large doses of vitamin C and A and highly variable amounts of vitamin E exceeding recommended intakes (e.g., supranutritional) but less than safe upper intake levels. Some experimental designs included placebo or control groups for comparison of supplement effects.

Consumption of supplemental vitamins C and E (tocopherols) consistently elevates indicators of oxidative damage after various types of physical activity. Triathletes consuming self-prescribed vitamins C and E supplements (1,100 mg and 314 mg, respectively) for prolonged periods as compared with non-supplement users had significantly increased concentrations of postrace lipid peroxidation assessed with plasma malonaldehyde (MDA) (91). Trained cyclists with adequate daily intakes of vitamins C and E (91 and 16 mg, respectively) received daily vitamin E (400 IU or 268 mg), vitamin C (1,000 mg), combined vitamin C (1,000 mg) and vitamin E (200 IU or 134 mg), or placebo for three weeks in a crossover design (21). After a bout of prolonged exercise, vitamin E supplementation significantly decreased postexercise MDA whereas vitamin C supplementation significantly increased MDA at rest and after exercise, compared with placebo. The combined vitamins C and E supplement elicited similar MDA levels as placebo. Ultra-endurance runners supplemented daily for two months with high dose vitamin E (800 IU) or placebo before competition (123). Compared with placebo treatment, vitamin E significantly increased postrace plasma F2-isoprostane, an indicator of lipid peroxidation, and biomarkers of inflammation with no effect on performance. In a double-blind, placebo-controlled crossover study, pre- and postexercise MDA concentrations were significantly increased in athletes supplemented daily for 12 to 14 days with an antioxidant mixture of vitamin E (107 IU), vitamin C (450 mg), β-carotene (36 mg), and selenium (100 mcg) (95). Similarly, compared with placebo, a six-week daily supplementation treatment with a complex blend of antioxidant and other nutrients (vitamin C, 400 mg; vitamin E, 268 mg; B$_6$, 2 mcg; folic acid, 200 mcg; zinc, 5 mg; B$_{12}$, 1 mcg) elicited a significant increase in postexercise F2-isoprostane, cortisol, and inflammatory cytokines in men (5). These findings consistently demonstrate that supplementation of antioxidant vitamins promotes exercise-induced oxidative stress.

Adverse Effects on Adaptation to Training

Chronic exposure to oxidative stress elicits protective cellular responses to attenuate tissue damage and promote recovery. These defensive responses include increased expression of trace-element-dependent antioxidant enzymes, such as superoxide dismutase (SOD), catalase (CAT) and glutathione peroxidase (GPx), heat shock proteins (HSP), and inflammatory cytokines in exercised muscle, other cells, and blood (140). Untrained men randomized to receive either vitamin C (500 mg/day) or placebo for eight weeks underwent a single bout of controlled exercise (89). Supplemental vitamin C upregulated basal (preexercise) expression of SOD, CAT, HSP60 and HSP70 in lymphocytes that was diminished during in vitro exposure to oxidants. Muscle HSP70 increased with vitamin C supplementation but did not increase after exercise. Physically active men were randomized and received a daily supplement containing 400 to 420 IU of vitamin E isomers (α and γ) plus vitamin C (400 mg) for 28 days and then performed prolonged knee extensor exercise (47). Indicators of postexercise oxidative stress significantly decreased with the α-isomer (a potent antioxidant and the predominant form in tissues and blood) combined with vitamin C. But the γ-isomer (a weaker antioxidant found in plant foods) plus vitamin C was associated with significantly reduced expression of HSP72 mRNA in muscle and blood. Untrained men were randomly assigned to either vitamin C (1,000 mg) or placebo before a bout of downhill running and then continued supplementation for the following 14 days (26). Whereas both groups self-reported delayed muscle soreness, only the placebo-treated men had significantly increased MDA whereas the vitamin C-treated group reported delayed recovery. Kayakers with sufficient intakes of antioxidant vitamins and minerals received either placebo or a supplement with supranutritional levels of vitamins C and E, lutein, β-carotene, zinc, selenium, and magnesium for four weeks and then participated in a race (166). Supplementation neither improved performance nor diminished postrace plasma levels of lipid peroxidation and inflammatory cytokines, which led to the conclusion of no benefit on recovery.

Reactive oxygen species can enable physiological process fundamental to circulatory responses during exercise. One key aspect is vasodilation, which enables greater blood flow and thus boosts delivery of oxygen and removal of metabolic by-products to working muscle, after supplementation with antioxidants. Richardson and colleagues (143) provided healthy young men with one dose containing vitamin E (200 IU) and vitamin C (500 mg) plus the antioxidant lipoic acid (30 mg) followed by another supplement capsule with similar content but more vitamin E (400 IU) or placebo. The researchers then administered a submaximal graded hand-grip exercise test. The antioxidant mixture, compared with placebo, significantly decreased free radical content of the blood at rest and after exercise (98% and 85%, respectively). Noteworthy, however, was a 300% decrease in brachial artery vasodilation in the antioxidant-supplemented group. Using a similar acute antioxidant supplementation protocol, vasodilation and vascular reactivity was assessed in older men after knee extensor training (35). The antioxidant supplement similarly reduced circulating free radical levels and decreased vasodilation. A follow-up study compared circulatory responses in healthy young and older men after acute antioxidant supplementation (185). Supplementation had no effect in either group on increased blood flow after 5 minutes of forearm occlusion but paradoxically improved flow mediated vasodilation only in the older men. This finding confirms the observation of an adverse effect of the antioxidant mixture at supranutritional levels on vasodilation in young men and indicates a potential diminution of a beneficial training effect on circulatory function. Aging is associated with increased levels of oxidative stress indicators and reduced blood vessel function. The observation that acute supplemental supraphysiological doses of antioxidants may improve blood vessel endothelial function is an opportunity for future research.

Antioxidant supplementation impairs insulin sensitivity in response to exercise training. Trained and untrained men received either antioxidant supplement (vitamin C: 1,000 mg and vitamin E: 400 IU) or placebo daily for four weeks while undergoing muscular endurance training (144). Exercise training increased ROS and improved insulin sensitivity. Antioxidant supplementation decreased ROS in muscle and attenuated the insulin sensitivity. The exercise-induced increase in ROS upregulated expression of specific transcription factors and antioxidant enzymes associated with increased insulin sensitivity, whereas antioxidant supplements had a detrimental effect on insulin sensitivity. These findings demonstrate that supplementation with antioxidant vitamins blunts the adaptative response of exercise training on insulin sensitivity.

No Benefit of Antioxidant Supplementation on Performance

Evidence of an ergogenic effect of antioxidant supplementation is lacking. Swimmers supplemented with vitamin E (400 IU) had no performance improvement compared with placebo-treated swimmers (149, 150). Similarly, daily supplementation with vitamin C (1,000 mg) did not improve aerobic endurance performance of adults (56, 86, 99, 169). Supplementation of vitamin C in athletes with subclinical vitamin C deficiency, however, increases physical performance and diminishes oxidative stress (127).

Vitamin C supplementation significantly decreased mitochondrial biogenesis and reduced adaptation to training. Compared with placebo treatment, supplementation of men with vitamin C (1,000 mg) daily for eight weeks attenuated the gain in peak oxygen uptake (60). A companion study in rodents revealed a significant reduction in expression of SOD, GPx, and, importantly, cytochrome c and regulatory transcription factors for mitochondrial biogenesis in skeletal muscle of vitamin C-repleted animals.

Young women received either an antioxidant supplement or placebo (vitamin C: 1,000 mg and vitamin E: 400 IU) and participated in resistance training for 10 weeks. Self-reported daily intakes of vitamin C were adequate (>90 mg), but vitamin E intakes were less than the recommended intake (3 to 4 mg compared with 15 mg). Antioxidant vitamin supplementation did not improve strength gain, but the increase in lean muscle mass was significantly greater for the placebo group (4% versus −0.7%, respectively) (38). Elderly men with adequate vitamins C and E intakes were stratified by strength measures and then randomized and treated with supplemental vitamin C (500 mg) and vitamin E (~200 IU) or placebo consumed as two doses before and two doses after daily resistance training for 12 weeks (14). Antioxidant-supplemented men gained significantly less lean muscle mass (1.4% versus 3.9%, respectively), had smaller increases in rectus femoris size (10.9% versus 16.2%, respectively), and had no differences in strength gain. These findings demonstrate that antioxidant vitamin supplementation does not improve athletic performance, muscular endurance, or strength gain.

Evidence of the mechanism for the lack of a benefit of antioxidant vitamin supplementation on training outcomes is emerging. Vitamin C and E supplementation (1,000 mg and 400 IU daily) provided within a few hours, compared with placebo, during four weeks of muscular endurance training provided no performance benefit to young men. It neither reduced skeletal muscle levels of indicators of lipid peroxidation nor increased markers of mitochondrial biogenesis of young men after prolonged exercise (118). Paulsen and colleagues (129) used a similar dose and timing of ingestion of these vitamins and found no effect of supplementation, compared with placebo, on peak work capacity and running performance (20 m shuttle) of muscular-endurance-trained young adults. The authors reported a significant decrease in mitochondrial cytochrome c protein content and cytosolic proteins. Young men and women supplemented with a similar dose of vitamins C and E while participating in resistance training program had smaller gains in some strength measures but similar increases in lean muscle mass compared with placebo-treated participants (130).

Supplementation, however, significantly decreased expression of signaling pathways for muscle hypertrophy. These findings provide evidence that supplemental vitamins C and E interfere with signaling processes and thus reduce training adaptations for muscular endurance and muscle hypertrophy.

Professional Applications

Vitamins and minerals function in the human body as metabolic regulators, influencing several physiological processes important to exercise or sport performance. For example, many of the B-complex vitamins are involved in processing carbohydrate and fat for energy production, an important consideration during exercise of varying intensities (181). Several B vitamins are also essential to help form hemoglobin in red blood cells, which is a major determinant of oxygen delivery to the muscles during aerobic endurance exercise. Additionally, vitamins C and E function as antioxidants, which are important for enhancing immune function but of limited value in preventing oxidative damage to cellular structure and function during exercise training and optimizing exercise-induced adaptation to training (28).

Minerals are important to athletes because they are involved in muscle contraction, normal heart rhythm, nerve impulse conduction, oxygen transport, oxidative phosphorylation, enzyme activation, immune functions, antioxidant activity, bone health, and acid–base balance of the blood (159, 182). Because many of these processes are accelerated during exercise, adequate amounts of minerals are necessary for optimal functioning. Athletes should obtain adequate amounts of all minerals in their diet because a mineral deficiency may impair optimal health, and health impairment may adversely affect sport performance (182).

Because vitamins and minerals cannot be produced by the body, but rather must be consumed in the diet, athletes and physically active people must consume a balanced diet. A balanced diet is one that contains adequate amounts of all the necessary nutrients required for healthy growth and activity. To help ensure a balanced diet, athletes should adopt a "food first" approach and regularly ingest the following types of foods:

- Lean meats (e.g., poultry, fish, low-fat pork, low-fat beef)
- Fruits (e.g., apples, bananas, grapes, oranges, pineapple, blueberries)
- Vegetables (e.g., broccoli, spinach, green beans, carrots)

This list of foods that athletes should ingest on a daily basis is not comprehensive; rather, it summarizes the types of food choices they should make frequently and consistently. An athlete or physically active person who does not consistently eat these types of foods as part of the diet should take a multivitamin to prevent deficiencies. This recommendation has been advanced by the American Medical Association (48) and professional organizations (167). Athletes who consistently restrict food intake are at greater risk for nutrient deficiencies. Athletes who participate in gymnastics, ballet, cheerleading, and wrestling are typically the types of athletes who restrict food intake and would benefit from a multivitamin supplement.

Some athletes and coaches believe that ingesting a vitamin and mineral supplement will confer athletic advantages, but scientific investigations have not supported this theory. Several studies have provided multivitamin–mineral supplements over prolonged periods and shown no significant effects on either laboratory or sport-specific tests of physical performance (156, 179). In a long-term study, Telford and colleagues (165) evaluated the effect of seven to eight months of vitamin–mineral supplementation (100 to 5,000 times the RDA) on exercise performance of nationally ranked athletes in training at the Australian Institute of Sport. They reported no significant effect of the supplementation protocol on any measure of physical performance when compared with results for athletes whose vitamin and mineral RDAs were met by normal dietary intake (165, 179).

Physically active people should not self-supplement with vitamin D and vitamins C and E. Coaches should encourage athletes to seek counseling from a sport nutritionist that involves an assessment of nutrient intakes and, when appropriate, biochemical assessment of nutritional status (96). Supplementation is indicated only when deficiency is present. Recent equivocal evidence indicates that vitamin D supplementation boosts performance in athletes (126). Because new and compelling evidence supports the essential role of free radicals as messengers for intracellular signaling pathways that facilitate adaptations to exercise training, supplementation with vitamins C and E to quench free radicals is not recommended. To avoid any ill effects of a megadose of antioxidant vitamin supplements, athletes are encouraged to implement a "food first" dietary approach to obtain the vitamins and minerals necessary to support training and recovery and to optimize performance (114).

In summary, vitamin and mineral supplements will not improve performance when dietary intake of these nutrients is adequate. But if a vitamin or mineral deficiency is present (as is the case more commonly in weight-control sports), a vitamin and mineral supplement could improve performance by eliminating the deficiency.

Summary Points

- Vitamins and minerals cannot be produced by the body and thus must be consumed in foods and beverages.
- The content of vitamins and minerals in food is small (micrograms to milligrams) compared with that of protein, carbohydrate, and fat (up to hundreds of grams).
- Vitamins and minerals are not direct sources of energy, but they facilitate energy production and use from carbohydrate, fat, and protein; transport oxygen and carbon dioxide; regulate fluid balance; support immune function; and protect against oxidative damage.
- Subclinical deficiencies of some vitamins and minerals occur in physically active people.

- Vitamins are characterized into two main groups: water soluble and fat soluble. The water-soluble vitamins include the B vitamins and vitamin C. The fat-soluble vitamins are vitamins A, D, E, and K.
- Minerals are classified as either major minerals or trace minerals. Major minerals are those needed by the body in amounts greater than 100 mg/day. Trace minerals are those required in daily quantities of less than 100 mg.
- Vitamin supplements are not necessary for an athlete on a balanced diet, but health professionals may recommend them to athletes if their diet is not balanced, if they are on a very low-calorie diet, or for other special dietary needs.
- Athletes should use a "food first" approach to meet their nutritional needs.

Chapter 8

Strength, Size, and Power Supplements

Colin Wilborn, PhD, FNSCA, CSCS, FISSN

Tim N. Ziegenfuss, PhD, CSCS, FISSN

Different sports place unique metabolic requirements on bioenergetic systems, and these differences alter the nutritional requirements among athletes involved in various types of strength and power sports. Particularly important to the strength and power athlete are

- increasing lean muscle mass that translates into functional sport-specific strength,
- increasing power and speed over short distances, and
- increasing explosiveness.

These goals typically drive strength–power athletes to seek various options in their training methodologies to maximize the training stimulus. Besides intense training, a proper nutrition program is needed to maximize the performance of a strength–power athlete. More specifically, precise nutritional supplementation can provide the impetus for maximizing lean muscle mass, power, speed, and explosiveness. Therefore, any nutritional program (including sport supplements) that enhances lean muscle mass, power, speed, and explosiveness, when combined with a proper training program, has a high likelihood of augmenting exercise and sport performance.

The author would like to acknowledge the significant contributions of Bill I. Campbell to this chapter.

To stay on the cutting edge of nutritional supplementation, it is important to identify supplements that have been shown to be effective and safe when ingested appropriately. Many experts in the field have identified and separated the leading sport supplements into categories, ranging from those that are safe to those that have harmful side effects or those whose effectiveness has not been demonstrated in the literature. A comprehensive analysis of the sport supplements that may benefit the strength and power athlete can be based on three simple questions:

- Is the sport supplement legal and safe?
- Does scientific evidence show that the sport supplement can improve health or exercise performance?
- Is there a sound scientific rationale for beneficial effects?

Claims of enhanced exercise performance have been advanced for hundreds of sport supplements. Rather than address every sport supplement with claimed **ergogenic** (i.e., work-enhancing) potential, this chapter covers the most popular sport supplements that have been demonstrated to be safe, effective, and legal relative to increasing lean muscle mass, strength, and power. These supplements are creatine, HMB, protein, and beta-alanine.

Note that some argue against the use of sport supplements. People who hold this position often cite ethical considerations relating to unfair advantage during competition. Inherent in this viewpoint is the belief that athletes who would normally refrain from using sport supplements feel pressured to use them just to stay on equal footing with their competitors (45). The intent of this chapter is not to address those concerns but instead to focus on those few sport supplements with demonstrated safety and effectiveness.

Creatine

The sport supplement creatine monohydrate (creatine) has been the gold standard with which other nutritional supplements are compared (35) because it improves performance, increases lean muscle mass and strength, and has an excellent safety profile when consumed in recommended dosages (35). Creatine is one of the most widely researched sport nutrition supplements on the market. Although several methods of ingestion can be used, the most common is to mix creatine as a powder into a drink. Creatine is also commonly ingested in the form of a capsule, tablet, or gummy.

Chemically, creatine is derived from the amino acids glycine, arginine, and methionine; it is obtained from the ingestion of meat or fish and is also synthesized in the kidney, liver, and pancreas (1, 39). When creatine enters the muscle cell, it accepts a high-energy phosphate and forms phosphocreatine. Phosphocreatine is the storage form of high-energy phosphate, which is used by the skeletal muscle cell to rapidly regenerate adenosine triphosphate (ATP) during bouts of maximal muscular contraction (40). The conversion of ATP into adenosine diphosphate (ADP) and a phosphate group generates the energy needed by the muscles during short-term, high-intensity exercise. The energy for all-out maximal-effort exercise lasting up to approximately 6 seconds (typical duration of activity for a strength and power athlete) is primarily derived from limited stores of ATP in the muscle. Phosphocreatine availability in the muscles is vitally important in energy production because ATP cannot be stored in excessive amounts within the muscle and is rapidly depleted during bouts of exhaustive or high-intensity exercise.

Oral creatine monohydrate supplementation has been reported to increase muscle creatine and phosphocreatine content by 15% to 40%, enhance the cellular bioenergetics of the **phosphagen system** (the quickest and most powerful source of energy for muscle movement), improve the shuttling of high-energy phosphates between the mitochondria and cytosol through the creatine phosphate shuttle, and enhance the activity of various metabolic pathways (57). Relative to dosage, most published studies on creatine supplementation divided the typical dosage pattern into two phases: a loading phase and a maintenance phase. A typical loading phase comprises 20 g of creatine (or 0.3 g/kg body weight) in divided doses four times a day for two to seven days; this phase is followed by a maintenance dose of 2 to 5 g daily (or 0.03 g/kg body weight) for several weeks to months at a time.

Scientific studies indicate that creatine supplementation is an effective and safe nutritional strategy to promote gains in strength and lean muscle mass during resistance training—both important attributes for the strength and power athlete (34, 57, 58, 99, 117). Creatine does this using at least four separate mechanisms of action: (1) by increasing the rate of ATP regeneration (which reduces fatigue during intense, repeated exercise bouts and thus allows more high-quality work to be performed), (2) by promoting greater secretion of intramuscular IGF-1 concentrations (an intramuscular growth factor), (3) by increasing muscle fiber protein content, and (4) by increasing several myogenic regulatory factors (i.e., proteins that activate gene expression in muscle). Specific to lean muscle mass, creatine supplementation has been shown to be effective in several cohorts, including males, females, and the elderly (6, 7, 15, 60, 112). Short-term creatine supplementation increases total body weight by approximately 0.8 to 1.7 kg (1.8 to 3.7 lb). Longer-term creatine supplementation (e.g., six to eight weeks) in conjunction with resistance training increased lean muscle mass by approximately 2.8 to 3.2 kg (~7 lb) (23, 35, 61, 100).

Unequivocally, one of the most visible effects of creatine supplementation is a rapid increase in body weight, particularly if athletes undergo a loading phase. This effect has traditionally been attributed to acute osmotic stimulation of intra- and extracellular water retention. For the strength and power athlete, however, an increase in body weight will impart benefit only if the weight gain is in the form of lean tissue. Fortunately, several scientific investigations have demonstrated that long-term gains in body weight are mostly attributable to actual increases in the cellular protein content of muscle tissue (116, 125).

Creatine can also be advantageous to strength athletes given its ability to enhance strength gains during training. Studies indicate that creatine supplementation during training can increase gains in 1RM strength and power. Peeters, Lantz, and Mayhew (79) investigated the effect of creatine monohydrate and creatine phosphate supplementation on strength, body composition, and blood pressure over a six-week period. Strength tests performed were the 1RM bench press, 1RM leg press, and maximal repetitions on the seated preacher bar curl with a fixed amount of weight. Subjects were matched for strength and placed into one of three groups—a placebo, creatine monohydrate, or creatine phosphate group. All subjects performed a standardized resistance training regimen and ingested a loading dosage of 20 g/day for the first three days of the study, followed by a maintenance dose of 10 g/day for the remainder of the six-week supplementation period. Significant differences were noted between the placebo group and the two creatine groups for changes in lean muscle mass, body weight, and 1RM bench press. Eckerson and colleagues (24) also studied the effects of two and five days of creatine loading on anaerobic working capacity using the critical power test. Ten physically active women randomly received two treatments separated by a five-week washout period: (a) 18 g dextrose as placebo or (b) 5 g creatine plus 18 g dextrose taken four times a day for five days. Ingesting the placebo resulted in no significant changes in anaerobic working capacity, but creatine ingestion significantly increased anaerobic working capacity by 22.1% after only five days of loading.

Elsewhere, Kreider and colleagues (60) conducted a study in which 25 National Collegiate Athletic Association Division IA football players supplemented their diet for 28 days with creatine or a placebo during resistance and agility training. Before and after the supplementation protocol, the football players performed a maximal-repetition test on the isotonic bench press, squat, and power clean and performed a high-intensity cycle ergometer sprint test. The creatine group showed significantly greater gains in bench press lifting volume; the sum of bench press, squat, and power clean lifting volume; and total work performed during the first five 6-second cycle ergometer sprints. Ingestion of creatine promoted greater gains in lean muscle mass, isotonic lifting volume, and sprint performance during intense resistance and agility training.

The studies reviewed here are only a few among dozens that have reported an increase in strength, power, and high-intensity performance. Combined, these three studies indicate that creatine supplementation can increase maximal strength, high-intensity exercise performance, and lifting volume.

In its original review on creatine supplementation and position stand, the International Society of Sports Nutrition (10) stated the following:

- Short-term adaptations include increased cycling power; total work performed on the bench press and jump squat; and improved sport performance in sprinting, swimming, and soccer (69, 70, 78, 85, 92, 104, 106, 117, 128).

- Long-term adaptations when creatine monohydrate supplementation is combined with training include increased muscle creatine and PCr [phosphocreatine] content, lean muscle mass, strength, sprint performance, power, rate of force development, and muscle diameter (60, 109, 116).

- In long-term studies, subjects taking creatine monohydrate typically gain about twice as much body weight, lean muscle mass, or both (i.e., an extra 2 to 4 lb [0.9 to 1.8 kg] of lean muscle mass during 4 to 12 weeks of training) as subjects taking a placebo (48, 54, 74, 97).

- The only clinically significant side effect reported in the research literature is weight gain (62, 63), but many unsubstantiated, anecdotal claims of other side effects, including dehydration, cramping, kidney and liver damage, musculoskeletal injury, gastrointestinal distress, and anterior (leg) compartment syndrome, still appear in the media and popular literature. Although a minority of athletes who take creatine monohydrate may experience those symptoms, the scientific literature suggests that athletes have no greater, and a possibly lower, risk of these symptoms or adverse effects than those not supplementing with creatine monohydrate (36, 63).

The International Society of Sports Nutrition position stand also included the following statement: "The tremendous numbers of investigations conducted with positive results from creatine monohydrate supplementation lead us to conclude that it is the most effective nutritional supplement available today for increasing high-intensity exercise capacity and building muscle mass" (p. 4). Two recent studies from Taiwan have reported that creatine supplementation can reduce postactivation potentiation (PAP) time of the lower (122) and upper (123) body after only six days of supplementation at 20 g per day. PAP is the increase in muscle force or rate of force development that occurs as a result of previous muscle action. In the first study, 30 explosive athletes completed a 1RM back squat before determining their individual PAP time for the lower body. In the second study, 16 canoeists performed a bench row 1RM before doing similar PAP testing for the upper body. In both cases, creatine increased strength and improved (i.e., shortened) the athletes' PAP time. Strength and conditioning coaches who use PAP training with their athletes should keep these studies in mind.

HMB

β-Hydroxy-β-methylbutyric acid, or HMB, is a **metabolite** (substance produced by, or taking part in, a metabolic reaction) of the essential amino acid leucine. HMB has been shown to play a role in the regulation of protein breakdown in the body. HMB helps inhibit proteolysis, which is the natural process of breaking down muscle that occurs during and especially after high-intensity activity. HMB is typically available as a powder (in the calcium salt form) that is mixed with water, as well as in capsule form (usually the "free acid" form that is better absorbed). HMB supplementation appears to have a protective effect on muscle and may help the body get a head start on the recovery process, mainly by minimizing the amount of protein degradation during and after intense exercise. Therefore, the theoretical rationale behind HMB supplementation is that it could slow the breakdown of muscle protein in the body, thus increasing lean muscle mass and strength (35) adaptations during resistance training. Many of the early scientific investigations on HMB were conducted in animal models, with results such as the following:

- Enhanced growth rates in pigs (71)
- Increased lean muscle mass and decreased body fat in steers (111)
- Improvement in several markers of immune function in chickens (80, 81)

Extending the work of those early findings, subsequent researchers investigated the effects of HMB supplementation during training in humans to determine its effects on inhibiting protein degradation and increasing muscular strength and lean muscle mass. Nissen and coworkers (73) conducted the first research study to highlight the anticatabolic potential of HMB. Untrained subjects ingested one of three levels of HMB (0, 1.5, or 3.0 g/day) and two protein levels (117 or 175 g/day) and resistance trained three days per week for three weeks. Among other markers of muscle damage, protein breakdown was assessed through measurement of urinary 3-methyl-histidine. After the first week of the resistance training protocol, urinary 3-methyl-histidine increased by 94% in the control group and by 85% and 50% in the individuals ingesting 1.5 and 3 g of HMB per day, respectively. During the second week, urinary 3-methyl-histidine levels were still elevated by 27% in the control group but were 4% and 15% below basal levels for the groups taking 1.5 and 3 g HMB per day. Interestingly, urinary 3-methyl-histidine measures at the end of the third week of resistance training were not significantly different between the groups (73). Other studies demonstrating an **anticatabolic** effect or suppression of muscle damage have supported these findings (55, 114).

Van Someren and colleagues (114) instructed their male subjects to ingest 3 g of HMB in addition to 0.3 g **alpha-ketoisocaproic acid** (an intermediate in the metabolism of leucine) daily for 14 days before performing a single bout of eccentric-dominant resistance exercise. This supplemental intervention including HMB resulted in a significant reduction of plasma markers of muscle damage. Gallagher and associates (30) evaluated the effects of HMB supplementation (0.38 and 0.76 mg per kilogram body weight per day) during eight weeks of resistance training in previously untrained men. The researchers reported that HMB supplementation promoted significantly less muscle creatine kinase excretion and greater gains in lean muscle mass (in the 0.38 mg per kilogram body weight per day group only) than in subjects taking a placebo. Collectively, these findings support contentions that HMB supplementation may lessen catabolism, leading to greater gains in strength and lean muscle mass during resistance training.

HMB supplementation may suppress protein breakdown and markers of muscle damage, but does this anticatabolic effect *always* lead to gains in lean muscle mass? The scientific literature on this topic is quite polarized and equivocal. In a second arm of the study by Nissen and colleagues (73), male participants ingested 3 g of HMB or a placebo for seven weeks in conjunction with resistance training six days per week. Lean muscle mass increased in the HMB-supplemented group at various times throughout the investigative period but not at the end of the study (the seventh week). Vukovich and coworkers (118) reported that HMB supplementation (3 g/day for eight weeks during resistance training) significantly increased lean muscle mass, reduced fat mass, and promoted greater gains in upper and lower extremity 1RM strength in a group of elderly men and women initiating training.

Not all studies have shown that HMB ingestion results in an accretion of lean muscle mass (41, 59, 75, 93, 105). In studies not showing this effect, subjects received approximately the same amount of HMB as in the studies demonstrating increases in lean muscle mass.

One of the greatest concerns with the literature on the effectiveness of HMB supplementation in strength athletes is that many of the studies have not used trained populations (30, 73, 113, 114). In addition, some studies used elderly populations (27). Extrapolating research findings in an untrained population to a trained population is unwise given the variance in training adaptations among these groups. To further convolute the data, many of the studies using trained populations were not effective at enhancing training adaptations (41, 59, 75).

Taking these observations into account, Hoffman and colleagues (41) stated that if HMB supplementation has any ergogenic benefit in attenuating muscle damage, it is likely to be most effective in untrained people, who have the greatest potential for muscle damage during exercise. In relation to safety, no side effects have been reported in human studies using as much as 6 g/day (30, 31). In conclusion, it appears that HMB may be beneficial (relative to increasing lean muscle mass) for a person beginning a resistance training program, but not for athletes who are already resistance trained. Note that the potential benefits of HMB on strength and hypertrophy are diminished when athletes are ingesting optimal amounts of high-quality dietary protein. Conversely, some have speculated that HMB may be of particular benefit during periods of caloric restriction as well as during recovery from injuries that result in muscle atrophy (e.g., ACL reconstruction and rotator cuff surgery) because of the associated elevation in muscle protein breakdown that accompanies those scenarios.

Prohormones

Prohormones or hormone precursors are naturally derived precursors to the synthesis of testosterone. Prohormones include DHEA or dehydroepiandrosterone, androstenedione, 4-AD, 1-AD, Nor-diol, and other analogs. The rationale for supplementing with prohormones is to aim to increase the body's ability to synthesize testosterone, which could lead to increases in lean muscle mass, strength, and bone density and improvements in body composition (89, 127). Although clinical studies on prohormones are scarce, one study showed no anabolic or ergogenic effects with 344 mg/day over an eight-week period of prohormone supplementation (110). Most studies indicate that they do not affect testosterone and that some may increase estrogen levels. Despite the rampant claims associated with taking prohormones, research does not support the assertions, and prohormones are thought to have no benefit on strength and body composition (9, 49, 86). Several reports have shown that supplementing prohormones can significantly elevate estrogen (8, 53), which can have negative effects on body composition and strength.

In addition, prohormones are steroid-like compounds, so most athletic organizations have banned their use. One of the most popular and common prohormones is DHEA. DHEA is a steroid that is produced naturally by the adrenal glands and serves as a precursor to the sex hormones, testosterone and estradiol. The conversion of DHEA to estradiol would not be advantageous for athletes considering its anabolic effect on fat cells (i.e., increases fat cell size). The conversion of DHEA to testosterone, however, may have potential performance-enhancing effects. Although testosterone is a potent anabolic hormone that promotes skeletal muscle protein accrual, the ergogenic effects and influence of DHEA supplementation on testosterone have been questioned. Wallace and colleagues (120) investigated the effects of a 12-week resistance training program and DHEA supplementation (100 mg per day) in a group of healthy middle-aged men and reported no significant changes in the DHEA group for upper and lower body strength. In addition, another study, employing three weeks of DHEA supplementation and resistance training in healthy adults, reported no significant changes in lean muscle mass or strength gains (72). But other studies employing DHEA supplementation in elderly men and women have demonstrated significant improvements in immune function, muscle strength, lean muscle mass, and quality of life (115). To date, DHEA appear to be more effective for elderly people, who have physiologically low levels. The benefits for the tactical athlete appear to be low.

Protein and Amino Acids

For years, many have believed that extra protein intake is necessary for optimal muscle growth in response to resistance training (35). Skeletal muscle hypertrophy occurs only when muscle protein synthesis exceeds muscle protein breakdown. The body is in a continuous state of protein turnover as old proteins are destroyed or degraded and new proteins are synthesized. When synthesis of contractile proteins is occurring at a faster rate than their degradation, the net result is a positive protein balance (i.e., myofibrillar hypertrophy). At rest, in the absence of an exercise stimulus and nutrient intake, net protein balance is negative (3, 83, 84, 119).

Resistance exercise is essential for creating the stimulus needed for skeletal muscle hypertrophy to occur. But when resistance exercise is performed in the absence of nutritional or supplemental protein or amino acid intake, net protein balance will not increase to the point of becoming anabolic. Specific nutrients and supplements (nitrogen-containing compounds) are needed in conjunction with the resistance training for net protein balance to become positive and growth to occur.

This knowledge makes it clear that protein or the building blocks of proteins—amino acids—need to be available to ensure attainment of a positive balance. Amino acids are made available from the amino acid pool. The amino acid pool is a mixture of amino acids available in the cell that is derived from dietary sources or the degradation of protein. Amino acids enter this pool in three ways:

- During digestion of protein in the diet
- When body protein decomposes
- When carbon sources and amino groups ($-NH_2$) synthesize the non-essential amino acids

The amino acid pool exists to provide individual amino acids for protein synthesis and oxidation, and it is replenished only by protein breakdown or amino acids entering the body from the diet. Thus, the free amino acid pool provides the link between dietary protein and body protein in that both dietary protein and body protein feed into the free amino acid pool.

Protein Intake

One of the most controversial debates that has pervaded the science of sport nutrition involves protein intake. The main controversy has centered on the safety and effectiveness of protein intake above the Recommended

Dietary Allowance (RDA). Currently, the RDA for protein in healthy adults is 0.8 g of protein per kilogram body weight per day. This recommendation accounts for individual differences in protein metabolism, variations in the biological value of protein, and nitrogen losses in the urine and feces. When determining the amount of protein that must be ingested to increase lean muscle mass, many factors must be considered, such as the following:

- Protein quality
- Total energy intake
- Carbohydrate intake
- Fat intake
- Amount, type, and intensity of the exercise training program
- Timing of protein intake
- Age

Although 0.8 g of protein per kilogram body weight per day may be sufficient to meet the needs of nearly all non-resistance-trained people, it is clearly not sufficient to provide substrate for lean tissue accretion or for the repair of exercise-induced muscle damage (102) during exercise training. In fact, many clinical investigations indicate that people who engage in physical activity or exercise require higher levels of protein intake than 0.8 g per kilogram body weight per day, regardless of the mode of exercise (e.g., aerobic endurance or resistance) (28, 29, 64, 68, 82) or training state (i.e., recreational, moderately trained, or well trained) (35, 65, 67, 103).

So, the question remains: How much protein is required for people who engage in resistance training and want to increase lean muscle mass? As stated in chapter 4, a general recommendation relative to protein ingestion is 1.4 to 1.7 g per kilogram body weight per day of high-quality protein (11, 66). More specifically, it is recommended that those engaging in strength or power exercise ingest levels at the upper end of this range.

At the cellular level, studies have found that dietary protein amino acids increase the rate of muscle protein synthesis. Biolo and colleagues (4) evaluated the interactions between resistance training and amino acid supplementation and the corresponding effects on protein kinetics. Six untrained men served as subjects in this study. Each participant was infused with a mixed (phenylalanine, leucine, lysine, alanine, glutamine) amino acid solution. Samples were taken at baseline and after resistance training (5 sets of 10 leg presses; 4 sets of eight Nautilus squats, leg curls, and leg extensions). The results demonstrated increased protein synthesis and no change in protein degradation.

Although researchers have concluded that pre- or postexercise amino acid supplementation have a positive effect on protein synthesis, amino acid infusion is not a practical means of obtaining amino acids. Hence, Tipton and colleagues (108) investigated the effects of orally administered amino acids;

subjects received 40 g mixed amino acids (essential and nonessential), 40 g essential amino acids only, or 40 g of a carbohydrate placebo. The investigators also sought to determine whether the anabolic effect of amino acid supplementation would be different if they used a mixed amino acid source or essential amino acids alone. Their findings indicated that postexercise amino acid supplementation elicits a positive protein balance as compared with the negative balance seen with resistance training alone. The authors also concluded that supplementation with the essential amino acids alone is equivalent to a mixed amino acid supplement. In other words, nonessential amino acids are not required to stimulate muscle protein synthesis.

Elsewhere, Esmark and colleagues (26) investigated the timing of protein intake after exercise on muscle hypertrophy and strength. This study used a milk and soy protein supplement (10 g protein from skim milk and soybean), 7 g carbohydrate, and 3.3 g of lipid instead of an amino acid mixture. Although the investigators did not calculate acute changes in muscle protein synthesis, they did measure long-term effects on muscle hypertrophy. The results indicated that skeletal muscle hypertrophy significantly increased after resistance training when subjects took the mixed macronutrient supplement containing 10 g of protein.

Ingesting between 1.4 and 1.7 g of protein per kilogram body weight per day is not the only parameter to consider, however, because not all protein sources are the same. One simple way to classify proteins is by whether they contain adequate amounts of the essential amino acids. **Complete protein** sources that contain greater amounts of essential amino acids generally have higher protein quality. Complete proteins are typically found in sources such as beef, eggs, turkey, chicken, pork, milk, and cheese, whereas **incomplete proteins** lack one or more essential amino acids. Examples of incomplete protein sources are plant foods like rice, nuts, lentils, beans, grains, and seeds. Note, however, that some plant foods are sources of complete protein, namely soy, quinoa, seitan, and buckwheat.

Common Types of Protein in Sport Supplements

Three of the most common types of protein found in protein supplements are whey, casein, and egg protein. Each of these types of protein is a complete protein, and all are classified as high quality (for an in-depth discussion of the classification of the quality of various proteins, refer to chapter 4) and can be administered as a powder. Whey protein, derived from milk protein, is currently the most popular source of protein used in nutritional supplements. Of the three common types of protein found in protein supplements, whey protein has been investigated most thoroughly relative to its effects on muscle protein synthesis and lean muscle mass accretion. Cribb and colleagues (18) investigated the differential effects of whey versus casein protein on strength and body composition. Subjects ingested either whey or casein (1.5 g per kilogram body weight per day) for 10 weeks while following a structured resistance training program; the whey protein group experienced significantly greater gains in strength and lean muscle mass than the casein group.

Casein, also a milk protein, is often characterized as a slower-acting protein (5, 19). In comparison with whey protein, casein takes longer to digest and absorb. The reason is most likely that casein takes more time to leave the stomach (5). Although casein stimulates muscle protein synthesis, it does this to a lesser extent than whey protein (5). Unlike whey, casein helps decrease muscle protein breakdown (20) and therefore has anticatabolic properties. Indeed, a recent study by Kouw and colleagues (56) demonstrated that ingesting a 40 g dose (but interestingly, not a 20 g dose) of casein before bed increased muscle protein synthesis during sleep. As such, this nutritional strategy should be considered by athletes wishing to increase their total daily protein intake or augment gains in lean muscle mass and strength during resistance training.

Given the findings that whey protein stimulates protein synthesis and casein helps decrease muscle breakdown, some supplement manufacturers include both whey and casein in their formulations. An investigation by Kerksick and colleagues (52) illustrated the effectiveness of the combination. Subjects performed a split body resistance training program four days a week for 10 weeks. They received 48 g of carbohydrate, 40 g of whey and 8 g of casein, or 40 g of whey, 5 g of glutamine, and 3 g of branched-chain amino acids. After 10 weeks, the group that received both whey and casein had the largest increase in lean muscle mass. Willoughby and colleagues (126) investigated the effect of a combination whey and casein protein on strength, lean muscle mass, and markers of anabolism. Their findings agree with those of Kerksick and associates in that the whey and casein combination elicited a superior response in strength and lean muscle mass compared with placebo. A combination protein mixture appears to be adequate to stimulate protein synthesis and promote positive training adaptations (52, 107, 126).

Egg protein is typically derived from whole eggs and is considered a high-quality protein source. Eggs are low in lactose, cholesterol, and fat and are a good source of riboflavin and biotin. Egg also has the advantage of being miscible (it mixes easily in solution) (21). Egg protein supplements, however, generally do not smell or taste good and are typically more expensive than other protein supplements. For these reasons, along with the availability of other high-quality protein sources such as whey and casein, egg protein is not as popular a supplement as whey and casein.

In a review, Rennie and colleagues (88) concluded that increasing amino acid concentration by intravenous infusion, meal feeding, or ingestion of free amino acids clearly increases muscle protein synthesis. The magnitude of the increase in essential amino acid concentrations in blood (which is largely determined by digestibility) appears to determine how effective a certain protein is for building muscle. Therefore, to optimize the muscle protein synthetic response to resistance exercise, essential amino acids (whether from intact protein sources or as free-form essential amino acids) need to be consumed. Readers are referred to chapter 4 for a more thorough discussion of this topic.

Beta-Alanine

Over the past few years, beta-alanine has continued to gain notoriety in the sport nutrition market. Beta-alanine is typically administered as capsules or as a powder that is mixed with a liquid (usually water). Although several clinical trials have reported increases in markers of exercise performance, body composition, and strength with beta-alanine, others have demonstrated no ergogenic benefits. This section discusses beta-alanine as a sport supplement, beginning with its parent compound carnosine.

Carnosine is a dipeptide composed of the amino acids histidine and beta-alanine. Carnosine occurs naturally in the brain, cardiac muscle, kidney, and stomach, as well as in relatively large amounts in skeletal muscles (primarily type II muscle fibers). These type II muscle fibers are the fast-twitch muscle fibers used in explosive movements like those in resistance training and sprinting. Athletes whose performance demands extensive anaerobic output have higher concentrations of carnosine.

Carnosine contributes to the buffering of hydrogen ions, thus attenuating (slowing down) a drop in pH associated with anaerobic metabolism. This point is important because the accumulation of H^+ in muscle has been shown to disrupt the resynthesis of phosphorylcreatine, inhibit glycolysis, and disrupt the functioning of the muscle contractile machinery (90). Along with this critical role in regulating intracellular pH, carnosine also has important roles in reducing reactive oxygen species, reactive nitrogen species, and advanced glycation end products in muscle. For hard-working athletes who need to tolerate and compete with high levels of lactate in skeletal muscle and blood, carnosine is believed to be one of the primary intracellular buffering substances in skeletal muscle. In theory, if carnosine could attenuate the drop in pH noted with high-intensity exercise, an athlete could possibly exercise at high intensities for a longer duration. When carnosine is ingested, however, it is rapidly degraded into beta-alanine and histidine as soon as it enters the blood by the enzyme carnosinase. Thus, ingesting carnosine directly appears to offer little advantage. Instead, independent ingestion of beta-alanine and histidine allows these two compounds to be transported into the skeletal muscle and to be resynthesized into carnosine. Beta-alanine appears to be the amino acid that most influences intramuscular carnosine levels because it is the rate-limiting substrate in this chemical reaction (22). In fact, studies have demonstrated that 28 days of beta-alanine supplementation at a dosage of 4 to 6 g/day resulted in an increase of intramuscular levels of carnosine by approximately 60% (37, 129).

Over the past 10 or more years, researchers have begun extensive research in beta-alanine supplementation for strength athletes. Stout and colleagues (98) examined the effects of beta-alanine supplementation on **physical working capacity at fatigue threshold** (PWCFT) in untrained young men. PWCFT, often obtained using a cycle ergometer test, can identify the power output at the neuromuscular fatigue threshold. The participants ingested 6.4 g of beta-alanine for six days followed by 3.2 g for three weeks. The results revealed a significantly greater increase in PWCFT in the beta-alanine group as compared with the placebo group. Stout and colleagues (101) then investigated the effects of 90 days of beta-alanine supplementation (2.4 g/day) on the PWCFT in elderly men and women. They found significant increases in PWCFT (28.6%) from pre- to postsupplementation for the beta-alanine treatment group but no change with the placebo treatment. In a study using collegiate American football players, Hoffman and colleagues (42) found that subjects supplementing with beta-alanine (4.5 g) increased training volume significantly over 30 days compared with subjects taking a placebo. Elsewhere, Hoffman and associates (44) investigated the effect of 30 days of beta-alanine supplementation (4.8 g/day) on resistance exercise performance and endocrine changes in resistance-trained men. The beta-alanine group experienced a significant 22% increase in total number of repetitions as compared with the placebo group at the end of the four-week intervention. There were no significant differences between groups in hormonal responses.

Several studies have investigated the effects of supplementing creatine and beta-alanine together (43, 98, 129). The proposed benefit would increase work capacity and increase time to fatigue. Hoffman and colleagues (43) studied the effects of creatine (10.5 g/day) plus beta-alanine (3.2 g/day) on strength, power, body composition, and endocrine changes as collegiate American football players underwent a 10-week resistance training program. Results demonstrated that creatine plus beta-alanine was effective at enhancing strength performance. Creatine plus beta-alanine supplementation also appeared to have a greater effect on body composition (i.e., more lean muscle mass, less fat mass) than creatine alone. But Stout and colleagues (98) found that creatine did not appear to have an additive effect over beta-alanine alone.

Although many studies have highlighted the positive results of beta-alanine supplementation, several other investigations have shown no improvements. In the study of collegiate American football players already mentioned, Hoffman and colleagues (42) examined the effects of 30 days of beta-alanine supplementation (4.5 g/day) on anaerobic performance measures. Supplementation began three weeks before preseason football training camp and continued for an additional nine days during camp. Results showed a trend toward lower fatigue rates during 60 seconds of maximal exercise, but three weeks of beta-alanine supplementation did not result in significant improvements in fatigue rates during high-intensity anaerobic exercise. Elsewhere, Kendrick and colleagues (50) assessed whole-body muscular strength and changes in body composition after 10 weeks of beta-alanine supplementation at a dosage of 6.4 g/day. Participants included 26 healthy male Vietnamese physical education students who were not currently involved in any resistance training program. The authors reported no significant differences between the beta-alanine group and a placebo group in whole-body strength and body composition measures after 10 weeks of supplementation.

Beta-alanine supplementation is relatively new and is a potentially useful ergogenic aid. Note that interindividual responses to beta-alanine supplementation are highly variable and that only a few well-designed clinical investigations have been completed on this compound. Thus, the published results to date have been somewhat equivocal, particularly when low doses of beta-alanine are ingested. Indeed, much of the research has been positive when the dosing regimen provides subjects with at least 3 to 6 g/day for at least four weeks. With respect to side effects and dosage, research from Harris and colleagues (38) has revealed that in most people relatively high single doses of beta-alanine are responsible for unpleasant symptoms of paresthesia (burning and tingling sensations in the neck and face) that may last up to an hour. This sensation can be reduced if the maximum single dose is kept to approximately 10 mg/kg body weight, which corresponds to an average of 800 mg of beta-alanine in a single dose (38), by using time-released versions of beta-alanine, or by using newer technologies that are capable of attenuating this response.

Arginine

Arginine is a conditionally essential amino acid found in meat, seafood, nuts and soy that has numerous functions in the body. It is used to make compounds in the body such as nitric oxide, creatine, glutamate, agmatine (a signaling molecule that enhances blood flow), and proline, and it can be converted to glucose and glycogen if needed. In large doses, arginine also stimulates release of growth hormone and prolactin. Arginine has been purported to be advantageous for strength athletes, but the research on arginine shows conflicting results. Although some evidence indicates that arginine supplementation can increase strength, lean muscle mass, and growth hormone levels (2, 12, 25), evidence is currently insufficient to support its use.

Glutamine

Glutamine is the most abundant amino acid in the body, representing about 60% of the amino acid pool in muscles. It is considered a conditionally essential amino acid because it can be manufactured in the body, but under extreme physical stress, the demand for glutamine exceeds the body's ability to make it. Glutamine serves a variety of functions in the body including cell growth, immune function, and recovery from stress. Research has shown that under severe circumstances, glutamine contributes to the prevention of muscle breakdown, increases growth hormone, increases protein synthesis, and improves immune function (13, 14, 124). Most research demonstrating these benefits, however, has not been done on resistance-trained athletes, and it does not appear at this time that glutamine increases strength–power or improves body composition in these athletes. But because of its well-established effects on improving intestinal and immune system health, glutamine may be useful under certain stressful scenarios to keep athletes healthy.

Branched-Chain Amino Acids (BCAAs)

BCAAs refers to three essential amino acids: leucine, isoleucine, and valine. BCAAs are unique among amino acids because they are the only ones that bypass the liver and are metabolized directly in skeletal muscle. Some studies have reported that BCAAs can decrease muscle soreness when compared with an isocaloric amount of carbohydrate (91). Leucine is the most important BCAA for muscle growth, but even in combination with isoleucine (which helps regulate blood sugar and synthesize hemoglobin) and valine (which has mild stimulant properties) at doses of 5.6 g, BCAAs have been shown to increase muscle protein synthesis by only 22% (46). To put these effects in proper perspective, this increase is approximately half as much as a typical 20 to 25 g serving of whey protein, which ironically contains approximately 5 g of BCAAs. Notably, this study demonstrates that to optimize the muscle protein synthetic response, all essential amino acids need to be ingested at the same time. For this reason, BCAA supplementation is not routinely recommended unless athletes are not ingesting at least 1.4 to 1.7 g per kilogram body weight per day of high-quality protein.

Preworkout Supplements

Multi-ingredient preworkout supplements have become increasingly popular. Formulations include several ingredients, such as creatine, caffeine, BCAAs, whey protein, nitric oxide precursors, and other isolated amino acids. Although many of these ingredients have been reviewed in other areas of this text, comparing one product with another is difficult because of the varying type and amount of ingredients in these products. A recently published review (47) analyzed the top 100 preworkout supplements for ingredients and amounts. The study found that the following percentage of products included these ingredients: beta-alanine 87%, caffeine 86%, citrulline 71%, tyrosine 63%, taurine 51%, and creatine 49%. Nearly half (44.3%) of all ingredients were included as part of a proprietary blend with undisclosed amounts of each ingredient. Thus, with such a range of ingredients and formulations, drawing conclusions is difficult. Nevertheless, several studies have been done on various formulations. When ingested acutely before exercise, these multi-ingredient supplements have been shown to improve muscular endurance (32), running time to exhaustion (121), and power output (32). Some studies have documented improvements in subjective feelings of energy and focus (96, 121), whereas others (32) have not. When taken chronically for a period of four to eight weeks, multi-ingredient preworkout supplements have been shown to increase measures of strength (51, 96), power output (76), and lean muscle mass (77, 95). Smith and colleagues (94) investigated the effects of a preworkout supplement containing caffeine, creatine, and amino acids during three weeks of high-intensity exercise on aerobic and anaerobic performance. Subjects did high-intensity interval training 3 days per week for three weeks. After three weeks subjects taking the preworkout supplement had a significantly greater increase in $\dot{V}O_2$max, critical velocity, and lean muscle mass as compared with the placebo group.

Although many preworkout supplements have positive data supporting their use, caution should be used when using these supplements. As previously noted, many of these supplements do not disclose the amounts of given ingredients in the supplement. Thus, ascertaining whether the supplements include efficacious doses of an ingredient may be impossible. The amount of research done on many of the ingredients has not been significant enough for them to be considered a stand-alone product. Ingredients such as caffeine, creatine, beta-alanine, and whey protein, however, all have significant support in the literature for their effectiveness (16, 17, 33, 87). Ultimately, when choosing a preworkout supplement, look for ingredients that have solid scientific support, demonstrating safety and efficacy (e.g., creatine, beta-alanine, and others).

Professional Applications

Athletes whose performance requires high levels of strength and power spend considerable time training to improve those performance characteristics. A proper nutrition program is also helpful for maximizing the performance of a strength–power athlete. In addition to optimal training techniques and sound nutritional principles, certain sport supplements have been shown to enhance muscular strength and power. The four sport supplements that may benefit the strength–power athlete are protein, creatine, HMB, and beta-alanine.

Protein can be ingested from whole food sources, but modern technology has enabled manufacturers to isolate some of the highest quality sources of protein (i.e., whey, essential amino acids, and casein). In addition, supplemental protein is often more convenient for athletes who travel and must ingest protein several times throughout the day. Protein supplements make ingesting the recommended 1.4 to 1.7 g per kilogram body weight per day a manageable task for many athletes who are busy with training and competitive schedules. In addition to whole protein products, individual and amino acid blends are sold to support protein synthesis and potentially improve performance. The most

(continued)

Professional Applications *(continued)*

common of the amino acids are glutamine, arginine, and BCAAs. Although sound scientific rationale supports use in each of the categories, the same support does not appear to be found in the literature as it pertains to athletic populations. Thus, athletes should focus on protein intake from complete protein sources or essential amino acid blends.

The other three sport supplements discussed in this chapter—creatine, HMB, and beta-alanine—have different levels of scientific support and reported benefits in relation to athletic and exercise performance. Creatine monohydrate has been scientifically demonstrated to improve performance and increase lean muscle mass in resistance-trained athletes. This finding is important: Even if an athlete has been resistance training for several years, when creatine monohydrate is introduced at recommended doses (20 g/day for approximately one week followed by a maintenance dose of 2 to 5 g daily), resistance training performance will likely improve. Therefore, strength–power athletes can ingest creatine at any time during the training year—in the off-season (to increase lean muscle mass) and during the season (to maintain lean muscle mass).

In contrast, HMB supplements (typically dosed at 3 g/day) have not consistently demonstrated effectiveness in improving strength and increasing lean muscle mass in resistance-trained individuals. But in untrained athletes (athletes beginning a resistance training program) or in athletes who are significantly increasing their training volume, HMB supplementation may accelerate the regenerative capacity of skeletal muscle, inhibit protein degradation, reduce markers of muscle damage, and increase strength and lean muscle mass. HMB supplementation appears to be more effective when (1) total daily protein intake is not optimized (i.e., athletes fail to ingest 1.4-1.7 g per kilogram body weight per day) and (2) the potential for muscle damage during exercise is greatest, as is the case for an athlete beginning a resistance training program or during periods of a competitive season when training volume and intensity are both elevated.

In some scenarios, creatine and HMB supplementation can potentially be cycled to maximize strength and performance. For instance, American football involves three distinct periods over the year—the off-season, preseason, and the competitive season. During the off-season, sport-specific skill acquisition training decreases, and emphasis is on maximizing strength and lean muscle mass. During this period, ingesting a creatine supplement in addition to the athlete's training program would likely result in muscular strength and lean muscle mass gains above those that would be elicited by the training program. After the off-season at the end of the summer, the American football player enters the preseason. The preseason is associated with an enormous amount of training and conditioning. Football players commonly have practices multiple times per day (which include conditioning drills) and are still expected to resistance train. During this time when training volume drastically increases (and the potential for muscle damage increases), HMB supplementation may be a wise choice to limit the amount of muscle damage incurred. After the preseason, the American football season begins; this period typically lasts three or four months and involves daily practices and one competitive game per week. To maintain the strength, lean muscle mass, and power improvements attained during the off-season, the athlete may want to supplement with creatine again as the volume of resistance training decreases because of the practice and game schedule.

Another supplement discussed in this chapter, beta-alanine (typically dosed at 3-6 g/day), does not improve maximal strength but has been shown to improve short-term, high-intensity exercise, particularly of 1 to 4 minutes duration. More specifically, beta-alanine has the demonstrated ability to delay fatigue, increase power, and improve muscular endurance during high-intensity exercise. This attribute can be advantageous for athletes such as sprinters (800 m), rowers, mixed martial artists, short-distance swimmers, and other athletes engaged in high-intensity conditioning aimed at optimizing metabolic adaptations, regardless of the sport. The absolute increase in muscle carnosine levels appears to determine the benefit on performance, however, and higher doses (i.e., beta-alanine "loading") may therefore be needed to achieve peak or greater effects.

The final product discussed in this chapter was preworkout multi-ingredient supplements. Most preworkout supplements contain caffeine and beta-alanine, which are well supported in the literature as being efficacious. Thus, athletes may gain some benefit by taking a preworkout supplement. The difficulty is that most of the preworkout supplements contain several ingredients and varying amounts of each ingredient. Therefore, making a general recommendation about safety or effectiveness of preworkout supplements as a category is nearly impossible.

Summary Points

- Although nothing can replace a nutrient-dense diet, the judicious use of certain sport supplements can help maximize training adaptations, leading to increased strength, power, and lean muscle mass.

- Creatine monohydrate has been shown to increase strength, lean muscle mass, and sprint performance; no other supplement is supported by the same level of positive research.

- High-quality protein and amino acids (especially essential amino acids) are required to optimize protein balance and promote gains in lean muscle mass.

- Several clinical investigations have shown that HMB acts as an anticatabolic supplement, but more research is needed.

- Beta-alanine appears to improve certain aspects of high-intensity exercise performance.

- A final consideration with these sport supplements is the fact that each has been found to be safe when ingested at the recommended dosages.

Chapter 9

Aerobic Endurance Supplements

Laurent Bannock, DProf, MSc, CSCS, FISSN, RNutr, SENr

Before considering whether to use an ergogenic aid, athletes and their advisors should consider the cost-to-benefit ratio of its use, taking into account the safety, legality, and efficacy of the supplement in question. Nutrition supplements are designed to be added to a person's normal or typical eating program. These supplements are both popular and widely available. They can also be found in many forms, including pills, powders, drinks, gels, chews, and bars. Some aerobic endurance supplements are evidence based and can therefore be justified as part of a well-chosen strategy (1), whereas many others are either not evidence based or are marketed on weak or poorly translated evidence. This chapter discusses the relevant evidence-based supplements that have been shown to support aerobic endurance training and performance.

Sport Drinks as Ergogenic Aids

Research on sport drinks originated in the 1960s when a then assistant football coach at the University of Florida (UF) (the "Florida Gators"), who was also a former UF and National Football League player, asked a UF kidney specialist why the football players lost a significant amount of weight during practice but did not urinate much. Although the answer was simple, the question led to the development of the sport drinks category in the market, which is now a multibillion-dollar industry. The players lost so much fluid

The author would like to acknowledge the significant contributions of Bob Seebohar to this chapter.

through sweat that they did not have the need to urinate. The scientists found that after practice, the players they tested had low total blood volume, low blood sugar, and alterations in their electrolyte balance. The scientists then went to work developing a drink to replace fluid, sodium, and sugar. Over the next few years, the drink formula was tweaked and was made available on the sidelines of all UF football games and practices. This drink, which at the time propelled UF to outperform teams in the second half of games, eventually became known as Gatorade. Since the development of Gatorade, many research studies performed at university laboratories all over the world have examined various sport drink formulations and their ergogenic potential (95). A significant amount of this research indicates that consuming fluids, electrolytes, and carbohydrate is of benefit to athletes in events lasting longer than 1 hour—making sport drinks potential ergogenic aids for athletes.

The main purpose of a sport drink is to help maintain body water, carbohydrate stores, and electrolyte balance (3, 48, 77). A drastic decrease in body water or an alteration in electrolyte balance could lead to serious medical conditions such as heat exhaustion, heatstroke, and hyponatremia. In fact, just a 1% decrease in body weight from fluid losses can increase stress to the cardiovascular system by raising the heart rate and reducing the ability to transfer heat from the body to the environment (81). In addition, a 2% loss in body fluid may impair aerobic endurance performance (73). On a practical level, research shows that many athletes can lose 2% to 6% of their body weight in fluids during exercise in the heat (81). Therefore, the effect of fluid replacement on preventing aerobic endurance performance decrements may be greater in exercise lasting longer than 1 hour as well as in extreme environmental conditions such as heat.

Maintaining Carbohydrate Stores

In addition to optimizing hydration, sport drinks have been shown to help athletes fuel their performance with carbohydrate (30,46,47). Consuming carbohydrate during prolonged aerobic endurance exercise has been shown to improve performance while also reducing the potential for exercise-induced stress and suppression of the immune system (68). Initially, during prolonged strenuous aerobic endurance exercise, the main storage form of carbohydrate in the body, muscle glycogen, provides most of the carbohydrate needed to fuel activity. Muscle glycogen stores are limited, however, and as they become depleted their contribution to fueling performance also declines (66). In fact, the trained athlete typically has only enough muscle glycogen to fuel a few hours of exercise at most (39). Therefore, blood **glucose**, maintained by carbohydrate from a supplement, such as a sport drink or gel, becomes a potentially important strategy for providing the necessary energy to help maintain activity (66). In addition to increasing the likelihood of reduced performance, low levels of muscle glycogen are associated with protein degradation, reduced muscle glycogenolysis, and impaired excitation–contraction coupling (the process that enables a muscle cell to contract) (36).

Sport drinks increase levels of blood glucose, improve carbohydrate oxidation, and may help reduce fatigue during aerobic endurance training (81). Improved carbohydrate oxidation (metabolism) reduces the reliance on the limited bodily stores of carbohydrate (39), which becomes more relevant in prolonged aerobic endurance exercise activities that last beyond several hours (such as in ultra-endurance training and competition). Therefore, the more carbohydrate that athletes can oxidize, the more they can benefit from supplemental carbohydrate consumption through sport drinks, energy gels, and bars while sparing muscle glycogen.

The important components of a sport drink that can influence fluid consumption before, during, and after exercise are the type of carbohydrate and electrolytes, color, temperature, palatability, odor, taste, and texture (81). People should consider both the scientific and practical aspects of all these factors when choosing a sport drink. Athletes' needs vary considerably, so the choice of a sport drink should be individualized as much as possible. Sufficient effort should be made to determine the best fit for an athlete's physiological needs and personal preferences.

Carbohydrate added to a sport drink may facilitate rehydration and improve the intestinal uptake of water and sodium (84). A carbohydrate concentration between 6% and 8% is considered ideal for providing the required fuel for performance without unduly slowing down the rate of gastric emptying (9, 54, 59). Gastric emptying refers to how quickly fluids leave the stomach. A delay in gastric emptying indicates a delay in the absorption of the contents of the drink, increasing the risk of gastrointestinal distress (59). Beverages up to 2.5% carbohydrate will leave the stomach as rapidly as water. As the carbohydrate content increases, the gastric emptying rate slows, and a carbohydrate concentration of even 6% has a gastric emptying rate significantly slower than that of water, though obviously faster than that of more concentrated drinks (59).

In addition to the total amount of carbohydrate, the type of carbohydrate has been shown to have a significant effect on prolonged aerobic endurance performance and carbohydrate oxidation rates. Research indicates that during exercise, consuming **multiple transporter carbohydrates** (MTCs) such as a drink containing more than one kind of carbohydrate source (such as glucose and fructose), may be preferential to consuming a drink with just one type of carbohydrate (i.e., just glucose). In one study examining carbohydrate oxidation rates, eight well-trained cyclists cycled on three separate occasions for 150 minutes each time. Glucose and **fructose** were fed at a rate of 108 g/hour (2-4 g/minute), which led to 50% higher carbohydrate oxidation rates in comparison with the ingestion of only glucose at the same rate (23). A previous study by the same authors showed that a mixture of glucose, sucrose, and fructose resulted in high peak carbohydrate oxidation rates

(43). Each carbohydrate type has its own intestinal transport mechanism; therefore, the researchers concluded that after the glucose-only transporter becomes saturated, carbohydrate oxidation cannot increase if glucose is the only carbohydrate ingested.

This research on MTCs is of interest to the aerobic endurance athlete because it demonstrates that the body can absorb more total carbohydrate when a combination of various types of carbohydrate are consumed versus a single type of carbohydrate (23, 44). Using a combination of carbohydrate types will increase the rate of carbohydrate oxidation; as already mentioned, this could help preserve the precious body stores of carbohydrate. Note as well that fructose is more slowly absorbed than either sucrose or glucose. Therefore, the aerobic endurance athlete should avoid ingesting high amounts of fructose, because accumulation in the gastrointestinal tract may lead to gastrointestinal distress during exercise (78).

The relevance and subsequent recommendations for use are thus dictated by the type and duration of exercise. MTCs are most likely going to benefit aerobic endurance performance in training sessions and events lasting longer than 3 hours (i.e., ultra-endurance) by reducing the rate of perceived exertion and increasing time to exhaustion (44). The use of MTCs in shorter duration events, therefore, is not warranted because saturation of gastrointestinal carbohydrate transporters is unlikely.

Electrolyte Replacement

The five main electrolytes are sodium, chloride, potassium, calcium, and magnesium. Sodium is considered the most important because it is lost to the greatest extent during exercise yet is vital for maintaining hydration and plasma volume (84). When sodium levels are low, fluid loss through urine may increase, leading to negative fluid balance (81, 84). Typical sweat sodium levels range from 10 to 70 mEq/L, and chloride ranges from 5 to 60 mEq/L, although these levels can vary tremendously and are increased by sweat rate and decrease with training adaptations and heat acclimation. Note that a large amount of sodium is typically found in people with correspondingly high sweat rates, so these people may need to be especially cognizant of their sodium consumption.

The risk of sodium deficiency increases with longer-duration exercise and with increased intakes of fluid low in sodium (81, 84). Potassium sweat loss ranges are only 3 to 15 mEq/L, followed by calcium at 0.3 to 2 mEq/L and magnesium at 0.2 to 1.5 mEq/L (14). Potassium deficiency is rare with fluid loss from exercise (84). In fact, 8 to 29 times more sodium is lost compared with potassium (58, 63, 71).

Sport drinks should contain about 176 to 552 mg sodium per fluid liter (83), and if potassium is present, it should be in significantly smaller quantities because it is not excreted in great amounts in sweat. During ultra-endurance exercise, an even greater concentration of sodium ranging from 552 to 920 mg per fluid liter may be warranted (83). To remain in positive fluid balance, people need to consume more sodium than they lose through sweat (83, 84). Aerobic endurance athletes seldom consume enough fluids to replace sweat losses. According to one research study, athletes consumed less than 0.5 L/hour of fluid while their sweat rates ranged from 1.0 to 1.5 L/hour (69). Thus, sodium becomes of utmost importance and can help reduce cardio-vascular strain when ingested with fluid. Additionally, when combined with water, sodium can assist in decreasing fluid deficits seen during exercise (80).

The American College of Sports Medicine recommends consuming 0.5 to 0.7 g of sodium per liter of fluid per hour; other researchers recommend an even higher range, 1.7 to 2.9 g per liter of fluid per hour (58). Regardless of the quantities suggested by research, athletes need to determine individualized sweat sodium losses during training of different durations and intensities and in varying environmental conditions, ideally with the support of a qualified sport nutritionist or sport scientist. Electrolyte needs vary among athletes and can exceed 3 g/hour (64). Regular sodium intake is important for improving cardiovascular functioning and performance because it replaces lost sodium, continues the thirst response, and enhances voluntary drinking (4).

Amino Acids and Protein for Aerobic Endurance Athletes

Some researchers believe that protein requirements for aerobic endurance athletes are higher than those for nonaerobic-endurance-trained individuals (19, 45, 52) because branched-chain amino acids (BCAAs) are oxidized in greater amounts during exercise than at rest. Although some research supports this theory, other evidence shows that training does not have this effect on leucine (98) or BCAAs (52). Additionally, some scientists believe that exercise increases protein efficiency, which eliminates the need for additional protein in the diet (16). In contrast, other investigations using the questionable nitrogen balance technique (97) have found that athletes require more protein than the average 0.8 g per kilogram body weight per day recommended for nonexercising people (56). Precisely how much protein aerobic endurance athletes should consume is not clear, but 1.0 to 1.6 g of protein per kilogram body weight per day seems most likely (55).

Perhaps more important, having adequate dietary protein appears to help prevent sickness and infection in athletes. A study conducted on trained cyclists undergoing two weeks of high-volume, high-intensity training and divided into either a high-protein diet (3 g per kilogram body weight per day) or a normal-protein diet (1.5 g per kilogram body weight per day) found that the increased training volume depressed the immune system. During the normal protein diet, cyclists reported increased symptoms of upper respiratory tract infection (URTI) than during the high-protein diet; in addition, having higher protein intake maintained superior white blood cell function (96).

Protein exhibits a high satiety response; in athletes seeking weight loss or weight maintenance, intakes up to 2.0 g per kilogram body weight per day could prove useful in curbing hunger (35, 53). But a protein intake over 2.0 g per kilogram body weight per day did not elicit any performance advantage for aerobic endurance athletes (88). What is certain is that people who participate in aerobic endurance exercise must consume enough protein to support both training adaptations and recovery relative to the training demands placed on the body. If training volume and intensity fluctuate throughout the year with different aerobic endurance and resistance exercise goals, readjusting the diet and protein intake accordingly makes sense (26). Research in aerobic endurance athletes has examined the effect of both BCAAs and different types of protein on performance and recovery from exercise.

Branched-Chain Amino Acids

Amino acids are the building blocks of protein and can serve as an energy source for skeletal muscle (70, 97). Although mounting evidence suggests that dietary supplements of branched-chain amino acids (BCAAs) alone do not act as stimulators of muscle protein synthesis (72), BCAA supplements have become more popular in aerobic endurance exercise because of their potential benefits for aerobic endurance performance. Recent research suggests that BCAA supplementation with aerobic endurance training may enhance adaptations in muscle power and postexercise recovery in well-trained aerobic endurance athletes (6, 43). The BCAAs include leucine, isoleucine, and valine. The skeletal muscle can oxidize them to provide the muscles with energy. The average BCAA content of food proteins is roughly 15% of the total amino acid content (28); therefore, people who regularly consume high-quality protein-rich foods (such as meat, fish, eggs, and dairy products) are most likely consuming adequate amounts of BCAAs to support daily body protein needs. In aerobic endurance athletes who consume primarily low-quality protein food sources, such as vegans and vegetarians, co-ingestion of BCAA supplementation with their regular meals may help rescue the protein quality needed to provide the associated benefits attributed to high-quality protein sources.

During aerobic endurance exercise, the availability of all amino acid precursors from the free intracellular pool is important. The free intracellular pool is maintained through muscle protein breakdown (90, 97), which makes it especially important that the body remain in protein balance. In longer-duration aerobic endurance exercise, the oxidation of BCAAs in skeletal muscle usually exceeds their supply from protein. This process causes a decline of BCAAs in the blood and may facilitate the progression of "central fatigue." According to the central fatigue hypothesis, central fatigue occurs when tryptophan crosses the blood–brain barrier and increases the amount of serotonin forming in the brain (70), resulting in perceptions of fatigue and subsequent reductions in performance. The hypothesis predicts that during exercise, free fatty acids (FFAs) are mobilized from fat tissue and transported to the muscles to be used as energy. Because the rate of FFAs being mobilized is greater than their uptake in the muscles, the concentration of FFAs in the blood increases. Free fatty acids and the amino acid tryptophan compete for the same binding sites on **albumin** (a water-soluble protein found in many animal tissues). Because FFAs are present in high amounts in the blood, they bind to albumin first, thus preventing tryptophan from binding and leading to an increase in free tryptophan concentration in the blood. This increases the free tryptophan-to-BCAA ratio in the blood, resulting in an increased free tryptophan transport across the blood–brain barrier. After free tryptophan is inside the brain, it is converted to serotonin, which plays an important role in mood and the onset of sleep (5). Thus, a consequence of more serotonin production in the brain may be central fatigue, forcing athletes either to stop exercise or to reduce the intensity.

Research has been conducted to determine if oral intake of BCAAs may reduce this tryptophan uptake into the brain and subsequently delay fatigue (67). Although several studies show a drop in BCAA concentration in the blood and although BCAAs may help with mental performance during or after exhaustive exercise, supplementation appears to have little if any effect on actual aerobic endurance performance. A few studies have examined changes in amino acid concentration after exhaustive exercise. Researchers in one study examined these changes in 22 subjects participating in a marathon and eight subjects participating in a 1.5-hour army training program. Both groups experienced a significant decline in their plasma concentration of BCAAs. No change was noted in the concentration of total tryptophan in either group, although the marathon subjects showed a significant increase in free tryptophan leading to a decrease in the free tryptophan-to-BCAA ratio (11). Other studies also show a decrease in BCAA concentration and increase in free or total tryptophan after exhaustive exercise (12, 86). In a double-blind examination of the direct effect of BCAAs on tryptophan, 10 aerobic-endurance-trained males cycled at 70% to 75% maximal power output while ingesting drinks that contained 6% sucrose (control) or 6% sucrose and one of the following: 3 g tryptophan, 6 g BCAAs, or 18 g BCAAs. Tryptophan ingestion resulted in a 7- to 20-fold increase in brain tryptophan levels, whereas BCAA supplementation resulted in an 8% to 12% decrease in brain tryptophan levels at exhaustion. No differences were noted in exercise time to exhaustion, indicating that the changes in amino acid concentrations did not affect aerobic endurance exercise performance (92, 93).

In addition to studying changes in amino acid concentration, examining whether a subsequent change occurs in cognitive performance makes sense. In a study examining the central fatigue hypothesis and changes in cognition, subjects received either a mixture of BCAAs in carbohydrate or a placebo drink. The investigators measured cognitive performance before and after a 30 km (18.6 mi) cross country race. Subjects given BCAAs showed an improvement from before to after the run in certain parts of a color-word test; the placebo group showed no change. The BCAA-supplemented group also maintained their performance in shape rotation and figure identification tasks, whereas the placebo group showed a significant decline in performance in both tests after the run. The authors noted that BCAA supplementation had a greater effect on performance in more complex tasks (37). In another study of cognitive functioning after exhaustive exercise, participants ran a 42.2 km (marathon distance) cross country race during which they were supplemented with either BCAAs or placebo. The BCAA supplementation improved running performance in the slower runners only. What is more interesting is that the BCAAs appeared to have a positive effect on mental performance. The BCAA-supplemented group showed significant improvement in the Stroop color and word test postexercise compared with preexercise (13).

Branched-chain amino acid supplementation can also influence recovery from exercise. Prolonged exercise will reduce the body's amino acid pool; thus, maintaining higher levels, specifically BCAA levels, is important to suppressing cell-signaling cascades that promote muscle protein breakdown (88, 97). Creating an anabolic environment through BCAA use may assist in faster recovery from exercise. Branched-chain amino acids also appear to have a positive effect on lessening the degree of muscle damage. In one study, untrained men performed three 90-minute cycling bouts at 55% intensity and consumed a 200 kcal beverage consisting of carbohydrate, BCAA, or placebo before and at 60 minutes during exercise. The BCAA-supplemented beverage trial lessened the amount of muscle damage resulting from the exercise session compared with the placebo trial at 4, 24, and 48 hours after exercise and the carbohydrate trial at 24 hours after exercise (34).

Protein and Recovery

Studies examining the effect of protein combined with carbohydrate on glycogen resynthesis are equivocal; some indicate that protein combined with carbohydrate is more effective (although some of these studies also provided more total calories), and others show no difference. One study showed that postworkout protein consumption with carbohydrate in a 3:1 or 4:1 ratio of carbohydrate to protein appears to accelerate the replenishment of muscle glycogen (10). This finding is of relevance for aerobic endurance athletes who train the same muscle groups during each training session (e.g., marathon runners), athletes with multiple training sessions per day, and for multiday competitions. Although commonplace in popular culture, postworkout protein consumption for the purposes of increasing muscle is actually of less importance. In another small study, six male cyclists received an **isocaloric** liquid carbohydrate–protein supplement (0.8 g/kg carbohydrate, 0.4 g/kg protein), a carbohydrate-only supplement (1.2 g/kg carbohydrate), or placebo immediately, 1 hour, and 2 hours after a 60-minute cycling time trial. Six hours after the initial trial, the cycling protocol was repeated. Although cycling performance in the subsequent time trial was not different between groups, muscle glycogen resynthesis was significantly greater in the carbohydrate and protein group versus the carbohydrate-only or placebo group during the 6 hours of recovery (8).

Although these results seem promising, a few studies indicate that the addition of protein to carbohydrate may not further augment muscle glycogen synthesis. In a small study, five subjects received either 1.67 g/kg body weight sucrose or 1.67 g/kg body weight sucrose and 0.5 g/kg body weight whey protein hydrolysate immediately after intense cycling and every 15 minutes for 4 hours during the recovery period. No significant differences were found in glycogen resynthesis rates between the carbohydrate-only and carbohydrate in combination with protein groups (93). One weakness of this study was that it did not use a crossover design as in the other studies (8). A crossover design uses the same subjects for all treatments, which allows the researchers to make more robust statements about the effectiveness of a given nutrient intervention.

Another investigation in six men yielded similar results. In this crossover study, the men performed two bouts of running on the same day (with a 4-hour recovery period between bouts) and repeated this protocol 14 days later. At 30-minute intervals during the recovery period, the subjects consumed either carbohydrate only (0.8 g/kg body weight) or carbohydrate (0.8 g/kg body weight) and whey protein isolate (0.3 g/kg body weight). Muscle glycogen resynthesis was not different between groups. During the second run, however, whole-body carbohydrate oxidation (use of carbohydrate) was significantly greater in the carbohydrate and protein treatment group, indicating a potential benefit of this combination (10).

Although the effect of protein added to carbohydrate on muscle glycogen resynthesis is unclear, the addition of protein to a carbohydrate beverage may increase net protein balance, which in turn may help prevent muscle soreness and damage and thereby promote recovery. In a crossover study examining this question, eight aerobic-endurance-trained athletes ingested carbohydrate (0.7 g per kilogram body weight per hour) every 30 minutes during 6 hours of aerobic endurance exercise, and protein and carbohydrate (0.7 g carbohydrate per kilogram body weight per hour and 0.25 g protein per kilogram body weight per hour) every 30 minutes during a subsequent 6-hour exercise bout. Whole-body protein balance during exercise with carbohydrate only was negative, whereas the ingestion of carbohydrate and protein resulted in either positive balance or less negative balance (depending on the tracer used to examine whole-body protein balance) (51).

Including protein or BCAAs in the postexercise nutrition plan may enhance muscle recovery and decrease the effect of muscular damage sometimes seen after heavy aerobic endurance exercise. Researchers observed significant reductions in creatine kinase, a blood marker of muscle damage, when cross country runners consumed a beverage with vitamins C and E and

0.365 g of whey protein per kilogram body weight versus a carbohydrate-only beverage (57). Another study showed that feeding 12 g of BCAAs for 14 days before aerobic endurance exercise as well as immediately afterward reduced creatine kinase levels (21). Other research has also reported that pre-exercise BCAA ingestion positively influences anabolic hormone responses postexercise (18).

Although these studies highlight positive results from the addition of protein or BCAAs postexercise, other researchers have found no benefit to adding protein to the postworkout nutrition plan as evidenced by no changes in the level of markers of muscle damage. In one study showing no performance benefit to adding protein to a 4-hour recovery feeding, subjects cycled, recovered, and then cycled the next day. This crossover design study used a small sample and used the subjects as their own controls; subjects received a protein-enriched recovery feeding in the first part of the experiment, followed by a two-week washout period and an isocaloric recovery feeding in the second phase (79). Additionally, in a study looking at the addition of protein to a carbohydrate drink postexercise in an eccentric exercise model that induced muscular injury, protein did not have a significant effect on returning creatine kinase levels to normal after 30 minutes of downhill running (33).

Combined, these studies indicate that protein or amino acids (particularly BCAA supplements) may or may not benefit aerobic endurance athletes when consumed postexercise because little research has provided evidence of the role of protein on aerobic endurance training adaptations and performance (29, 82, 89). Further, the bulk of those studies concern resistance training (50, 62). Nevertheless, with all this taken into account, aerobic endurance athletes should consume at least 1.0 to 1.6 g protein per kilogram body weight per day to ensure an adequate pool of amino acids that the body can rely on during times of need to reduce the catabolic effects of prolonged aerobic endurance exercise, especially if training or competing for 90 or more minutes.

Caffeine

Caffeine, one of the most widely used stimulants in the world, can be found in tea, coffee, soft drinks, energy drinks, chocolate, and a variety of other foods as well as in supplemental form. It acts as a stimulant to the central nervous system, which causes heart rate and blood pressure to increase. Caffeine is a multifaceted supplement that has been used in sport for more than 40 years. It remains one of the most popular among aerobic endurance exercisers because its ingestion has been shown to reduce perception of fatigue and to enable exercise to be sustained at optimal intensity and output for extended periods (2, 15, 87). The actual mechanisms by which caffeine helps improve aerobic endurance is, however, unclear. Despite this, the evidence is clear that caffeine has many potential sport applications. Studies show that doses of 4 mg caffeine per kilogram can increase mental alertness and improve logical reasoning, free recall, and recognition memory tasks (85). In addition, caffeine can help increase time to exhaustion in aerobic endurance exercise bouts (7, 20, 25), decrease ratings of perceived exertion during submaximal aerobic endurance exercise (24), and improve physical performance during periods of sleep deprivation (60). Caffeine also has the potential to decrease muscle soreness and augment glycogen resynthesis (74).

Despite the many uses of caffeine, research is equivocal regarding caffeine and improved sport performance. This conclusion, however, may be attributable to study design factors such as the caffeine dose, the form of caffeine (pill, coffee, or with carbohydrate sources), normal dietary use of caffeine, timing and pattern of caffeine intake before exercise, and the environment in which the exercise testing takes place (31).

Caffeine ingestion affects many body targets including the central nervous system by crossing the blood–brain barrier and antagonistically binding to adenosine receptors, causing a decrease in adenosine bound to those receptors and a subsequent increase in circulating dopamine activity (27). According to one theory, this mechanism affects the perception of effort and neural activation of muscular contractions. This is the most popular of the main theories aimed at explaining the ergogenic effect of caffeine and has the most value in terms of scientific support and field validation with exercisers. Another theory surrounding the benefits of caffeine involves a muscle performance effect on enzymes that control the breakdown of glycogen. Most of the support for this theory has come not from in vivo (within the body) but from in vitro (outside the body) research, so drawing any formal conclusions related to the theory is difficult. Finally, caffeine can acutely increase **lipolysis** (the breakdown of fat stored in fat cells) and **thermogenesis** (the production of heat) and potentially increase both over time. In addition, it may exert a glycogen-sparing effect (31). Caffeine is thought to enhance the enzymes that break down fat or increase the levels of **epinephrine** (also known as adrenaline), which can mobilize stored fat (15, 31, 32). Research examining this theory, however, is not conclusive (15, 31). The current consensus lends more support to the effect on the central nervous system and the reduced perception of effort. Support also comes from athletes undergoing training sessions and competitions encompassing various modes of activity. Caffeine is rapidly absorbed and can reach a maximum level in the plasma within 1 hour. Because it is broken down slowly (half-life of 4-6 hours), concentration can usually be maintained for 3 to 4 hours (31).

Ergogenic benefits of caffeine have been shown with doses ranging from 3 to 9 mg/kg body weight (about 1.5-3.5 cups of automatic drip coffee in a 70 kg [154 lb] person) (42). The performance effects are usually evident when caffeine is consumed within 60 minutes before exercise but are also noticeable when it is consumed during prolonged exercise (31, 32, 99).

Researchers have also looked at the effect of caffeine on carbohydrate absorption and the effects of consuming caffeine combined with a carbohydrate source. Caffeine increases carbohydrate absorption in the intestine. This process has been observed with small amounts (1.4 mg/kg body weight) (14, 94) and larger amounts (5 mg/kg body weight) of caffeine intake. Further, caffeine ingestion has been shown to increase carbohydrate oxidation rates by 26% during the last 30 minutes of a 2-hour exercise bout (99). Taken together, these data indicate that caffeine could have a positive effect on carbohydrate use in the body through faster delivery to the working muscles. Additional research has confirmed the improvement of work capacity (15%-23%) and lower ratings of perceived exertion when caffeine is consumed with a carbohydrate beverage (22). Caffeine has long been thought to act as a diuretic, but the addition of caffeine to a sport drink does not influence fluid delivery or produce any adverse fluid balance or thermoregulation issues during moderate- to high-intensity exercise (62), and recent research has shown no evidence of dehydration with moderate regular daily caffeine intake in the form of coffee (49).

Although it is considered a drug, caffeine appears to be safe when used properly, and for most aerobic endurance sports, an ergogenic benefit is seen in doses ranging from 3 to 9 mg/kg body weight taken about 1 hour before exercise. Concerns regarding use primarily relate to the potential side-effects when consumed in high doses or at inappropriate times and include tremors, anxiety, increased heart rate, and sleep disturbances (2, 15, 87), all of which can result in detrimental effects to performance and recovery. Caffeine is permitted for use by the International Olympic Committee and is on the National Collegiate Athletic Association (NCAA) restricted list (urine concentrations of caffeine must not exceed 15 mcg/ml) (65, 91).

Sodium Bicarbonate and Citrate

Sodium bicarbonate has been of interest to athletes and researchers for some time. Sodium bicarbonate is an antacid that is used as a muscle buffer. A decrease in pH, resulting in a buildup of acid, is associated with fatigue, and this can have negative performance implications such as increased ratings of perceived exertion and reduced force production (38). Nutritional muscle buffers, such as sodium bicarbonate, have been used for many years thanks to the strong positive effect they have on exercise performance in events that would otherwise be limited by acid–base disturbances associated with high rates of anaerobic glycolysis. Such events include high-intensity efforts of 1 to 7 minutes, repeated high-intensity sprints, and capacity for high-intensity sprints during aerobic endurance exercise. Note that these muscle buffers are potentially effective only when taken as an acute dose preexercise, due to increasing extracellular buffering capacity (17). The use of these buffering agents is more beneficial in higher-intensity, short-duration exercise that entails larger muscle groups and faster motor unit recruitment (61). In equally high-intensity but longer-duration exercise, results on the efficacy of these products have been conflicting and have not provided sufficiently robust evidence of their performance enhancement capabilities (17, 76). The recommended dosing protocol for sodium bicarbonate is 0.3 g/kg body weight ingested approximately 60 to 90 minutes before short-duration, high-intensity exercise performance (41, 61) and tried during practice before using it as a precompetition aid.

Although sodium bicarbonate has historically been the most frequently used buffering agent, sodium citrate has been proposed as a potentially better option because of its lower incidence and risk of gastrointestinal distress, but the evidence for this is mostly negative. Sodium citrate is not a base, but it is also able to increase blood pH without the associated gastrointestinal distress commonly seen with sodium bicarbonate use. With regard to an evidence-based dosing protocol for sodium citrate, more research is needed. Fortunately, better implementation protocols using sodium bicarbonate, such as including ingestion timing (40), have helped resolve some of the gastrointestinal discomfort issues associated with this supplement.

Because the results of research studies have been mixed, many athletes and their advisors opt for ergogenic aids such as beta-alanine (discussed in more detail in chapter 8), which has a great deal more research evidence behind it to justify its use. Current evidence indicates that sodium bicarbonate can be useful in sports using different energy systems but is likely most beneficial to performance of shorter, higher-intensity bouts. Sodium bicarbonate, therefore, should be considered with caution because of the increased risk of gastrointestinal upset, which will result in performance impairment (17).

Professional Applications

Advising athletes on supplements must be done with great care and with full consideration of their health status, medications, other supplement usage, and personal preferences. When making recommendations for aerobic endurance athletes, practitioners must always keep in mind three important factors related to performance nutrition: hydration, electrolyte balance, and carbohydrate intake.

Aerobic endurance events can be won or lost by a matter of minutes, so ergogenic aids are tempting and popular tools among athletes. The ergogenic aids discussed in this chapter are those that have the strongest and most promising evidence in relation to potential benefits for aerobic endurance performance.

Sport drinks are one of the most widely used ergogenic aids among aerobic endurance athletes. Why consider a sport drink over plain water? As first

(continued)

Professional Applications *(continued)*

discovered on the American football field at the University of Florida in the 1960s, consuming water only may not suffice when it comes to optimizing performance. Sport drinks can help maintain body water, carbohydrate stores, and electrolyte balance. Athletes are also more likely to consume a greater quantity of a fluid that they perceive as tasting good in comparison with water. Athletes engaging in strenuous exercise, especially in the heat, can lose 2% to 6% of their body weight in fluid. They will not only overheat when they lose this much fluid but also are more likely to experience a significant drop in performance. Sport drinks have been shown to be effective in blunting this potential reduction in performance.

Ideally, an athlete who consumes a sport drink should opt for a 6% to 8% carbohydrate solution and consume 3 to 8 fluid ounces (90 to 240 ml) every 10 to 20 minutes during aerobic endurance exercise lasting longer than 60 to 90 minutes. Athletes who choose not to consume a sport drink but instead opt for water will need to consume carbohydrate both during and immediately after training and competition. In addition, they should consume a source of electrolytes, especially sodium. Although recreational athletes who walk or jog a marathon can likely get away with consuming a variety of whole foods during competition with little stomach upset, most competitive athletes will opt for the convenience and ease of digestibility of various sport nutrition products, including gels and gummies.

Aerobic endurance athletes should aim for 30 to 60 g of carbohydrate per hour while exercising, although those consuming multiple types of carbohydrate can consume as much as 90 g of carbohydrate per hour. Athletes should also aim to consume approximately 0.8 to 1.2 g carbohydrate per kilogram body weight postexercise, depending on the intensity and duration of the exercise and the amount of carbohydrate consumed during exercise. In addition, athletes will benefit from ingesting some protein, approximately 0.3 to 0.4 g/kg body weight with their carbohydrate postexercise to facilitate muscle repair.

Ideally, athletes will consume their postworkout snack within 30 to 60 minutes. Delaying this consumption can decrease the rate of glycogen resynthesis, because subsequent bouts of exercise (especially if the rest period is <24 hours) may become compromised. Typically, athletes can replenish glycogen stores within 24 hours, although this may not be the case with prolonged exhaustive exercise. Even trained athletes have enough stored carbohydrate, in the form of glycogen, to fuel them for only a few hours. In addition to potential performance decrements, low levels of muscle glycogen are associated with protein degradation, which could result in the breakdown of muscle tissue, especially if the athlete is not consuming enough total protein and calories.

Excellent examples of postworkout snacks that meet the criteria for a 150-pound (68 kg) athlete are 20 fluid ounces (600 ml) of low-fat chocolate milk or a blended shake made with 1 cup of sliced strawberries, 1 cup of grapes, 1 banana, and 1 scoop of whey protein powder in water. Athletes can use a variety of combinations to refuel themselves, including cereal with skim milk, salted crackers with low-fat cheese, or combinations of sport supplement products and food (a sport drink followed by nonfat yogurt with fruit on the bottom, for instance).

Athletes who opt for water should also consider their electrolyte needs (75). Every athlete loses a different amount of the electrolytes (sodium is the electrolyte lost in the greatest quantity). The sport nutrition professional should help athletes determine approximate sweat sodium needs for different durations of training and in different environments. Unless otherwise told by their physician, aerobic endurance athletes should not follow the general recommendations to the public—1,500 to 2,000 mg sodium per day. Instead, they should consume about 500 to 700 mg sodium per liter of fluid during exercise. From a practical standpoint, however, some athletes need quite a bit more than this and will still cramp and lose too much fluid even if they consume the upper limit of this range. Again, the sport nutrition professional can work with athletes to find a range that better suits their needs. After exercise, athletes should consume at least 500 mg sodium for every pound (0.45 kg) of water weight they lose.

Aside from fluid, electrolytes, and carbohydrate, athletes looking to get an edge on their competition may look toward a variety of other ergogenic aids to help them perform better and enhance recovery. Branched-chain amino acids may help decrease central fatigue so that the aerobic endurance athlete can perform well on mental tasks immediately after exercising (this is helpful for a college athlete who must study for a test after a long run). For athletes consuming primarily low-quality sources of protein, supplementing the diet with branched-chain amino acids may also help rescue the protein quality and potentially help mitigate muscle soreness and inflammation, thereby speeding up recovery from long bouts of exercise. Studies have used anywhere from 6 to 12 g of BCAAs for this purpose, although it is unclear exactly how much should be given and whether BCAAs should be dosed based on per kilogram body weight, on the intensity and duration of exercise, or both.

Although BCAAs may help mitigate soreness and inflammation postexercise, some athletes looking to buffer muscular fatigue during exercise may look to try sodium bicarbonate. Even though the evidence shows that sodium bicarbonate may work in certain situations, it is not a recommended ergogenic aid because of the significant potential for gastrointestinal upset. The cost-to-benefit ratio associated with the use of an ergogenic aid or supplement must be considered because its use may come at the risk of impairing health or performance. A better option is beta-alanine, which is discussed in detail in chapter 8.

One of the best ergogenic aids for aerobic endurance athletes is caffeine. In doses of 3 to 9 mg/kg body weight (about 1.5-3.5 cups of automatic drip coffee in a 70 kg [154 lb] person) consumed either before exercise (typically 60 minutes) or during prolonged exercise, caffeine is ergogenic. It can decrease feelings of perceived exertion, improve work capacity, and increase mental alertness. This quantity of caffeine does not produce any harmful changes in fluid balance or lead to dehydration. Athletes who try caffeine typically notice an immediate difference.

The use of nutrition supplements with aerobic endurance athletes is widespread, but they vary widely in their efficacy and safety. Many do not have

(continued)

Professional Applications (continued)

scientific or field evidence to support their proposed mechanisms of action or efficacy of use in training or competition. Others are not backed by research, but some athletes swear by them. The sport nutrition professional should pay particularly close attention to the safety and legality of sport supplements because testing for banned substances has become much more frequent in collegiate, professional, and Olympic athletes. It is always wise to conduct an extensive background check on supplement companies, their manufacturing process, and standards of quality assurance before recommending any supplement to an athlete. Supplements for NCAA athletes and the means of procuring them (whether they are provided by the school or purchased by athletes themselves) should be in accordance with NCAA regulations. Each professional sport governing body recognizes specific certification organizations (such as the NSF International and Informed Choice). Before considering any ergogenic aid, an athlete should become informed or seek advice from an appropriately qualified sport nutrition professional about the safety, legality, and efficacy of the supplement, and where there is any doubt to avoid them. And finally, nutrition supplements are designed only to supplement or optimize a well-balanced diet as part of a well-chosen evidence-based decision-making process, ideally with the support of an appropriately qualified sport nutrition or health care professional. The athlete should trial new nutritional supplements and ergogenic aids well in advance of competition, to avoid experiencing any unwanted side effects on the day that would impair performance.

Summary Points

- Sport drinks can improve performance by increasing levels of blood glucose, improving carbohydrate oxidation, and reducing perception of fatigue.
- A sport drink with a carbohydrate concentration between 6% and 8% is ideal for faster gastric emptying rates.
- Consuming multiple sources of carbohydrate, specifically glucose and fructose in a 2:1 ratio, leads to improvement in prolonged aerobic exercise endurance performance when compared with the use of a single source of carbohydrate. This practice, however, is most likely going to benefit aerobic endurance performance in training sessions and events lasting greater than 3 hours.
- Electrolyte needs vary among athletes. Regular electrolyte consumption during aerobic endurance exercise, specifically sodium and especially in hot environments, is important for improving cardiovascular function and performance by replacing lost sodium, continuing the thirst response, and encouraging voluntary drinking.
- BCAAs may help decrease markers of muscle damage, but this is likely to be of real-world value only to those in an energy deficit (i.e., making weight) and in aerobic endurance athletes consuming a primarily plant-based diet.

- Caffeine can be used as an effective ergogenic aid in doses ranging from 3 to 9 mg/kg body weight. The performance effects are usually seen with consumption of caffeine within 60 minutes before exercise but are also noticeable with consumption during prolonged exercise. Dosing and timing of caffeine requires careful consideration to avoid potential side effects.

- Buffering agents such as sodium bicarbonate may benefit athletes participating in high-intensity, short-duration exercise such as track and field events but are unlikely to be of any practical value to aerobic endurance athletes, who have an increased risk of gastrointestinal distress.

Chapter 10

Nutrient Timing

Chad M. Kerksick, PhD, FNSCA, FISSN, CSCS*D, NSCA-CPT*D

Shawn M. Arent, PhD, CSCS*D, FISSN, FNAK

Timed administration of nutrients can facilitate physiological adaptations to exercise and may promote optimal health and performance. Nutrient timing recommendations vary among athletes within a particular sport as well as between sports. Specific recommendations are modified relative to the travel, competition, and training demands throughout the year as well as the volume, intensity, and purpose of the work performed. The dynamic nature of nutrient timing makes it important for all athletes and coaches to develop a firm foundation of knowledge regarding energy, macronutrient, fluid, and micronutrient consumption. This chapter offers a detailed description of the nutritional considerations that are supported by the scientific literature, helping the reader to understand how and when to employ timing strategies and how to implement such strategies to deliver the necessary levels of energy and nutrients to sustain human performance and promote recovery.

This chapter emphasizes when to consume specific nutrients or supplements. Many research studies have illustrated that the timed ingestion of specific macronutrients and select amino acids may significantly affect the adaptive response to exercise. Depending on the type of training, these responses can include improved glycogen resynthesis, maintenance of blood-based fuels, muscle growth, and improvements in performance, body composition, immune system functioning, and mood.

Historically, the first consideration of nutrient timing involved delivering a source of carbohydrate before or during the exercise bout. In fact, reports indicate that athletes consumed sugary snacks or foods before the 1928 Olympic marathon. Starting in the 1960s, researchers began to explore the impact of carbohydrate status, and the concept of carbohydrate loading was born. Carbohydrate loading increases the storage of carbohydrate in the liver and muscles (20, 68, 100, 119), and it can help sustain normal glucose (carbohydrate) levels in the blood during prolonged exercise (25, 68). Later, preexercise ingestion of carbohydrate, amino acids, protein, and creatine (Cr) was studied for the ability of these substances to stimulate further adaptations to exercise training (23, 27, 75, 110, 117) and prevent the breakdown of muscle tissue (75, 114). Alternatively, strategies have been explored to heighten intramuscular adaptations in athletes while restricting carbohydrate intake or through the performance of multiple sessions in one day. These approaches are generally classified as "train low, compete high" approaches whereby robust changes in intracellular content of key metabolic enzymes or proteins occur (53). Most recently, studies involving minerals, amino acids, and other nonnutrients demonstrate the need for more research to improve understanding of the potential outcomes involving the timing of nutrients (102).

Nutrient Timing and Aerobic Endurance Performance

To sustain life, the human body primarily burns three compounds—carbohydrate, fat, and protein—to generate the energy necessary to drive hundreds of chemical reactions. Carbohydrate is the preferred fuel source for exercising muscles, but unfortunately, carbohydrate supply in the muscle and liver is limited (25). During prolonged moderate- to high-intensity exercise (65% to 85% $\dot{V}O_2$max), internal carbohydrate stores become depleted (51, 105), often resulting in decreases in exercise intensity (25), reductions in performance (115), breakdown of muscle tissue (94), and a weakened immune system (43, 93).

At rest, intramuscular glycogen levels of most trained athletes are considered adequate to meet the physical demands of moderate-intensity exercise bouts lasting anywhere from 60 to 90 minutes (33). Assuming no appreciable amount of muscle damage, a carbohydrate intake of 8 to 10 g per kilogram body weight per day combined with adequate rest between sessions (~24 hours) can maintain adequate glycogen levels in the muscle for up to several days. Another recommendation, which also facilitates adequate maintenance of glycogen levels, is to ingest 55% to 65% of daily caloric intake as carbohydrate. This recommendation, however, assumes that the athlete is consuming an adequate number of calories relative to body size and physical activity level, and for this reason a recommendation based on an athlete's body weight is preferred. For athletes who regularly ingest this level of dietary carbohydrate based on adequate caloric intake, simply taking a day or two off (or markedly reducing volume and intensity of exercise) before competition will allow restoration of **muscle glycogen** (the storage form of carbohydrate in the liver and skeletal muscle; estimated to be approximately 250-300 g of carbohydrate). Unfortunately, many athletes

Protocols for Rapid Repletion of Intramuscular Glycogen Stores

- Approach 1: 0.6 to 1.0 g of carbohydrate per kilogram body weight within 30 minutes with repeated doses occurring every 2 hours for the next 4 to 6 hours
- Approach 2: 1.2 g of carbohydrate per kilogram body weight every 30 minutes for 3.5 hours after completion of the training bout

do not consume adequate levels of carbohydrate (18); therefore, practitioners should weigh the practicality of providing daily recommendations of high carbohydrate intake against more aggressive feeding approaches. As such, strategies have been developed to help athletes quickly achieve maximal levels of glycogen in their muscle.

Carbohydrate Loading

Carbohydrate loading is a practice that athletes use to significantly increase their endogenous stores of muscle glycogen before longer-duration events that typically lead to depletion of glycogen stores. Traditional carbohydrate loading studies conducted on untrained people incorporated a three- or four-day depletion phase in which athletes ingested a low-carbohydrate diet and completed a high volume of exercise training to "deplete" the internal stores of glycogen (8). This phase was followed by a three- or four-day period of high carbohydrate ingestion (>70% carbohydrate or 8 to 10 g carbohydrate per kilogram body weight per day) and a decrease in exercise volume to facilitate supersaturation of muscle glycogen. Using this approach, early studies reported an ability of athletes to maintain their pace of training for significantly longer periods (67).

A series of studies in well-trained runners (99, 100) suggested that a reduction in exercise training volume along with a high-carbohydrate diet (65% to 70% dietary carbohydrate) over a minimum of three days can elevate muscle glycogen levels. These conclusions were well received as a much more practical approach to maximizing muscle glycogen. Another strategy that maximized intramuscular glycogen required trained runners to consume a high-carbohydrate diet (10 g carbohydrate per kilogram body weight per day) for three days while completely refraining from exercise (20). Additionally, a high-carbohydrate (8.1 g carbohydrate per kilogram body weight per day or 600 g carbohydrate per day) diet significantly elevated preexercise glycogen stores versus a low-carbohydrate (1.4 g carbohydrate per kilogram body weight per day or 100 g carbohydrate per day) diet given to trained individuals for three days before completion of a 45-minute bicycle ride at 82% $\dot{V}O_2$peak.

Interestingly, a dose–response effect may be evident regarding the amount of carbohydrate that needs to be ingested when no depletion phase occurs to promote maximal levels of muscle glycogen. For example, baseline muscle glycogen was notably higher after ingestion of 10 g carbohydrate per kilogram body weight per day for one to three days when compared with ingesting 8 g per kilogram body weight per day for three days. Currently, this effect has not been investigated further, because initial carbohydrate-loading studies that incorporated depletion phases and longer intakes of high carbohydrate reported higher levels of muscle glycogen (7). For this reason and for simplicity, it is commonly recommended to have athletes who desire to maximize muscle glycogen stores to ingest as much carbohydrate as they are able and to achieve a minimum of 10 g of carbohydrate per kilogram body weight per day while simultaneously reducing the volume of their training (18).

Nutrient Intake Before Aerobic Endurance Exercise

The hours before an aerobic endurance exercise bout or competition are an important consideration, because athletes can take many steps to ensure provision of optimal doses of carbohydrate and other fuel sources. This period has been further divided into two phases: (a) 2 to 4 hours preexercise and (b) 30 to 60 minutes preexercise (33, 70, 71). Collectively, research involving single carbohydrate feedings before exercise suggests that it is possible to achieve higher levels of muscle glycogen and an improvement of **blood glucose** maintenance **(euglycemia)**. Euglycemia is a state in which blood glucose levels are in normal ranges, often considered values between 80 and 100 mg/dl (4.4-5.5 mmol/L). Notably, changes in performance have been equivocal with regard to single carbohydrate feeding in the hours before the initiation of exercise (26, 33, 34, 37, 39). To optimize carbohydrate use, preexercise meals should consist largely of high-carbohydrate foods or liquids. This practice becomes even more important when athletes make poor recovery efforts (e.g., low energy intake, especially low dietary carbohydrate intake, failure to rest or reduce training volume, or both). In this situation, or when an athlete has fasted overnight (i.e., sleeping), a high-carbohydrate meal ingested 4 hours before an exercise bout causes significant increases in both muscle and **liver glycogen** levels (26). See figure 10.1 for the effect of preexercise feedings on muscle glycogen levels.

Similarly, when subjects either consumed no carbohydrate or ingested a large carbohydrate meal (~300 g carbohydrate) 4 hours before completing a standardized bout of cycling exercise, participants who ingested carbohydrate were able to significantly reduce the amount of time required to complete the session (98). Other studies have supported these findings, demonstrating that ingestion of a carbohydrate-rich meal (200 to 300 g) 3 to 4 hours before exercise can improve aerobic endurance or work output compared with no carbohydrate ingestion (82, 118). For this reason, it is commonly

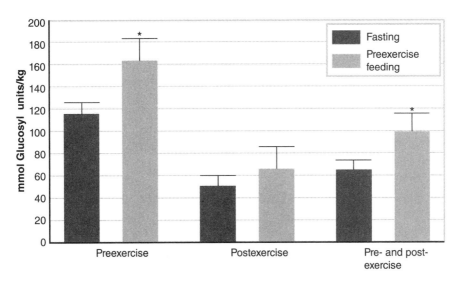

FIGURE 10.1 Effect of preexercise feedings on muscle glycogen levels. Preexercise feeding of a high-carbohydrate meal significantly increased muscle glycogen levels before exercise and reduced the extent to which these glycogen stores were depleted after exercise. This study provided the first documented evidence that feeding preexercise affects glycogen status. The need to sustain glycogen levels during exercise or competition largely serves as the basis for preexercise nutrient timing and the need for carbohydrate before exercise or competition.

* = Different from preexercise feeding.

Data from Coyle et al. (1985).

recommended that aerobic endurance athletes ingest snacks or meals high in carbohydrate at a dosage of 1 to 4 g carbohydrate per kilogram body weight several hours before exercise (105).

Ingestion of a high-carbohydrate meal 2 to 4 hours before an exercise bout becomes extremely important when the exercise bout begins in the early morning hours. The time spent sleeping is similar to a fasting period, which often results in a reduction of liver glycogen stores. Ultimately, lower liver glycogen stores will affect carbohydrate availability after the exercise bout begins. From a practicality standpoint, however, ingesting key nutrients 4 hours (or even 2 hours) before an exercise bout may not be feasible because of the start time of the practice, training session, or competition. Morning start times may complicate the decision between optimal fueling and an additional hour or two of sleep. In these situations, the athlete must not overwhelm the storage capacity of the stomach in an attempt to fuel the body (with less digestive time) and end up causing gastrointestinal distress in the process. This consideration emphasizes the importance of proper planning by the athlete and coach to make sure that neither component (i.e., sleep or fueling) is compromised. In this scenario, the athlete needs to overcome the lack of available carbohydrate by working harder to ingest optimal carbohydrate levels during the first hour of exercise or, alternatively, they could consider eating a large snack or small meal of foods containing predominantly carbohydrate before going to bed. Although many food choices can provide carbohydrate, athletes need to experiment during training sessions to figure out what foods work for them without causing gastrointestinal distress.

Although it is widely recommended that ingestion of carbohydrate be completed before an exercise bout to help ensure maximal storage of muscle and liver glycogen, much controversy and misinformation exist regarding the extent to which the type of carbohydrate can positively or negatively influence the metabolic response to ingestion and subsequent exercise performance. Ingestion of carbohydrate results in a concomitant increase in insulin levels, a pancreatic hormone that increases the uptake of glucose into the body's cells and decreases the level of glucose in the blood. This physiological response may lead to hypoglycemia (<3.5 mmol/L), which has been purported to reduce exercise intensity and increased feelings of fatigue from exercise. Furthermore, this effect may be exacerbated by the exercise itself because of additional glucose uptake from activation of GLUT-4 transporters. Collectively, this effect is often referred to as "rebound hypoglycemia." Additionally, increases in insulin levels decrease the breakdown of adipose tissue and increase the rate of **carbohydrate oxidation** (the amount of carbohydrate that can be broken down or used in a given period) when compared with fasted conditions.

Foster and colleagues (41) conducted the first study to report a rebound hypoglycemia response to ingesting carbohydrate before (<60 min) exercise. Though this response has not been consistently reported in the scientific literature (50), it continues to be widely reported anecdotally and is an area of concern for athletes and coaches. Glucose and insulin changes immediately after carbohydrate ingestion exhibit inconsistent patterns, which makes it challenging to offer universal recommendations for all athletes. During exercise, though initial hypoglycemia may be reported, this response has not been shown to negatively affect performance in several studies. In fact, most studies report that after 20 to 30 minutes of exercise, or even a sufficient warm-up, glucose levels return to normal with no untoward effects on the athlete (81). In addition, variability among people is considerable, because not everyone experiences this hypoglycemic response. A review by Hawley and Burke (50) revealed that providing some form of carbohydrate within 60 minutes before exercise has no negative effect on performance and may, in fact, increase performance anywhere from 7% to 20%.

Nonetheless, some athletes do have negative responses to preexercise carbohydrate ingestion, but a consensus is still unavailable on why this response occurs. Further, the extent to which the glycemic index of a carbohydrate source alters glucose and insulin kinetics, glycogen use and subsequent performance has received much consideration. Initially, it was reported that lower-glycemic carbohydrate sources such as fructose may be preferred to avoid the hypoglycemic rebound and subsequently improve performance. Research, however, does not entirely support this theory. Febbraio and Stewart (39) showed that ingestion of a high-glycemic meal 45 minutes before 135 minutes of cycling exercise was not responsible for changes in muscle glycogen use or performance when compared with a low-glycemic meal or water.

Additional studies have shown that altering the glycemic index of a preexercise carbohydrate source has no effect on subsequent performance (34, 38). Further research indicates that fructose ingestion may be responsible for gastrointestinal distress and may have a negative effect on performance (35). For this reason, a common recommendation is that athletes avoid ingesting fructose as a primary carbohydrate source before and during exercise or that they combine it with other carbohydrate sources to take advantage of multiple transporters.

In summary, athletes should ingest a diet high in carbohydrate (8-10 g carbohydrate per kilogram body weight per day), especially during the days before competition. High dietary intake of carbohydrate along with a brief reduction in training volume can maximize glycogen stores. Ingesting a carbohydrate meal (200 to 300 g) 2 to 4 hours before exercise helps to maximize glycogen stores and performance. As commencement of the training bout or competition draws near, regular consumption of a carbohydrate beverage containing 6% to 8% carbohydrate can help to maintain glucose levels in the blood, stimulate liver glycogenesis, and prevent hypoglycemia. Athletes should be cautious about ingesting too much food volume before exercise and should limit fructose because of the potential for gastrointestinal upset with ingestion of large quantities of fructose.

Nutrient Intake During Aerobic Endurance Exercise

Nutrient considerations during exercise have largely focused on aerobic endurance exercise because of the increased energy demands placed on aerobic endurance athletes. Initially, research efforts focused on carbohydrate administration to sustain blood glucose levels and spare internal stores of glycogen (37, 74, 84, 115). More recent strategies have combined carbohydrate sources and added varying amounts of amino acids during aerobic endurance exercise to improve performance, heighten recovery, and mitigate muscle damage.

Providing Carbohydrate During Aerobic Endurance Exercise

Although some studies suggest that carbohydrate ingestion before or during exercise may have negative metabolic consequences (e.g., reactive hypoglycemia) (41), an overwhelming majority of the published studies support the contention that carbohydrate ingestion improves (or at least sustains) performance (37, 79, 84, 115). The metabolic demand for carbohydrate can be quite high during exercise. Providing carbohydrate to the muscle before exercise may slow down the rate at which muscle glycogen is broken down (35, 46). But this conclusion is not universally accepted, because other studies have reported that the rate of muscle glycogen breakdown is not affected by carbohydrate feedings (26, 40). The biochemistry within the body during exercise (specifically the active muscle) suggests that ingestion of carbohydrate at this time may facilitate performance by providing a readily available supply of glucose and therefore sparing muscle and liver glycogen stores (16, 25, 26).

Carbohydrate Oxidation Rate   The rate at which carbohydrate is oxidized, whether it comes from blood glucose, liver glycogen, or muscle glycogen, is an important consideration. It has been widely accepted that regardless of the source of carbohydrate (high or low glycemic, except for fructose), the peak rate of carbohydrate oxidation during prolonged moderate-intensity exercise is around 1 g carbohydrate per minute (60 g/hour) (66). *Carbohydrate oxidation* refers to the amount of carbohydrate that can be broken down or used in a given period. When feeding schedules are altered, the rate of carbohydrate oxidation does not appear to be influenced, leading some to conclude that a limiting factor may be the rate at which carbohydrate is absorbed throughout the digestive system and subsequently made available in the bloodstream (49).

Although peak carbohydrate oxidation rates are well established, a research group led by Jeukendrup studied the effect of mixing various forms of carbohydrate in an attempt to increase peak carbohydrate oxidation rates (58, 59, 61-63, 65). Different types of carbohydrate have different transport mechanisms; therefore, providing more than one type of carbohydrate may increase the amount of carbohydrate in the bloodstream and thus provide more carbohydrate for oxidation as a fuel source. For example, a 21% increase in carbohydrate oxidation (1.2 g carbohydrate per minute) was seen during moderate-intensity exercise after ingestion of a mixture of glucose and sucrose (59). Similarly, a combination of maltodextrin and fructose resulted in a peak carbohydrate oxidation rate of 1.5 g carbohydrate per minute, which was approximately 40% greater than ingestion of maltodextrin alone during prolonged cycling at 60% to 65% $\dot{V}O_2$max (113).

Indeed, findings from this research team have regularly shown enhanced carbohydrate oxidation rates, from 1.2 to 1.75 g carbohydrate per minute, when mixtures of carbohydrates have been ingested (58, 59, 61-63). More recently, this same group reported an 8% improvement in time-trial performance after a 120-minute ride at 55% maximum power with ingestion of a combination of glucose and fructose during exercise (30). During exercise, aerobic endurance athletes may benefit from consuming a mixture of carbohydrate types. This is especially true if they start exercise without having consumed a high-carbohydrate meal over the last few hours (or days); the resulting reductions in stored glycogen can negatively affect performance.

Frequency and Timing of Carbohydrate Intake   Other research efforts have focused on changing the frequency of feedings or the timing of feedings within an exercise bout to determine if favorable metabolic adaptations or an increase in performance occurs during exercise (40, 79). Fielding and colleagues (40) reported that a more frequent intake of carbohydrate (10.75 g every 30 minutes) versus one large feeding (21 g every hour) over a 4-hour cycling ride better maintained blood glucose levels, but this difference did not influence how much muscle glycogen was used during the exercise trial. Performance in an exhaustive time trial at the end of the 4-hour exercise bout was found to be significantly improved with more frequent ingestion of carbohydrate. A 4-hour exercise session is substantially longer than most training or competitive exercise sessions, except for Ironman or half-Ironman triathlons, marathons, or ultra-endurance races. The ability of carbohydrate administration to continue delivering adequate blood glucose for this extended period to facilitate improvements in performance is a significant finding that supports the utility of the delivery of carbohydrate during exercise. In any case, the frequency or size of carbohydrate feeding does not appear to influence glycogen changes (40), but it may affect performance after a long bout of exercise.

In a study by McConell and colleagues (79) on the effect of carbohydrate supplementation during exercise, endurance-trained males participated in two time trials in which they cycled to volitional exhaustion. The cyclists consumed either 250 ml of an 8% carbohydrate solution or an artificially flavored and sweetened placebo immediately before and every 15 minutes during exercise. The cyclists given carbohydrate throughout the entire trial increased time to fatigue by 30% (47 minutes) compared with the placebo group.

Febbraio and colleagues (37) also reported the benefit of consuming carbohydrate throughout exercise. In this study, cyclists completed a 120-minute bout of cycling at 63% of their peak power under four conditions:

1. Noncaloric placebo 30 minutes before and during exercise
2. Noncaloric placebo 30 minutes before and 2 g carbohydrate per kilogram body weight in a 6.4% solution during exercise
3. 2 g carbohydrate per kilogram body weight in a 25.7% solution before exercise and noncaloric placebo during exercise
4. 2 g carbohydrate per kilogram body weight in a 25.7% solution before exercise and 2 g carbohydrate per kilogram body weight in a 6.4% solution during exercise

Changes in blood glucose oxidation throughout the exercise bout and performance in the time trial were improved only when carbohydrate was provided during exercise. The authors concluded that preexercise ingestion of carbohydrate improves performance only when carbohydrate ingestion continues throughout the exercise bout and that the ingestion of carbohydrate during 120 minutes of cycling with or without a preexercise carbohydrate feeding can improve subsequent time-trial performance (37). See figure 10.2.

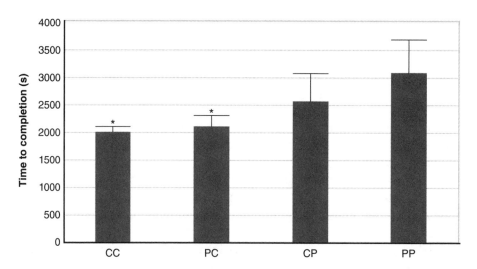

FIGURE 10.2   Effect of carbohydrate provision before and during exercise. The study showed that providing carbohydrate during exercise was of greatest importance; providing carbohydrate before exercise affected performance only when carbohydrate was provided throughout the exercise bout. CC = carbohydrate before and during exercise; PC = placebo before and carbohydrate during exercise; CP = carbohydrate before and placebo during exercise; PP = placebo before and during exercise.

* = Both CC (constant carbohydrate; 2 g/kg body weight of CHO in a 25.7% CHO beverage 30 minutes preexercise and 2 g/kg of CHO in a 6.4% CHO solution throughout the time trial) and CP (carbohydrate before the time trial followed by placebo during the time trial; 2 g/kg body weight of CHO in a 25.7% CHO beverage 30 minutes preexercise and placebo throughout the time trial) were different from either PC or PP (placebo consumed before and during the time trial).

Data from Febbraio et al. (2000).

Influence of Baseline Glycogen Levels

Both the Febbraio and colleagues (37) and McConell and colleagues (79) performed studies that clearly illustrate the importance of providing carbohydrate throughout exercise to sustain blood glucose and carbohydrate oxidation. The effect of glycogen status before beginning the exercise bout remains an undetermined factor. Widrick and colleagues (115) had cyclists complete 70 km (43.5 mi) self-paced time trials under four different conditions: (1) high intramuscular glycogen and carbohydrate beverage; (2) high intramuscular glycogen and noncaloric beverage; (3) low intramuscular glycogen and carbohydrate beverage; (4) low intramuscular glycogen and noncaloric beverage (115). The carbohydrate drink was ingested at the onset of exercise and every 10 km (6.2 mi) afterward, providing 116 ± 6 g carbohydrate per exercise trial. Carbohydrate administration adequately maintained blood glucose, while blood glucose declined significantly under the noncaloric conditions. Over the final 14% of the time trial (9.8 km [6.1 mi]), power output and pace were significantly less in the low glycogen and noncaloric condition compared with the other three conditions (figure 10.3a and b). Thus, baseline glycogen levels appear to be an important consideration before prolonged exercise, because carbohydrate

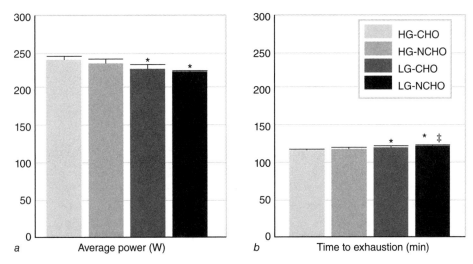

FIGURE 10.3   Effect of preexercise glycogen status and carbohydrate availability on power output (*a*) and time to exhaustion (*b*). Delivery of carbohydrate during exercise did not improve performance when muscle glycogen was high but did significantly improve performance when muscle glycogen was low before the start of the exercise bout, indicating the importance of starting exercise or competition with high glycogen levels.

* = Both LG-CHO (low levels of muscle glycogen preexercise with a carbohydrate beverage consumed before and during exercise) and LG-NCHO (low levels of muscle glycogen preexercise and a noncarbohydrate beverage consumed before and during exercise) had lower average power output and greater time to exhaustion when compared with HG-CHO (high levels of muscle glycogen preexercise and a carbohydrate beverage consumed before and during exercise).

‡ = LG-NCHO time to exhaustion was significantly greater than HG-NCHO.

Data from Widrick et al. (1993).

delivery during exercise did not improve performance when muscle glycogen was high but did significantly improve performance when muscle glycogen was low before the beginning of the exercise bout. Additionally, the combination of high intramuscular glycogen before the exercise bout and provision of carbohydrate throughout the exercise bout led to the greatest levels of performance.

As seen throughout this discussion, carbohydrate clearly influences performance. Most of these studies used prolonged (120 to 150 minutes) exercise bouts at a moderate intensity (65% to 70% $\dot{V}O_2$max). The results of one study suggested that carbohydrate delivery during a high-intensity intermittent running test of trained field players can also increase performance (84). In this study, subjects received either a 6.9% carbohydrate solution or a noncaloric placebo before exercise at a dose of 5 ml/kg body weight, as well as 2 ml/kg body weight every 15 minutes throughout exercise. The athletes who received carbohydrate were able to exercise significantly longer than the placebo group (84). Another study showed that a carbohydrate-gel preparation helped soccer players maintain blood glucose and enhanced performance during a high-intensity intermittent run compared with a placebo (86).

In summary, a great deal of research supports the notion that carbohydrate ingestion during exercise can sustain blood glucose levels, spare glycogen (119), and promote greater levels of performance (37, 84). Several reviews deal with this topic in more detail (33, 64, 65).

Providing Carbohydrate and Protein During Aerobic Endurance Exercise

In recent years, studies have examined the addition of protein to carbohydrate during aerobic endurance exercise. Initial findings suggested that the addition of protein or amino acids may facilitate improved performance and may help promote recovery or prevent the amount of damage that occurs to the exercising muscle tissue. In one study, participants completed 3 hours of cycling at 45% to 75% $\dot{V}O_2$max, followed by a time-to-exhaustion trial at 85% $\dot{V}O_2$max. During each session, participants consumed a placebo, a 7.75% carbohydrate solution, or a solution of 7.75% carbohydrate and 1.94% protein. Although the carbohydrate group increased time to exhaustion versus the placebo, the addition of protein resulted in even greater performance (56).

Saunders and colleagues (94) examined the effect of ingesting a carbohydrate and protein combination on performance and changes in muscle damage. Subjects completed an exhaustive bout of exercise at 75% $\dot{V}O_2$max before resting for 12 to 15 hours and then completed a second exhaustive exercise bout at 85% $\dot{V}O_2$max. Throughout both exercise bouts, cyclists ingested a consistent amount of either a 7.3% carbohydrate solution or a solution of 7.3% carbohydrate and 1.8% protein every 15 minutes. Immediately after exercise, they ingested identical solutions at a dose of 10 ml/kg body weight. Each group ingested identical amounts of carbohydrate, but energy intake was slightly different (because of the extra calories provided by the added protein). With the combination of carbohydrate and protein, performance (time taken to reach exhaustion) increased by 29% after the first bout of exercise and by 40% after the second bout (figure 10.4). Markers of muscle damage were also 83% lower, suggesting that the carbohydrate and protein combination, or the higher total calorie intake, helped attenuate the muscle damage associated with prolonged and exhaustive exercise (94).

The same group reported similar performance increases when subjects ingested a carbohydrate and protein combination in a gel composition rather than a liquid solution (95). Finally, Koopman and colleagues (74) recruited ultra-endurance athletes to compare the effect of consuming carbohydrate alone or a combination of carbohydrate and protein for changes in protein turnover and recovery after 6 hours of aerobic endurance exercise. With carbohydrate alone, **protein balance** became negative, which suggests that **protein breakdown** (likely muscle) was occurring at a rate greater than **protein synthesis**. Protein balance is generally defined as the balance between protein synthesis and protein breakdown. If rates of protein synthesis are greater than those of protein breakdown, protein balance is positive. When

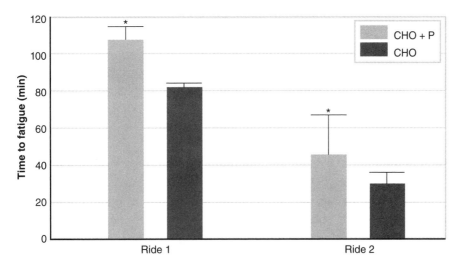

FIGURE 10.4 Time to fatigue during two rides to exhaustion with consumption of either carbohydrate or carbohydrate and protein. Ride 1 was at 75% VO$_2$max. Ride 2 was at 85% VO$_2$max, approximately 12 to 15 hours later. Supplementation with carbohydrate and protein every 15 minutes during exercise resulted in significantly greater performance during two exhaustion rides at 75% and 85% VO$_2$max. Key outcomes from this study indicated that a carbohydrate and protein solution may improve performance. Total calories were not controlled for, however, so it was unclear whether the increased total calories or addition of whey protein made the difference.

* = Time to exhaustion was significantly greater for the CHO and P (carbohydrate and protein) group when directly compared with the CHO (carbohydrate-only) group.

Data from Saunders, Kane, and Todd (2004).

protein was added to the carbohydrate in this study, net protein breakdown was reduced, and overall protein balance remained negative. The authors concluded that combined ingestion of protein and carbohydrate improves net protein balance at rest as well as during exercise and postexercise recovery (74).

In summary, the results from several studies (56, 74, 94) provide evidence that combining carbohydrate with protein before or after prolonged bouts of exercise can facilitate greater performance, and other studies (74, 94) show that this combination also reduces muscle damage.

Postexercise Considerations of Nutrient Intake and Recovery

Among studies on the various aspects of nutrient timing, postexercise investigations comprise most of the scientific literature. Collective findings from these studies suggest that various nutritional strategies can optimize specific aspects of the recovery process. Throughout this chapter and others, the importance of maintaining maximal glycogen levels is evident. Additionally, much interest exists in determining the extent to which providing certain nutrients (and in certain amounts or combinations) in the postexercise period will affect muscle protein balance. Finally, several studies have used prolonged resistance training programs with various nutrient timing strategies to determine the changes in resistance training adaptations such as improved strength and power as well as body composition parameters (1, 27, 36, 52, 96).

Carbohydrate and Glycogen Resynthesis

The recovery and maintenance of optimal levels of muscle glycogen are a key consideration for almost any type of athlete. A consistent finding in the literature is that athletes who rapidly ingest modest to high amounts of carbohydrates at hourly intervals (1.2 to 1.6 g carbohydrate per kilogram body weight) within the first few hours after completing a training bout or competition can stimulate rapid restoration of lost muscle glycogen (18, 19). Initial research first demonstrated that ingesting 1.5 g carbohydrate per kilogram body weight within 30 minutes after exercise promoted greater resynthesis of muscle glycogen than when carbohydrate is delayed by as little as 2 hours (54). Although many studies continue to explore the mechanisms associated with these increases, research has revealed that exercise stimulates insulin-independent increases of glucose uptake into skeletal muscle and enhances the muscle fiber's sensitivity to the hormone insulin, which increases markedly after carbohydrate ingestion (54). Multiple studies have agreed that solid or liquid forms of carbohydrate yield similar rates of glycogen resynthesis (69, 91, 105). Moreover, high levels of fructose ingestion are not advised because this form of carbohydrate is associated with lower levels of glycogen resynthesis than other forms of simple carbohydrate mainly because of the need for fructose to be transported first to the liver for conversion into glucose (24). An important consideration, which is highlighted in figure 10.5, is that delaying carbohydrate ingestion by as little as 2 hours can reduce muscle glycogen resynthesis by 50% (54).

If glycogen depletion occurs, which typically results from prolonged-duration (>90 minutes) moderate-intensity exercise (65% to 85% $\dot{V}O_2$max) but can also result from shorter durations of higher intensity or situations in which the athlete began the workout with less than maximal muscle glycogen levels, an aggressive regimen of carbohydrate administration is necessary. A carbohydrate intake of at least 0.6 to 1.0 g per kilogram body weight per hour during the first 30 minutes and again every 2 hours for the next 4 to 6 hours, can adequately replace glycogen stores (57, 60), though perhaps not optimally. A 165-pound (75 kg) athlete, for example, should ingest 45 to 75 g carbohydrate within 30 minutes of completing exercise and an identical dose every 2 hours after exercise for the next 4 to 6 hours.

Additional strategies have been investigated, and a slightly more aggressive approach has shown that maximal glycogen resynthesis rates can

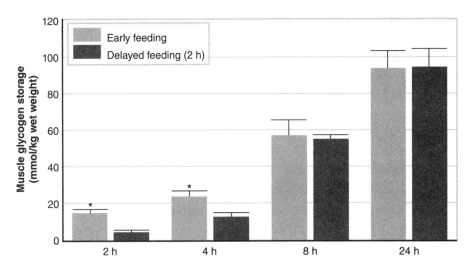

FIGURE 10.5 Postexercise glycogen values after early feeding of carbohydrate or feeding delayed by 2 hours. During short-term recovery (<4 hours), early feeding had a significant effect on recovery of muscle glycogen. An important point of emphasis is that if recovery is delayed by several more hours, immediate intake provides no further effect on glycogen recovery if total carbohydrate intake meets recommended guidelines. This finding demonstrates that early feedings replace glycogen faster, although this intake is not as important if the athlete does not need to perform again within 4 to 6 hours and successfully consumes the necessary amounts of carbohydrate in the diet.

* = Early feeding resulted in significantly greater muscle glycogen levels than delayed feeding.

Data from Ivy (1998).

be achieved if 1.2 g carbohydrate per kilogram body weight per hour is consumed every 30 minutes over a period of 3.5 hours (57, 112). Consequently, the most current and practical recommendation is for athletes to have frequent (every 1 to 2 hours) feedings of carbohydrate in high amounts over the 4 to 6 hours after exercise to ensure recovery of muscle and liver glycogen (66, 105).

An important consideration connected with these studies, however, is the practicality associated with the athlete's immediate need to recover. For example, if an athlete is participating in a sporting activity that requires a follow-up performance within this 2- to 4-hour time period (e.g., track and field events that have preliminary heats and semifinal and final heats, rugby 7s tournaments), then findings from these studies are of the utmost importance. If, however, the athlete does not need to recover in less than 4 hours, other studies illustrate that eating high-carbohydrate meals and snacks at regular intervals (but independent of distinct timing benchmarks) can also result in maximal muscle glycogen levels. Research has shown that maximal glycogen levels are restored within 24 hours if optimal levels of dietary carbohydrate are available (typically around 8 g carbohydrate per kilogram body weight per day) and the degree of glycogen depletion is not too severe (69). Another study suggested a carbohydrate intake of 9 to 10 g per kilogram body weight per day for athletes completing intense exercise bouts on consecutive days (83). Also, providing more immediate feedings in the form of carbohydrate may help to alter inflammatory or proteolytic (breakdown of protein) cascades or other untoward events that will ultimately delay optimal recovery in an exercising athlete.

Carbohydrate With Protein and Glycogen Resynthesis

The addition of protein to carbohydrate continues to command interest and has evolved into a dynamic area of research; studies suggest that this combination may heighten recovery of muscle glycogen muscle damage, particularly if the carbohydrate intake is less than 1.2 g per kilogram body weight per hour in the initial refeeding window.

Ivy and colleagues (55) instructed cyclists to complete a 2.5-hour bout of intense cycling before ingesting a supplement immediately after exercise and 2 hours postexercise. The aim was to determine whether the combination of carbohydrate, protein, and fat promoted greater restoration of muscle glycogen. Therefore, three variations were studied: (1) a small amount of carbohydrate combined with protein and fat (80 g carbohydrate, 28 g protein, 6 g fat), (2) a small amount of carbohydrate combined with fat (80 g carbohydrate, 6 g fat), and (3) a high amount of carbohydrate combined with fat (108 g carbohydrate, 6 g fat). Glycogen levels were similar between the two carbohydrate and fat conditions (low amount of carbohydrate and high amount of carbohydrate), but muscle glycogen levels were significantly greater in the carbohydrate, protein, and fat treatment. The authors concluded that a carbohydrate, protein, and fat supplement may be more effective because of a greater insulin response (54, 60, 120). Follow-up research compared the rates of muscle glycogen resynthesis after ingesting a modest amount of carbohydrate (1.2. g carbohydrate per kilogram body weight per hour), a high amount of carbohydrate (1.6 g carbohydrate per kilogram body weight per hour), a modest amount of carbohydrate (1.2 g carbohydrate per kilogram body weight per hour) combined with a modest dose of protein (0.4 g protein per kilogram body weight per hour), and a high dose of carbohydrate (1.6 g carbohydrate per kilogram body weight per hour) combined with a modest dose of protein (0.4 g protein per kilogram body weight per hour) (60). Results indicated that providing carbohydrate intake after exercise rapidly stimulates rates of muscle glycogen synthesis. Additionally, ingesting higher amounts of carbohydrate (1.6 vs. 1.2 g carbohydrate per kilogram body weight per hour) stimulated higher rates of muscle glycogen resynthesis. Adding a small amount of protein to moderate, but not higher, amounts of carbohydrate appears to stimulate greater rates of muscle glycogen resynthesis when compared with moderate carbohydrate ingestion alone. In summary, this study provides valuable advice to guide coaches and athletes regarding ingesting

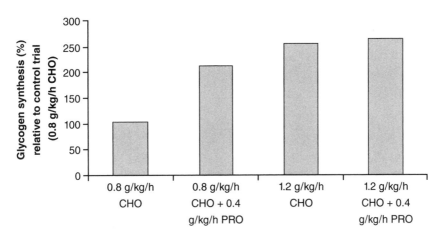

FIGURE 10.6   The rate of muscle glycogen synthesis after ingestion of various carbohydrate and carbohydrate–protein beverages. The synthesis rate for a drink that contains 0.8 g of carbohydrate per kilogram of body weight per hour is set at 100%, and all other synthesis rates are expressed relative to this baseline.

PRO = protein.

Reprinted by permission from A.E. Jeukendrup and M. Gleeson, *Sport Nutrition*, 3rd ed. (Champaign, IL: Human Kinetics, 2019), 165.

greater amounts of carbohydrate in the postexercise period to stimulate the fastest rates of muscle glycogen resynthesis, but if higher amounts of carbohydrate cannot be delivered (lack of access, carbohydrate taste fatigue), then adding a small amount of protein to lower amounts of carbohydrate can also stimulate elevated rates of muscle glycogen resynthesis (see figure 10.6).

Separate studies by Berardi and colleagues (5, 6) and Tarnopolsky and colleagues (104) had cyclists complete exercise bouts of 60 and 90 minutes, respectively, on separate occasions before ingesting either carbohydrate and protein or carbohydrate only. Both research teams concluded that carbohydrate ingestion increased muscle glycogen compared with placebo (6, 104). In addition to greater glycogen levels found in the 2006 study by Berardi and colleagues (6), their later work also reported increased levels of performance and work output (5) when the carbohydrate and protein combination was consumed postexercise. Furthermore, increasing the availability of the essential amino acids, possibly the branched-chain amino acids in particular, may influence the recovery process by optimizing protein synthesis and glycogen synthesis after exercise (15, 54, 55, 104, 120), but more research is needed to solidify these recommendations and its effect on both performance and recovery. An important practical point for an athlete or coach relative to promoting optimal glycogen recovery should be the time available before a subsequent training session or competition.

In summary, clear evidence exists that ingestion of carbohydrate as a single meal (1.5 g carbohydrate per kilogram body weight within 30 minutes after exercise) or as frequent feedings (0.6 to 1.2 g carbohydrate per kilogram body weight per hour every 30 to 60 minutes for up to 3 to 6 hours) can result in rapid restoration of muscle glycogen levels. Furthermore, the addition of protein to carbohydrate has been shown to result in greater glycogen resynthesis (and greater protein synthesis), but overall the absolute amount of carbohydrate ingested is the primary factor that facilitates recovery of muscle glycogen.

Nutrient Timing, Resistance Training, and Strength and Power Performance

Interest in the timing of nutrients surrounding resistance exercise has also begun to accumulate. These studies have explored how providing nutrients (carbohydrate and protein) during resistance exercise may alter muscle protein balance, anabolic hormone changes in the blood, recovery of muscle damage, inflammation or oxidative stresses, and modulation of strength or performance (3, 10-12, 45). Although this area of research continues to develop, nutrient timing strategies may be warranted for their ability to affect adaptations to resistance training or for athletes who desire to gain strength, power, or size.

Nutrient Intake Before and After Resistance Training

For many years, preexercise nutrient administration focused on delivering carbohydrate sources at various points before the start of exercise. Most of this initial research centered on aerobic endurance exercise, specifically cycling. In recent years, researchers have begun to explore the potential of ingesting protein, amino acids, or both (and sometimes in combination with carbohydrate) before exercise to enhance training adaptations to resistance exercise and to modulate the process of recovery to damaged muscle tissue.

Carbohydrate supplementation before resistance exercise is commonly advocated because of the known patterns of carbohydrate use that are observed in response to resistance exercise (85, 92). Although studies have clearly reported that resistance training can decrease intramuscular glycogen stores, the extent to which muscle glycogen is depleted is less than what is commonly observed for prolonged endurance exercise. But when carbohydrate supplementation was provided before resistance exercise, most studies have not reported an improvement in performance (31, 45, 78). When carbohydrate (35 g sucrose) and essential amino acids (6 g) were provided in combination either immediately before or immediately after the resistance training bout, ingestion immediately beforehand increased levels of muscle protein synthesis to a greater extent (110). A few years later, Fujita and investigators (42) completed a similar study using a slightly different isotope model and concluded that although rates of muscle protein synthesis were elevated, the timing of nutrient delivery did not affect the outcome. Later, the same authors compared the changes in muscle protein metabolism after ingesting 20 g whey protein immediately before, or immediately after, a single bout of resistance exercise. They found that whey protein ingestion (before or after) but not timing significantly increased the rate of muscle protein synthesis (107). Collectively, results from these two studies suggest that pre- or postexercise whey protein ingestion can stimulate significantly greater levels of muscle protein synthesis. But how these acute changes in protein synthesis relate to chronic adaptations, such as hypertrophy, has not been well established.

For athletes who are performing resistance training, increases in strength, power, or lean muscle mass are often the primary desired outcomes. A study by Kraemer and colleagues (75) suggested that preexercise ingestion of a multinutrient compound may modulate performance during explosive, powerful movements. In a double-blind format, subjects ingested a 25 kcal multivitamin mineral supplement containing 3 g creatine and other bioactives (e.g., 70 mg caffeine, 2 g arginine) or an isoenergetic maltodextrin placebo for seven days before reporting for two consecutive days of resistance training (75). On both exercise days, they ingested the supplement 30 minutes before the exercise bout. When compared with the placebo, the multinutrient supplement significantly improved vertical jump power and the number of repetitions performed at 80% 1RM while also increasing serum levels of hormones closely linked to muscle hypertrophy and enhanced training adaptations (i.e., growth hormone and free and total testosterone) (75). In this respect, multi-ingredient preworkout supplements (MIPS) such as those used in the study by Kraemer and colleagues have increased in popularity. Many of these formulations contain various blends or combinations of ingredients that have been purported to enhance performance. A narrative review by Harty (48) concluded that acute dosing of various MIPS can increase many indicators of performance and mood, whereas studies involving several weeks of exercise training and dosing differences are less clear and require more investigation.

Although acute studies provide detailed information about immediate responses, the additive effect of nutrient provision and several weeks of following a resistance training program are of the greatest practical interest. A small number of studies have used heavy resistance training programs over 8- to 12-week periods in conjunction with nutrient timing to determine the changes in strength and body composition. Longer-duration studies are more applicable to real-life training cycles in which athletes engage in preseason training and then lighten their training load during the season in favor of skill work and simulation of game-time situations. For example, Coburn and colleagues (23) reported that supplementation of 26 g whey protein and 6 g leucine before and after eight weeks of unilateral lower body resistance training resulted in greater increases in maximal strength (30.3% increase) over a six-week period than 26 g carbohydrate alone (22.4% increase). Similar conclusions were reached by Andersen and colleagues (1), who had healthy males resistance train for 14 weeks while supplementing with either 25 g protein or 25 g carbohydrate immediately before and again immediately after each workout. Although performance differences were modest, greater increases in markers of muscle growth were more apparent in the group that supplemented with protein.

Further research has examined the effects of protein (21, 117) taken before and after 8 and 10 weeks of resistance training, respectively. The Candow study (21) compared equal doses of whey protein and soy protein taken before and after each resistance training bout over an eight-week resistance training period. Both forms of supplementation increased strength and lean muscle mass when compared with a placebo, but no differences were found between the two sources of protein. Similarly, Willoughby and colleagues (117) had subjects resistance train four days per week for 10 weeks and ingest either 20 g protein or 20 g carbohydrate before and after each exercise bout for a daily total of 40 g. Impressively, protein supplementation increased body weight, lean muscle mass, strength, and several markers of muscle hypertrophy. Combined, these studies indicate that providing protein before and after resistance exercise is associated with greater improvements in strength, lean muscle mass, body fat percentage, serum levels of important anabolic (muscle building) hormones, and intramuscular markers of muscle hypertrophy. The additional impact of carbohydrate on these effects is somewhat unclear.

Cribb and Hayes (27) also investigated the effect of nutrient timing strategies over several weeks of supplementation and resistance training. Figures 10.7a and b show some of the results. Participants ingested equal quantities of a supplement containing protein, creatine, and carbohydrate either immediately before and immediately after each workout or in the morning and evening of each workout day. Significantly greater increases in lean muscle mass, 1RM strength, and type II muscle fiber cross-sectional area, as well as higher muscle creatine and glycogen levels, were seen when the supplements were consumed immediately before and after workouts (27). All these adaptations may allow an athlete to train harder over time, thereby contributing to better performance or greater resilience to training stress and injuries. The benefits gained, however, depend on the athlete; athletes in weight-restricted or aesthetic sports may need to consider whether strength gains are worth the increase in body weight.

In a follow-up to this study by Hoffman and colleagues (52), participants ingested 42 g of a hydrolyzed collagen before and after workouts over the course of several weeks. The authors reported no difference in strength, power, or body composition based on the timing strategies—an effect suggested to be linked to the already high protein intake of their participants, the lack of any carbohydrate source, and the relatively low quality of protein provided as part of the supplementation regimen.

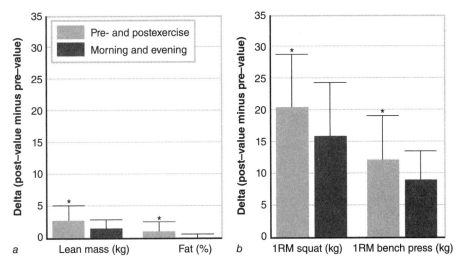

FIGURE 10.7 Effect of nutrient timing on resistance training adaptations. Nutrient ingestion (protein, creatine, and glucose) occurred either in the morning and evening on workout days or immediately pre- and postexercise. Pre and post ingestion was responsible for significant improvements in lean muscle mass, percent body fat (*a*), 1RM squat, and 1RM bench press (*b*). This investigation was the first resistance training study to focus solely on nutrient timing and show greater body composition adaptations in addition to performance improvements.

* = Different from morning and evening.

Data from Cribb and Hayes (2006).

Ingestion of essential amino acids or a whole protein source (e.g., whey), alone or in combination with carbohydrate, within 30 minutes before a bout of resistance training will significantly increase muscle protein synthesis (107, 108, 110). A complete protein source such as whey protein, however, increases protein synthesis to a similar degree whether it is ingested 1 hour before or 1 hour after a single bout of resistance exercise (17, 107). Adding carbohydrate (e.g., 35 g sucrose) to essential amino acids (e.g., 6 g) immediately before a resistance exercise will heighten the anabolic environment when compared with no feeding or carbohydrate-only feeding, and the magnitude of these outcomes are similar or greater to what may be observed if identical nutrients are consumed immediately postexercise (42, 110). Again, though, note that these acute changes in protein synthesis do not necessarily translate to chronic training responses.

The source of protein continues to be an area of inquiry, and without question, most of the supportive evidence is available with milk protein sources, in particular whey protein. Ingestion of soy protein has been shown to promote increases in lean muscle mass and strength (21), but the magnitude of observed adaptations is likely going to be less than if a whey protein source is consumed. Changes after only one bout of exercise are mechanistically important, but prolonged studies involving several weeks (8 to 12 weeks) of supplementation and resistance training reveal that any form of nutrients provided before and after exercise leads to significant improvements in body weight, lean muscle mass, body fat percentage, cross-sectional area, strength, and myofibrillar content (21, 23, 27, 75, 117).

Nutrient Intake During Resistance Training

A small number of studies have examined nutrient ingestion during resistance exercise or strength and power events. As with the aerobic endurance exercise studies, the data suggest that providing carbohydrate, or a combination of carbohydrate and protein, may help sustain muscle glycogen (45), prevent increases in serum cortisol and urinary markers of muscle breakdown (10, 12), and promote muscle hypertrophy (11).

Haff and colleagues (45) had resistance-trained males ingest either a noncaloric placebo or carbohydrate at a dose of 1 g/kg body weight before as well as during (every 10 minutes) a single bout of lower body resistance training. Muscle biopsies during each condition revealed that muscle glycogen levels were 49% higher when carbohydrate was consumed in comparison with when no carbohydrate was consumed. This initial study suggested that significant decreases in muscle glycogen were found throughout the resistance exercise bout and that providing carbohydrate during resistance exercise successfully promoted recovery and an overall greater volume of training (45). During competition in strength and power sports that last for extended periods and require high caloric expenditures, maintaining higher muscle glycogen levels could potentially attenuate any performance decrements later in the competition that could result in part from decreases in glycogen.

Later, researchers (11, 12) examined the extent to which a carbohydrate and protein combination could mitigate changes in protein degradation in the blood and urine during a single bout of resistance exercise. Thirty-two participants completed a 60-minute bout of resistance training while consuming either a 6% carbohydrate solution, a 6% carbohydrate and 6 g essential amino acid solution, or a placebo beverage. Blood cortisol levels (a crude indicator of protein breakdown) increased 105% in the placebo group from baseline, whereas increases in the carbohydrate and the carbohydrate and essential amino acid groups were only 11% and 7% elevated from baseline levels, respectively. Further, urinary levels of 3-methyl-histidine (an additional marker of muscle protein breakdown) decreased by 27% in the carbohydrate and essential amino acid group but increased by 56% in the placebo group (11, 12). Beelen and colleagues (4) presented similar conclusions when participants ingested a bolus of carbohydrate and protein before beginning a 2-hour bout of resistance training and at 15-minute intervals during the training session. The carbohydrate and protein combination lowered the rate of protein breakdown by 8.4% ± 3.6% and increased the protein synthesis rate by 49% ± 22%, resulting in a fivefold increase in protein balance.

Although immediate changes (in blood and urine markers) support the ingestion of a carbohydrate and protein combination during a single resistance training bout, the cumulative effect of this practice remained to be determined. Over a 12-week period, Bird and colleagues (11) had participants ingest a 6% carbohydrate solution, a 6% carbohydrate solution and 6 g of an essential amino acid solution, or a placebo during resistance training sessions. Serum insulin and cortisol, urinary markers of protein breakdown, and muscle cross-sectional area were measured, and as reported previously, carbohydrate and essential amino acid ingestion decreased protein breakdown by 26%, whereas the placebo group experienced a 52% increase in the same markers. Interestingly, muscle cross-sectional areas of the type I, IIa, and IIx fibers were increased with carbohydrate and essential amino acid ingestion compared with the placebo. The authors concluded that over a 12-week period ingesting a carbohydrate and essential amino acid combination during regular resistance training optimizes the balance between muscle growth and muscle loss, resulting in significant increases in the size of muscle fibers (11). Overall, the research supports the conclusion that the intake of carbohydrate alone or, perhaps more important, the combination of carbohydrate and protein during resistance training may help promote greater levels of muscle glycogen, increase muscle cross-sectional area, and decrease protein breakdown (10-12, 45).

Posttraining Nutrition and Protein Balance

A single bout of resistance training modestly stimulates protein synthesis but also stimulates protein breakdown, resulting in an overall negative protein balance after exercise (88, 89) in untrained individuals. As training continues, this balance shifts to the point that protein balance after an acute bout of resistance training (without provision of any form of nutrients before or after exercise) is neutral, meaning that no appreciable growth or breakdown of muscle is occurring (88). Providing amino acids (either by infusion or, more practically, through ingestion of amino acids as a dietary supplement, snack, or meal) increases plasma amino acid concentrations at rest or after resistance exercise (9, 15) and leads to increases in muscle protein synthesis. Consequently, increasing the concentration and availability of essential amino acids in the blood is an important consideration when attempting to promote increases in lean tissue and improve body composition with resistance training (9, 109).

A large dose of carbohydrate (100 g) 1 hour after completion of an intense bout of lower body resistance training causes only marginal improvements in the balance between protein synthesis and protein breakdown, resulting in an overall net negative protein balance (14). Regarding protein (muscle) changes, no studies have found carbohydrate to be detrimental, but it certainly is not the ideal nutrient (in isolation) to consume after resistance exercise. Its inclusion, however, is important for stimulating glycogen resynthesis and enhancing palatability (55, 104). Of primary interest has been the delivery of free amino acids (often just the essential amino acids) in dosages ranging from 6 to 40 g. These dosages have consistently been shown to stimulate rates of muscle protein synthesis (15, 80), and some evidence exists that adding carbohydrate to them may enhance this effect (110, 111). Within the first hour or two after competition, depending on the sport and the amount of time an athlete competes, consuming a combination of carbohydrate and protein can help facilitate glycogen restoration, minimize cortisol, promote protein synthesis, and facilitate tissue repair.

Consuming amino acids after resistance training (whether immediately after or up to 3 hours later) can increase muscle protein synthesis and blunt the increases commonly seen in protein breakdown (15, 80, 89). The optimal time point for supplementation has not yet been demonstrated and may not exist for all situations, but many sport nutrition researchers advocate consuming nutrients (whether just carbohydrate, just protein, or a combination) at some point relatively soon after completion of the exercise bout (55, 111). Notably, conclusions drawn from a combination of scientific studies suggest that when amino acids were provided with or without carbohydrate immediately, 1 hour, 2 hours, or 3 hours after exercise, similar increases in protein balance occurred (15, 55, 109-111).

To summarize, at present there is no universal recommendation about the dosage and ratio of essential amino acids and carbohydrate to apply to produce a maximal increase in protein balance. Studies using similar research methodologies and analytical techniques to measure protein kinetics during resistance exercise have used several nutrient combinations during the 2-hour postexercise period. Six grams of essential amino acids alone, 6 g essential amino acids and 6 g nonessential amino acids, 12 g essential amino acids alone, 17.5 g whey protein, 20 g casein protein, 20 g whey protein, 40 g of a mixed amino acid solution (essential and nonessential amino acids), and 40 g essential amino acids all have resulted in an increase in protein synthesis and protein balance (9, 109, 111).

Much research has addressed the effect of different types and dosages of protein (as either free amino acids or whole protein sources) on changes in muscle protein balance after resistance exercise. Results from these studies have led to practical recommendations that athletes ingest some form of nutrients as soon as possible after completing an exercise bout, and one study suggested that early consumption may help promote increases in muscle glycogen (54). Note that waiting to consume nutrients postexercise appears to provide no advantage.

Posttraining Supplementation and Training Adaptations

The postexercise considerations discussed thus far center on restoring muscle glycogen and the immediate changes in muscle protein synthesis during exercise, specifically resistance training. Although an optimal level of muscle glycogen is extremely important to an athlete who participates in a prolonged, continuous event that challenges muscle glycogen stores, it is less important for an athlete who resistance trains for 45 to 90 minutes to promote maximal strength and body composition changes. The immediate change in muscle protein synthesis after a bout of resistance training is much more important for a resistance training athlete than glycogen resynthesis, but the results from only one exercise session do not always extrapolate to what would occur after several weeks of resistance training and supplementation.

Researchers have investigated the effect of varying combinations of carbohydrate and protein after each exercise bout (1 to 3 hours postexercise) during resistance training over the course of several weeks (21, 27-29, 47, 72, 73, 106, 116, 117). As before, individual results from these studies differ, but the collective findings support the rationale for postexercise administration of carbohydrate and protein to facilitate improvements in body composition and strength. Staples and colleagues (101) suggested that the addition of carbohydrate offered no greater benefit toward improving strength and lean muscle mass accretion. Figures 10.8 and 10.9 show the changes in body composition and strength performance from the Cribb and Hayes (27) investigation using postexercise supplementation. Overall, results from these studies suggest that when 20 to 75 g protein is ingested alone or in conjunction with similar amounts of carbohydrate during resistance training, increases in strength and body composition can result. Finally, impressive amounts of popularity and

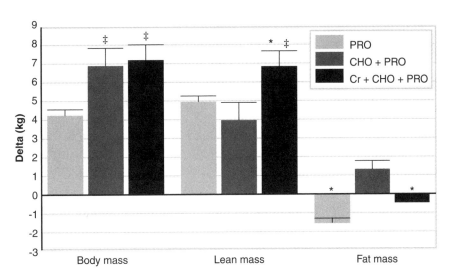

FIGURE 10.8 Changes in body weight, lean muscle mass, and fat mass after 10 weeks of resistance training with postexercise supplementation. These results show that long-term consistent nutrient administration after resistance exercise may favorably affect body composition.

* = Significantly different from CHO plus PRO.

‡ = Significantly different from PRO.

Data from Cribb and Hayes (2006).

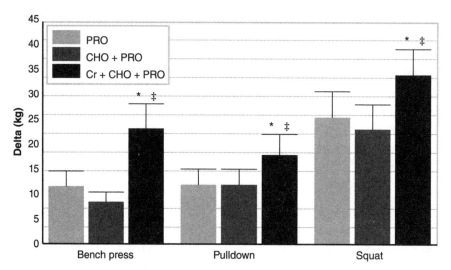

FIGURE 10.9   Delta value for changes in 1RM values for bench press, lat pulldown, and squat exercises after 10 weeks of resistance training with postexercise supplementation.

* = Significantly different from CHO and PRO.

‡ = Significantly different from PRO.

Data from Cribb and Hayes (2006).

fanfare arose surrounding the perceived need to ingest nutrients as soon as possible to deliver nutrients during a key "anabolic window." Critical reviews by Aragon and Schoenfeld (2) and Schoenfeld, Aragon, and Krieger (97) have since emphasized that employing this strategy for recreational bodybuilders may not afford the remarkable advantages initially considered, although no evidence exists to refute the potential for timing to heighten adaptations. Furthermore, as the level of training volume and specialization of training increases, it has been suggested that the potential benefit for timing may increase, but more research is needed to substantiate this consideration. Further research by Schoenfeld and colleagues (96) had resistance-trained males ingest a protein supplement either immediately before or immediately after their training bouts and determined that the timing of administration had no effect on strength and body composition changes.

Summary tables listing results from these studies are available in a comprehensive review devoted to the topic of nutrient timing (70, 71).

Whey and Casein

As with carbohydrate, researchers have investigated the effect of various protein sources on digestive and amino acid kinetics and resistance training adaptations (13, 32, 72, 73). In two studies, French researchers were the first to report on the differences in digestive and absorptive properties of the two primary forms of milk protein, whey, and casein. Their studies illustrated that whey protein is digested and absorbed into the bloodstream at a much greater rate than casein protein. This difference was associated with the greater propensity of whey protein (when compared with casein) to increase protein synthesis. Alternatively, casein protein was reported to be responsible for preventing the breakdown of muscle tissue, whereas whey protein exerted little to no influence over this parameter. When the two types of protein were compared in a head-to-head fashion, casein protein appeared to result in a greater overall improvement in whole-body protein balance (13, 32). Although whey and casein are commonly classified as "fast" and "slow," studies incorporating plant protein sources such as soy characterize the digestion speed of this protein as "intermediate" (87). Although amino acid uptake holds merit, stimulation of muscle protein synthesis or adaptations to weeks of training have greater practical meaning. In this respect, Tang and colleagues (103) examined the acute changes in muscle protein synthesis after ingestion of a single 20 to 25 g dose of a whey hydrolysate, micellar casein, and soy isolate. At rest and in response to acute exercise, whey protein stimulated the sharpest increases in muscle protein synthesis.

Wilkinson and colleagues (116) compared 18 g of a milk protein source with an equal dose of a soy protein source for their ability to increase net muscle protein accretion and protein balance after a single bout of resistance training. They concluded that the milk protein source was responsible for a greater increase in both net protein and muscle protein accretion when compared with soy and that a milk protein source would likely be responsible for an increase in lean muscle mass when combined with resistance training. Moreover, when this acute study was extrapolated over several weeks of training, people who consumed skim milk experienced significantly greater gains in lean muscle mass (47). Kerksick and colleagues (73) examined the influence of a "fast" protein source (40 g whey protein, 5 g glutamine, and 3 g branched-chain amino acids [isoleucine, leucine, valine]) compared with a blend of fast and slow proteins (40 g whey and 8 g casein), ingested postexercise over a 10-week period of resistance training. Subjects who ingested the blend of fast and slow protein showed significantly greater increases in lean muscle mass (+1.8 kg) compared with those who ingested the fast proteins (−0.1 kg). An additional study by this group demonstrated that daily ingestion of a 60 g blend of whey and casein protein over 12 weeks resulted in gains in lean muscle mass (+0.8 to +1.3 kg) similar to those seen in the previous investigation (72).

Creatine

Researchers have also examined adding creatine monohydrate to carbohydrate and protein combinations in subjects participating in a regular resistance training program for up to 10 to 12 weeks (28, 29, 72, 106). Creatine monohydrate is a popular dietary supplement that has been heavily researched for its ability to increase performance and facilitate positive training adaptations (76, 77). Tarnopolsky and colleagues (106) had previously untrained male participants follow an eight-week resistance training program while ingesting on a daily basis, 30 minutes after their assigned workout, either 10 g creatine and 75 g carbohydrate or 10 g protein and 75 g carbohydrate. The creatine and carbohydrate combination resulted in significantly greater gains in body weight (5.4% increase from baseline) than the protein and carbohydrate combination (2.4% increase from baseline). Lean muscle mass, muscle fiber area, 1RM, and isokinetic strength improved in both groups but were not different between the groups. Cribb and colleagues (28, 29) had participants resistance train for 11 weeks while consuming an isocaloric amount of creatine and carbohydrate, creatine and whey protein, whey protein only, or carbohydrate only. When compared with the carbohydrate-only group, all other groups showed greater improvements in maximal strength and muscle hypertrophy, but no differences were seen with the addition of creatine to the supplement.

In contrast, two studies suggest that the addition of creatine to a supplement may promote greater increases in muscle hypertrophy during resistance training over the course of several weeks (28, 72). Over a 10-week period, participants underwent a heavy resistance training program and ingested one of the following isocaloric supplements: protein; protein and carbohydrate; or creatine, protein, and carbohydrate. The investigators found that in contrast to their previous results, the addition of creatine appeared to elicit greater improvements in strength and muscle hypertrophy than the consumption of protein alone or protein and carbohydrate (28). Similarly, Kerksick and colleagues (72) had participants complete 12 weeks of resistance training and ingest a blend of either colostrum or whey or casein protein with or without creatine. Although all groups showed increases in strength and lean muscle mass, the groups ingesting creatine with a protein blend (regardless of the exact composition of the protein source) experienced greater gains in body weight and lean muscle mass. The mixed results from these studies suggest the need for additional research, but most of the available studies do indicate that adding creatine monohydrate to a postexercise regimen of carbohydrate and protein can maximally stimulate improvements in strength and body composition (28, 29, 72). Although creatine supplementation before *or* after exercise is effective, ingesting the creatine postworkout may offer a slightly greater benefit on hypertrophy (22).

Professional Applications

Timed administration of nutrients facilitates physiological adaptations to exercise and can promote optimal health and performance. Nutrient timing recommendations vary for athletes within a particular sport as well as between sports. Considerations will also vary for an individual athlete as demands related to travel, competition, and training change throughout the year. The dynamic nature of nutrient timing makes it important for all athletes and coaches to develop a firm foundation of knowledge regarding energy, macro-nutrient, fluid, and micronutrient consumption.

The current research on nutrient timing gives support to several recom-mendations that athletes can put into practice before, during, and after training and competition.

Before

- Athletes can maximize glycogen stores by following a high-carbohydrate diet (600 to 1,000 g or 8 to 10 g of carbohydrate per kilogram body weight per day) (20, 44, 105).

- A carbohydrate-rich meal 4 hours before exercise may increase perfor-mance, work output, or both (82, 98, 118). In general, athletes should ingest 1 to 4 g carbohydrate per kilogram body weight 1 to 4 hours before aerobic endurance exercise or competition (105).

- The type of carbohydrate consumed 60 minutes before exercise does not appear to have any negative effects on performance or glycemic status and in many cases may increase performance (50). If athletes are particularly sensitive to hypoglycemia, ingesting carbohydrates closer to the start of exercise will help in reducing hypoglycemic symptoms. For some athletes, manipulating the glycemic index of carbohydrate sources may help mitigate symptoms of hypoglycemia. Additionally, a proper warm-up can help restore euglycemia before competition (81).

- The glycemic index of a meal eaten before prolonged exercise does not appear to have a negative effect on performance or use of muscle glycogen (34, 38, 39), although certain carbohydrate sources (e.g., fructose) may have other unintended consequences related to gastro-intestinal upset.

- When combined with a regular resistance training program, ingestion of a combination of carbohydrate and protein or amino acids before and after training leads to improvements in strength, power, body weight, lean muscle mass, and intramuscular markers of muscle growth (23, 27, 75, 117).

During

- For exercise or events lasting longer than 60 minutes, athletes should consume a source of carbohydrate that provides 30 to 60 g carbohydrate per hour, typically by drinking 1 to 2 cups (8 to 16 fluid ounces) of a 6% to 8% carbohydrate solution (6 to 8 g carbohydrate per 100 ml of fluid) every 10 to 15 minutes (66).

- Mixing different forms of carbohydrate has been shown to increase muscle carbohydrate oxidation (58, 59, 61-63), an effect associated with an improvement in time-trial performance (30).

- Glucose, fructose, sucrose, and maltodextrin can be used in combina-tion, but large amounts of fructose are not recommended because of the greater likelihood of gastrointestinal problems.

(continued)

Professional Applications *(continued)*

- Ingesting carbohydrate alone, or in combination with protein, during resistance exercise can increase muscle glycogen stores (45) and facilitate greater training adaptations after acute (4, 10, 12) and prolonged periods of resistance training (11).

After

- Postexercise consumption of carbohydrate should occur within 30 minutes but minimally within 2 hours at a dose of 1.5 g carbohydrate per kilogram body weight to stimulate glycogen resynthesis (54).

- If an athlete does not need to replenish glycogen rapidly for repeated heats, trials, or events, a diet that provides high levels of dietary carbohydrate (>8 g carbohydrate per kilogram body weight per day) is adequate to promote peak levels of muscle glycogen (57, 105).

- Ingesting amino acids, primarily the essential amino acids, immediately after exercise until 3 hours postexercise can stimulate sharp increases in protein synthesis (15, 90, 109). Maximal improvements in muscular strength and body composition during resistance training over several weeks can be achieved by ingestion of a combination of carbohydrate and protein after exercise (73, 106, 117). Adding carbohydrate to protein, however, may not be necessary to promote maximal hypertrophy of skeletal muscle (101).

- The addition of creatine (0.1 g creatine per kilogram body weight per day) to a carbohydrate and protein supplement may facilitate even greater adaptations to resistance training (28, 72), but this finding is not universal (29).

Arguably one of the most important aspects of recovery and subsequent performance for the aerobic endurance athlete is the maintenance of maximal muscle glycogen levels. Although maximizing internal glycogen stores (e.g., liver and muscles) may not enhance maximal work output or speed, it will enable athletes to maintain their pace of training for a longer time. At rest, average intramuscular glycogen levels of trained athletes are adequate to meet the physical demands of events lasting anywhere from 60 to 90 minutes—significantly less than the amount of time needed to complete a marathon or an ultra-endurance event. Athletes can do four main things to maximize glycogen levels and adaptations to training: (1) consume carbohydrate immediately after training to refuel for the next exercise session, (2) load carbohydrate before an event, (3) consume carbohydrate during exercise, and (4) consume sufficient calories to allow optimal rates of adaptations and recovery.

To ensure maximum glycogen before an event, an athlete should consume 8 to 10 g carbohydrate per kilogram body weight per day and get adequate rest (do little or no training) before competition. To optimize carbohydrate use, preexercise meals should be largely composed of high-carbohydrate foods or liquids. This practice becomes even more important when the athlete makes poor recovery efforts (e.g., low dietary carbohydrate intake, failure to rest or reduce training volume, or both). In addition to eating a high-carbohydrate diet and reducing training volume, consuming a high-carbohydrate meal (200-300

g) 4 to 6 hours before exercise helps to maintain maximal muscle and liver glycogen levels.

Athletes who do not ingest an optimal amount of carbohydrate preexercise need to overcome the lack of available carbohydrate by working harder to ingest optimal carbohydrate levels during the first hour of exercise. Although many food choices can provide carbohydrate, athletes need to experiment during training sessions to figure out what foods work for them without causing gastrointestinal distress. Consuming a variety of types of sugar, maltodextrin, sucrose, and fructose, for example, may be more beneficial than consuming one type of sugar. This practice may enhance the amount of carbohydrate that the working muscle can oxidize. In addition to consuming different types of carbohydrate, athletes may benefit from ingesting carbohydrate at frequent intervals throughout exercise rather than a single large dose before exercise.

Results are equivocal whether or not adding protein to carbohydrate consumed during aerobic endurance exercise will enhance performance. Consistent evidence does indicate that this practice can boost recovery and minimize muscle damage to the exercising muscle tissue. Ingestion of protein with and without carbohydrate before or during resistance training sessions is a new area of research, but preliminary results suggest that greater improvements occur in strength, lean muscle mass, body fat percentage, serum levels of important anabolic (muscle-building) hormones, and intramuscular markers of muscle hypertrophy. How these strategies are practically employed across training sessions remain to be determined by athletes.

After aerobic endurance exercise, athletes should consume 1.5 g carbohydrate per kilogram body weight within 30 minutes of completing exercise, or 0.6 to 1.0 g carbohydrate per kilogram body weight per hour during the first 30 minutes and again every 2 hours for the next 4 to 6 hours, to replace glycogen stores adequately (and rapidly). Delaying delivery of nutrients by just 2 hours may cut muscle glycogen resynthesis rates in half.

The postexercise carbohydrate can be either solid or liquid but should not be high in fructose because this form of carbohydrate is associated with lower levels of glycogen resynthesis than other carbohydrate sources.

Athletes may benefit from adding protein to their postexercise carbohydrate meal. The addition of protein has been shown to result in greater glycogen resynthesis (and greater protein synthesis) compared with carbohydrate only. Typical dosages are 1.2 to 1.5 g carbohydrate per kilogram body weight and 0.3 to 0.5 g essential amino acids or whole protein per kilogram body weight. After regular resistance training, a common practice is to ingest a high-quality protein source (e.g., whey, casein, egg) in a dose that provides 10 to 12 g (2 to 4 g leucine) of the essential amino acids within 1 hour after completion of training. The necessity of feeding protein soon after finishing a workout has been an area of intense discussion. Additional research has indicated that athletes should first strive to meet their daily protein needs before placing high levels of importance on feeding protein immediately or soon after a workout. Note, however, that waiting to ingest protein postworkout appears to offer no advantage.

(continued)

Professional Applications *(continued)*

Table 10.1 provides an example of what all these timing recommendations would look like in practice for a 180-pound (82 kg) athlete performing regular aerobic endurance or resistance exercise. All athletes must consider their own training goals and adjust the nutrient timing plan to support those goals.

TABLE 10.1   Simplified Timing Recommendations for Aerobic Endurance and Resistance Athletes

	Aerobic endurance exercise	Resistance training
PREEXERCISE		
2 to 4 h before		
Recommendation	4 g CHO/kg	No specific recommendation
Intake	200-300 g CHO	Maintain continued delivery of carbohydrates
Foods	Whole-wheat bagel or toast, oatmeal, cereal, 24 fl oz (720 ml) sport drink	
30 to 60 min before		
Recommendation	1.2-1.5 g CHO/kg	No recommendation
Intake	60-80 g CHO	Maintain continued delivery of carbohydrates
Foods	Small energy or food bar, sport drink	
DURING EXERCISE		
Recommendation	6%-8% CHO solution	No specific recommendation
Intake	1.5-2 cups (12-16 fl oz [360-480 ml]) every 15-20 min	
Foods	Sport drink, gel packet with water	Sport drink, gel packet with water
POSTEXERCISE		
Recommendation	1.5 g CHO/kg within 30 min *or* 0.6-1.0 g CHO/kg in 30 min and again every 2 h	30-40 g carbohydrate and ~20-25 g protein delivering 8-12 g EAAs
Intake	123 g within 30 min *or* 49-82 g in 30 min and again every 2 h	30-40 g carbohydrate and ~20-25 g protein delivering 8-12 g EAAs
Foods	Sport drinks, bagels, fruits	Sport drinks, bagels, fruits, whey protein

Note: All "intake" values are developed using a 180-pound (82 kg) athlete. CHO = carbohydrate; PRO = protein. Actual amount depends on volume and intensity of training.

Summary Points

- Appropriate incorporation of science-based nutrient timing strategies takes a great deal of work and dedication on the part of the athlete and sometimes the coach or parent. Another key challenge regarding this area of research is that most topics and scenarios are shrouded in many layers of nuance that require practical, untethered attempts at building recommendations.

- The internal supply of carbohydrate is limited and will likely become depleted during any form of exercise at a moderate to high intensity continued for at least 60 to 90 minutes, particularly as duration extends past 90 minutes. For this reason, ingestion of high-carbohydrate meals at regular intervals during the postexercise period is recommended to stimulate maximal increases in muscle glycogen. During exercise, athletes should consume 10 to 15 fluid ounces (300-450 ml) of a carbohydrate–electrolyte solution that delivers 6 to 8 g carbohydrate for every 100 ml fluid (6% to 8% carbohydrate solution) every 15 to 20 minutes to sustain blood glucose levels, which ultimately should deliver 30 to 60 g of carbohydrate per hour. Athletes should consume more if intensity is higher and duration is prolonged.

- Many forms of carbohydrate are acceptable, but fructose is not easily digested and thus not recommended as a primary source because of its known relationship with gastrointestinal distress and low rates of glycogen resynthesis. Combining different forms of carbohydrate for ingestion during exercise is encouraged and may increase the rate of carbohydrate oxidation.

- A small amount of protein (0.15 to 0.25 g/kg body weight) added to carbohydrate at all time points is well tolerated and may facilitate heightened rates of muscle glycogen resynthesis. Maximal muscle protein synthesis can occur when 6 to 20 g of the essential amino acids is ingested within 3 hours (potentially with multiple feedings within this window) of completing a resistance training workout. Over the course of several weeks, postexercise ingestion of protein (0.25-0.30 g per kilogram per dose) is advised. Adding carbohydrate likely will not stimulate further increases in maximal strength and lean muscle mass accretion but may aid in glycogen recovery, attenuation of serum cortisol, and reduction of proteolytic activation.

- Postexercise protein timing considerations should derive their primary basis from the perspective of meeting daily protein needs because additional inquiry into a proverbial anabolic window suggests that timing considerations are less important than once believed.

- Milk protein (e.g., whey and casein) and some plant protein sources (e.g., soy) exhibit different digestion kinetics resulting in differences in delivery of amino acids into the bloodstream, which may affect accretion of lean tissue during resistance training.

- Adding creatine to nutrients in conjunction with regular resistance training may facilitate greater improvements in strength and body composition as compared with no creatine.

- Athletes should focus primarily on adequate availability and delivery of energy through appropriate proportions of the macronutrients (carbohydrate, protein, and fat) before using their financial resources for single ingredients (e.g., creatine monohydrate, essential amino acids) or multi-ingredient formulations. Irrespective of timing, regular snacks or meals should consist of adequate levels of carbohydrate and protein to sustain required work outputs and prompt recovery.

Chapter 11

Consultation and Development of Athlete Plans

Amanda Carlson Phillips, MS, RD, CSSD

The science of sport nutrition has uncovered nutrition and supplement strategies that improve aerobic endurance, speed, strength, focus, and concentration; reduce fatigue; and enhance recovery. But this body of scientific research is useless if athletes do not change their behavior. Therefore, creating a feasible plan that athletes can easily incorporate into their lifestyle is necessary if sound nutrition changes are to be made.

Those working with athletes can use a performance nutrition continuum model (figure 11.1) to build programs using an integrated approach. The concepts behind this approach are assess, educate, and implement. Across each concept is the need to evaluate, isolate, innovate, and then integrate across all levels of the athlete's training.

Providing nutrition advice and orchestrating a sport nutrition program are different. A sport nutrition program has many layers that need to work together. The surface layers encompass education and general guidance, and the center includes specific recommendations that are backed by science and integrated into the athlete's daily routine.

The goal of any nutrition program is to provide athletes with knowledge so that good nutrition practices become second nature, as well as to give them the tools to implement this knowledge. A good plan makes nutrition easy and incorporates foods to choose on days off as well as before, during, and

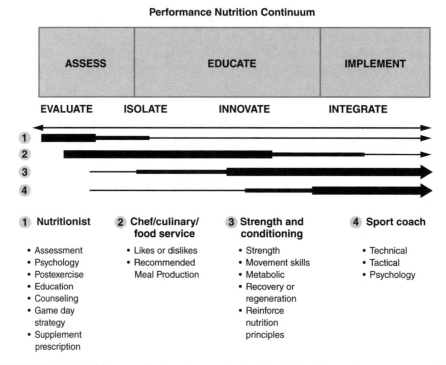

FIGURE 11.1   Many professionals may be involved in implementing a sport nutrition program across all stages of the performance nutrition continuum. The nutritionist, food service staff, strength and conditioning professional, and sport coach are all involved to a greater or lesser degree with each stage of the program. The thickness of the arrows in this figure shows the degree of involvement of each professional.

after practices and then around games, matches, or races. Nutrition should become a component of the athlete's training program, not just something else they need to do.

Providing Nutrition Knowledge

Many fitness professionals (certified personal trainers, conditioning coaches or professionals, athletic trainers, and strength coaches) are knowledgeable about athletes' physiology, the demands of a sport, and the role of nutrition in performance, but most are not qualified or legally allowed to deliver detailed nutrition information. Those who are qualified as **registered dietitians** can deliver personalized and specific nutrition information. Although a dietitian can focus on many specializations, the dietitian who works with athletes should have a background in sport nutrition.

According to the Academy of Nutrition and Dietetics, a **registered dietitian** (RD) or **registered dietitian nutritionist** (RDN) is a food and nutrition expert who has met the following criteria to earn the RDN credential:

- Completed a minimum of a bachelor's degree at a U.S. regionally accredited university or college and course work accredited or approved by the Accreditation Council for Education in Nutrition and Dietetics (ACEND) of the Academy of Nutrition and Dietetics.
- Completed an ACEND-accredited supervised practice program at a health care facility, community agency, or a food service corporation or combined with undergraduate or graduate studies. Typically, a practice program will run 6 to 12 months.
- Passed a national examination administered by the Commission on Dietetic Registration (CDR).
- Completed continuing professional educational requirements to maintain registration.

Many certifications and certifying bodies require that fitness professionals demonstrate a certain level of knowledge of basic nutrition before achieving certification status. This knowledge should equip them with the skills necessary to provide general nutrition recommendations and suggestions to athletes. Athletes should be referred to a registered dietitian, however, when medical nutrition therapy (for a disease state or eating disorder) is required or when the level of nutrition recommendations moves beyond general guidelines and into personalized recommendations. The sidebar lists several common nutrition certifications available in the United States and internationally.

Sport Nutrition Certifications

Board-Certified Specialist in Sports Dietetics (CSSD)

The Academy of Nutrition and Dietetics (AND) has taken steps to help distinguish qualified dietitians most knowledgeable in sport nutrition by creating a specialty certification, CSSD. The CSSD is offered by the Commission on Dietetic Registration (CDR) for registered dietitians who have specialized experience in sport dietetics. Being board certified as a Specialist in Sports Dietetics designates specific knowledge, skills, and expertise for competency in sport dietetics practice. CSSDs apply sport nutrition science to fueling fitness, sport, and athletic performance. Specialty certification differentiates sport dietitians from dietitians who are less qualified to provide sport nutrition services. Credibility, visibility, and marketability of sport dietitians are enhanced by specialty certification. Dietitians must meet strict eligibility requirements to sit for the CSSD exam. Minimum requirements for specialty certification are established and approved by the CDR. To be eligible to become a Board-Certified Specialist in Sports Dietetics, candidates must meet the requirements specified by the CDR.

(continued)

Sport Nutrition Certifications *(continued)*

Certified Sports Nutritionist From the ISSN (CISSN)

The International Society of Sports Nutrition (ISSN) offers the CISSN exam, incorporating core competencies in basic exercise physiology, integrated physiology, bioenergetics, nutrition, and sport psychology. The CISSN exam is not restricted to registered dietitians (2). To sit for the CISSN exam and obtain this certification, people must meet the requirements laid out on the ISSN website: www.theissn.org.

International Sports Sciences Association Sports Nutrition Certification

The sport nutrition certification from the International Sports Sciences Association (ISSA) emphasizes the importance of recommending a sound diet and nutrition regimen while teaching sport nutrition concepts. For more information, see ISSA's website: www.issaonline.com.

ACE Lifestyle and Weight Management Consultant Certification

This certification is offered through the American Council of Exercise. The ACE Lifestyle and Weight Management Consultant Certification provides knowledge to develop sound, balanced weight management programs that bring together the three critical components of long-term weight management success: nutrition, exercise, and lifestyle change. The organization's website gives information on the eligibility criteria needed to sit for this exam.

Remember that sport nutrition certifications do not override state or federal guidelines regarding nutrition practice.

The reason for this blurred scope of practice is that sport nutrition is a unique multidisciplinary field that requires many professionals to work together. Athletic trainers, strength and conditioning coaches, coaches, athletic directors, and food service providers all must come together to provide the most effective service, information, and guidance to the athlete. At the same time, professionals should be aware of the appropriate scope of practice for their credentials and of national or state laws that limit the types of assessment and counseling they can do. The sidebar on page 218 describes one example of this type of law.

Maintaining Confidentiality

When working with an athlete, the sport nutritionist is gathering, assessing, and analyzing personal health information. The confidentiality of medical information is protected by law in many countries, and professionals need to be aware of the applicable laws and handle medical information in a way that complies with those laws. In the United States, the **Health Insurance Portability and Accountability Act** (HIPAA) is legislation that was created to provide a national standard in the United States for handling medical information. The key to the privacy act is to ensure that a person's protected health information is not inappropriately distributed to others. The act broadly defines protected health information as individually identifiable information maintained or transmitted by a covered entity in any form or medium. The current law includes modifications that have been made since it was first passed:

1. Doctors, hospitals, and health care providers are allowed to share patient information with family members or others involved in the person's care without patient permission.

2. Health care providers must distribute a notice of their privacy practices to individuals no later than the date the service is provided. A health care provider with a direct treatment relationship must make a good faith effort to obtain the person's written acknowledgment of receipt of the notice. The requirement allows patients to request any additional restrictions on uses and disclosures of their health information or confidential communications. Health care providers may design an acknowledgment of the process best suited to their practices.

3. Patients must grant permission for each nonroutine circumstance in which the patient's personal health information is used or disclosed.

4. Covered entities must obtain authorization to use or disclose protected health information for marketing purposes.

5. Covered entities may use and disclose protected health information in the form of a limited dataset for research, public health, and health care operations. A limited dataset does not contain any direct identifiers of individuals but may contain other demographic or health information needed for research.

At times, an athlete's nutrition information is used in a collaborative effort with other members of the athlete's performance team. Sharing this information would fall under point 1 of the HIPAA modifications. In other cases, however, the sport nutritionist may be working with an athlete apart from the athlete's inner circle of coaches and strength and conditioning specialists. At these times, HIPAA points 2 and 3 come into play. The sport nutritionist should let the athlete know what they plan to do with the athlete's personal health information and receive permission from the athlete to communicate this information to other staff members when necessary. The best approach is always to err on the side of caution with the athlete's private information by getting a signed document.

The disclosing of a current weight or body fat percent to a coach, strength coach, or agent could result in a fine, a breach of contract by the athlete, or a negative perception about the athlete's lack of progress that may lead to untoward decisions about the athlete's playing time. The sport nutritionist should always disclose to the athlete what needs to be shared and why, and then get a signed document stating that the athlete acknowledges the disclosure of that information.

Nutrition Legality: The Louisiana Example

Like many states in the United States, Louisiana has clear definitions regarding the scope of nutrition practice. Only a licensed dietitian or nutritionist can perform nutrition assessment and counseling. Those in other disciplines, however, can provide nutrition education as long as the information is general and accurate and is offered to a person or group without individualization. For example, the educator cannot answer questions specific to a client's or participant's diet or nutrition status.

According to the Louisiana Board of Dietetics, nutritional assessment is "the evaluation of the nutritional needs of individuals and groups based upon appropriate biochemical, anthropometric, physical and dietary data to determine nutrient needs including enteral and parenteral nutrition regardless of setting, including but not limited to ambulatory settings, hospitals, nursing homes and other extended care facilities" (18a).

Nutrition counseling "provides individualized guidance on appropriate food and nutrient intake for those with special metabolic needs, taking into consideration health, cultural, socioeconomic, functional and psychological facts from the nutrition assessment. Nutrition counseling may include advice to increase or decrease nutrients in the diet; to change the timing, size or composition of meals; to modify food textures; and in extreme instances, to change the route of administration" (18a).

Athletic staff must know the laws of the state they are working in to determine the legality of their own scope of practice. If a member of the athletic staff is not a registered dietitian and is asked for specific nutrition information and advice, that person must find a registered dietitian well versed in sport nutrition whom they can trust and collaborate with. Checking the credentials and qualifications of staff who are providing nutrition recommendations is also important. These licensure laws exist to ensure that people are receiving specific nutrition information from qualified professionals.

Developing the Athlete's Nutrition Plan

The athlete's nutrition plan (figure 11.2) should include specific plans for both training days and game, competition, or race days. Plans should include guidance for nutrition, hydration, and recovery that the athlete can follow on a day-to-day basis. The design of a protocol of pre-, during, and postworkout nutrition should ensure adequate and timely protein and carbohydrate intake to enhance recovery from the training sessions. The third phase of program development is game or race day strategy. The game day strategy should focus on what is needed to fuel and hydrate the body and recover from the stress of competition. As the nutrition plan development begins, the sport nutritionist should take into consideration the athlete's desire to improve fueling for performance but also look at the athlete holistically. The best nutrition programs go beyond grams of carbohydrate, protein, and fat. The relationship that has been developed between the athlete and coaching staff sets up the athlete for successful nutrition improvement. Even with the help of a coach, nutritionist, trainer, and others, athletes may find themselves facing the same pitfalls as nonathletes: poor planning and poor implementation.

An athlete may want basic advice or a specific nutrition plan. A more specific nutrition plan that fits into an athlete's lifestyle (e.g., relying on fast food, cooking, cultural food preferences) and meets the athlete's needs is more beneficial than basic advice. But the athlete must be ready to receive and implement such a plan. A sport nutritionist can use the **stages of change model** to determine how ready an athlete is for making changes and whether

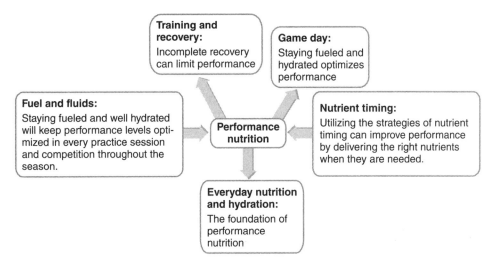

FIGURE 11.2 An athlete's nutrition plan should have good everyday nutrition as its base and include nutrition plans for training and recovery as well as competition.

to provide a detailed plan. The stages of change model is an approach to assessing a client's readiness to change. The stages are precontemplation, contemplation, preparation, action, maintenance, and relapse. Taking these into account and becoming more versed in behavioral science and psychology is an important piece to helping the athlete realize the recommendations. From a nutrition standpoint, the AND's nutrition care process is a good model to follow in working with an individual or team. The AND adopted the nutrition care process and model in 2003 in hopes of implementing a standardized process for providing high-quality care to patients. This same model is applicable to the development of a nutrition plan for athletes. These are the phases of the nutrition care process (17):

1. Nutrition assessment
2. Nutrition evaluation
3. Nutrition intervention and education
4. Nutrition monitoring and evaluation

Step 1: Assessment

Athlete assessment is the first step in creating an effective plan. This is the time to get to know the athlete and understand their situation and objective data. You can sit down with the athlete one on one or develop a questionnaire for the athlete to fill out by hand or electronically. You should gather the following information:

1. **Anthropometric data**: These data include measured height, weight, body fat, and circumference.
2. **Biochemical data**: Lab values can provide more detailed data, but the physiological state of the athlete when the blood is drawn is important. Both dehydration and intense training can cause changes in blood volume that can skew the interpretation of blood work. In addition, food and beverage intake can alter certain blood tests (cholesterol, triglycerides, and so on).
3. **Sport, position, and point in season or phase of training**: Prescribing correct nutrient and hydration recommendations will depend on the specific sport, position within the sport, and point in the athlete's season. Different positions within the same sport can have vastly different nutrient needs, such as a soccer goalkeeper compared with a forward on the same team. Long-distance runners have extremely different needs during the maximum-mileage weeks in comparison with the point in their training when they are in a building phase. The concept of altering athletes' food intake to correlate with where they are in their seasons is referred to as nutrition periodization, a term that corresponds with the concept of training periodization. A

football player in the beginning of the off-season will have decreased caloric needs as compared with those needs during the preseason with two-a-day practices. Recommendations for the athlete need to be individualized beyond just the sport.

4. **Nutrition knowledge**: A basic assessment of the athlete's foundational nutrition knowledge will provide a good idea about where to start with education and what concepts to focus on. Knowledge will empower the athlete and give them a greater understanding of nutrition recommendations.

5. **Stage of change and behavioral readiness**: The transtheoretical model (23) is useful for determining a nutrition counseling strategy (27). The goal is to help athletes get from stage to stage and help them permanently adopt a new positive behavior or extinguish a behavior that does not enhance performance. Moving too quickly through the stages or developing plans for athletes who are not ready will lead to noncompliance.

6. **Current dietary habits and intake**: A 24-hour or three-day diet recall will provide a snapshot of the athlete's current diet. In addition, questions about food habits should be asked. Questions that will elicit information about the athlete's nutrition habits include the following: How often do you grocery shop? How often do you eat out? How much water do you drink per day? How many meals do you eat per day? What do you typically snack on? How many days per week do you eat breakfast? What dietary supplements do you use, what is the dose size, and when do you take them? How consistent are you with these dietary supplements? Do you take anything (food or supplement) pre-, during, or postexercise?

7. **Allergies, dislikes, intolerances, cultural or religious considerations**.

8. **Medications**: The practitioner must check for drug–nutrient interactions to determine if the prescription or over-the-counter drugs interact with nutrients in food or supplements. For instance, an athlete who is taking blood thinners to prevent clots postsurgery needs to watch vitamin K intake through food and supplements and be aware of any supplements that may increase bleeding time.

9. **Injuries**: Acute injuries may affect training and activity load, but over-training injuries may be a sign of poor nutrition intake.

10. **Goals and time line**: Understanding the athlete's goals and time line will help shape the strategy for education and coaching. A National Football League draftee may be working on a tight time line to prepare for the draft; an elite figure skater may be looking for a plan to peak for a competition that is nine months away.

Step 2: Evaluation

This step involves the analysis of the assessment.

1. Determine the athlete's calorie needs. A way to do this is to measure the athlete's resting metabolic rate or use an energy expenditure equation and then account for activity. If the athlete is looking to gain or lose weight, add or subtract 500 to 1,000 kcal per day from the basal metabolic rate (BMR) and activity total. This number should produce a 1- to 2-pound (about 2-4 kg) weight loss or gain per week. Degree of weight loss or gain will depend on the athlete's genetic makeup, daily caloric deficit, number of rest and recovery days per week, and the type of training phase they are in (31).

2. Address the athlete's goals or issues (e.g., cramping, weight management, fatigue, soreness). When identifying something to work on with the athlete, be sure to state the issue consistently: (a) problem, (b) **etiology**, which is the cause of the issue, (c) signs and symptoms (24). For example: "Female tennis player has extreme fatigue and cramping toward the end of matches and practices, which is hindering performance. This is related to low daily energy intake that is not meeting nutrition needs, inadequate fluid intake during matches, and the lack of a carbohydrate/electrolyte drink while playing." Setting up the issues in this way will provide a clear path to additional recommendations beyond general needs for the athlete.

3. Figure out the athlete's carbohydrate, protein, and fat needs depending on sport, position, and stage of training. Create guidelines for everyday, specific recovery needs and for game or event days. The two ways to express those values are grams per kilogram body weight and percent of total calories. Grams per kilogram body weight gives the athlete a more exact recommendation and is advised. Critical thinking is key, and percentage of total calories is secondary to the athlete's total energy intake. For example, a 60 kg (132 lb) female aerobic endurance athlete at the high end of her training would fall into the 7 to 10 g/kg range, which would put her at 420 to 600 g carbohydrate ingestion per day. But if her total caloric intake is 2,800 kcal per day, carbohydrate would be 60% to 85% of her total calories. Although 60% makes sense, 85% of calories coming from carbohydrate is too much. Therefore, you must check macronutrient guidelines when you translate research-based recommendations into reality.

4. Determine the athlete's nutrient timing needs for training and for competition days. To do this, first look at the athlete's physique and training goals. Athletes who need to gain strength or size should incorporate a specific strategy for pre- and postworkout nutrition and possibly during-workout nutrition (depending on the duration and intensity of their training). For example, an athlete who needs to gain strength

and size while training for the NFL combine needs to consume calories during a 4-hour intense training sessions in addition to pre- and postworkout nutrition. After looking at physique and training goals, assess an athlete's performance, learn how they feel during training and performance, and consider this in conjunction with the current diet and supplement regimen. For instance, if a marathon runner tells you that the coach recently increased their mileage to 70 miles (113 km) per week and they have felt crummy ever since the change, you want to pay close attention to overall calorie intake, macronutrient distribution, and postexercise carbohydrate consumption (in addition to timing of the postexercise intake). Like all nutrition strategies, nutrient timing recommendations should be made on an individual basis and given to athletes within a context they can understand. You should not only tell athletes total grams of carbohydrate they need to consume after a 20-mile (32 km) run but also help them translate this number into quantities of the foods or sport nutrition products they typically consume.

Step 3: Intervention and Education

One might assume that athletes, especially highly trained athletes, have a vast knowledge of their own physiology and the nutrient demands of their sport and that coaches or others who work with them daily also have that knowledge. Often, however, this is not the case (33). When working with an athlete and developing a plan, start with the basics (general education) and then build into personalization and customization. Supplements are often the first thing athletes focus on because they are marketed as performance-enhancing aids. But athletes should focus first on their foundation nutrition and hydration, then add performance-based nutrition strategies, and then look at how supplements might help them. Just as athletes must develop foundational basics of their sport before moving on to highly refined tactical work, fine-tuning nutrition recommendations is difficult when the foundation knowledge is absent and the athlete's overall nutritional behaviors do not support optimal performance.

No matter how wonderful the information provided to or summarized for an athlete, the person may not be able to implement the strategies if the coach or dietitian does not take into account behavioral psychology and readiness for change. The behavior upgrade process converts thoughts to actions and actions to habits. The behavior upgrade process comprises distinct stages, and success across the stages is driven by a combination of intrinsic motivation, self-efficacy, and grit, empowering people to take responsibility for their own performance lifestyle (4, 11, 12).

The process should be personalized to be successful. Although this personalization is typically overlooked in current models, it has been shown to make a significant difference in program adherence. The science of upgrading behavior is supported by the evidence-based theories of the trans-theoretical model and the health belief model, the theory of reasoned action and planned behavior, the community ecological approach, the self-determination theory, B.J. Fogg's motivation wave, and motivational orientation (5, 13, 18, 19, 22, 23).

Intrinsic Motivation

Continuously connecting with desires or needs to make a change or upgrade can provide the necessary fuel to complete a journey from beginning to end. Without this connection, progress can stall or halt completely. Intrinsic motivation refers a person's underlying reasons for engaging in a behavior because of its intrinsic benefits. Identifying and reconnecting with internal motivators can help make the journey sustainable (1, 19, 26). An example of this approach relating to nutritional strategy is to connect an athlete's body composition goals with their deeper motivations, which may be more playing time, increased longevity, or making the world team.

Self-Efficacy

A person's trust and confidence in their ability and a positive outlook on the credibility of the proposed solution provides the foundation on which the entire journey is based. **Effectance**, the concept that what a person does makes a difference, is one of the most important factors in behavior upgrade. Without it, the person may remain in a state of ambivalence; the path to behavior upgrade may never start, and progress may come to a halt. Confidence, namely trusting oneself to perform based on appraisal of past successes, bolsters progress, but a lack of trust can derail the journey at any point. A history of failed attempts can erode the resolve to keep trying. All phases along the path of behavior upgrade provide opportunities to build trust in oneself and with the performance professional. Microgoals are the keys to making sacrifice manageable, enhancing overall self-efficacy, confidence, trust, and beliefs (4, 16, 30).

Grit and Resilience

The capacity to stay on track and not get derailed by setbacks or challenges is critical to meaningful change. Resilience is the capacity to exit from a period of challenge having gained and grown. Grit refers to the capacity to continue without experiencing immediate rewards because the future is valued over the present, suggesting that individuals' desires for long-term goals coupled with powerful motivation to achieve their objectives results in a tendency to persevere with the effort required to overcome challenges that lie in their way. Grit has relevance and implications for ambivalence, which is a limiting factor of behavioral upgrade. Over time, people can develop the habit of making an effort in the absence of immediate reward—this habit becomes more important as the complexity of activities increases. Resilience simply refers to a person's ability to thrive in the face of adversity, and deal effectively and grow, despite stressors, and in the absence of immediate reward (3, 9, 14, 25).

Athletes exude these qualities in relationship to developing skill and capacity with their sport, but often do not connect the same behavioral principles to lifestyle behavior and skills that will support their athletic goals. With an empathetic, evocative approach, the coach and the athlete can collaborate to enhance the strength of intrinsic motivation, self-efficacy, and grit and create the optimal path to achieve desired performance outcomes.

A sport nutritionist creates and implements a strategy to improve the opportunities identified during the assessment. The intervention should have the following components:

1. Education.
2. Nutrition and hydration plan for all phases of training and competition cycle.
3. Specific recommendations in grams per kilogram versus percent of calories (31).
4. A plan to help alleviate the problems identified during the diagnosis.
5. Discussion of supplement safety; many athletes are unaware that supplements may contain ingredients not identified on the label or that the labeling may be inaccurate. Check the respective governing body (National Collegiate Athletic Association, National Football League, Major League Baseball, World Anti-Doping Agency, and so on) to become aware of banned substance lists. Then find third-party testing organizations that the particular governing body supports. Finally, remind athletes that the responsibility falls on them and that if they take a supplement containing a banned substance, they will be held responsible and be reprimanded according to their governing body's specific rules. Useful websites for researching supplements include www.nsfsport.com, www.informed-sport.com, and www.bscg.org.
6. Set up realistic systems that will lead to success. Establish exact formulas and products or foods for during workouts, postworkout, and competition. Coordinate with food service to ensure that proper foods are selected or arranged for athletes or teams.
7. Set short-term and long-term goals.
8. Educate those who have personal relationships with the athlete (spouses, family members, others working with the athlete). All plans need to consider any food intolerances, allergies, religious beliefs, cultural influences, strong likes and dislikes, ability to cook, access to food, restaurants commonly visited, and socioeconomic status as the plan is being developed.

9. Develop a perfect day for the athlete in simple terms. The perfect day example in table 11.1 is for a gymnast who needs to eat a more nutrient-rich diet. Sample days can be used to help athletes see patterns of eating, nutrient timing (when they should eat in proximity to training), and incorporating good, healthy foods into their diet. The sport nutritionist should explain that the perfect day is an example; ideally, athletes will vary the types of foods they consume within each general category. For instance, instead of eating a plum with raw almonds every day for a snack, the athlete should consider a variety of nuts and fruit to get a wide variety of nutrients and antioxidants into the diet.

TABLE 11.1 Perfect Day Nutrition Plan

Time	Meal
5 a.m.	Wake up
5:15 a.m.	Whole-wheat toast with natural peanut butter, yogurt
6:00-7:15 a.m.	Workout
7:30 a.m.	Postworkout shake with carbohydrate and protein
9:30 a.m.	Oatmeal with berries and walnuts; egg whites scrambled with vegetables, low-fat cheese, and olive oil
12:30 p.m.	Turkey sandwich on whole wheat with large spinach salad and low-fat dressing
3:30 p.m.	Plum with raw almonds
6:30 p.m.	Grilled salmon, brown rice, steamed vegetables, large green salad with low-fat dressing
9:30 p.m.	Low-fat cottage cheese with berries

Step 4: Monitoring and Evaluation

An athlete who comes to see the nutritionist one time to get a plan and then never returns will not realize the same degree of success as one who is properly monitored. Athletes can be monitored in many ways:

- Weight monitoring: Daily or weekly body weights are tracked depending on the needs and mind-set of the athlete. Some athletes respond well to daily body weight measurement, whereas others become fixated on the number on the scale. The method of monitoring is up to the discretion of those working with the athlete (10).

- Body fat monitoring: Monthly body fat measures are a good way to track changes in lean muscle mass versus fat mass.

- Hydration monitoring: Weigh athletes before and after sessions to assess hydration practices.

- Habit monitoring.
- Energy monitoring.
- Intake monitoring.
- Personal contact and relationship building: The sport nutritionist must set up communication with the athlete. Staying in touch with athletes is critical to their success. Formal appointments or checkups can be effective, although sometimes time consuming. Use of technology can be extremely helpful. Email checkups are quick and easy, and a simple text message can be a great reminder to help keep the athlete on track. As much as possible, the sport nutritionist should attend the athlete's practice, games, training sessions, and strength and conditioning sessions.

The more the sport nutritionist is integrated into all parts of the athlete's life and sport, the greater influence they will have. The sport nutritionist should set realistic timelines to help athletes achieve their goals. For example, a healthy weight gain or weight loss is typically no more than 2 pounds (about 1 kg) per week (31). Using simple tools to allow the athlete to check in with their habits can be extremely helpful. The performance nutrition assessment in form 11.1 is a simple way to help athletes evaluate their own nutrition progress.

Performance Nutrition Assessment

Instructions: If the athlete thinks they are not doing well with a task, then mark a 1. If the athlete thinks they are doing great with a task, mark a 5.

Eating clean	1	2	3	4	5
Eating often	1	2	3	4	5
Keeping hydrated	1	2	3	4	5
Recovery	1	2	3	4	5
Mind-set	1	2	3	4	5

FORM 11.1 This performance nutrition assessment is a good tool to use at the beginning of a consultation and at consultations in the future. It helps the athlete think about how they are doing with their diet and helps the sport nutritionist see what the athlete actually thinks of their diet in comparison with what they are really doing.

From NSCA, *NSCA's Guide to Sport and Exercise Nutrition*, 2nd ed. (Champaign, IL: Human Kinetics, 2021).

Members of the athlete's training team should be informed of the athlete's nutrition performance plan as necessary. Sharing this information helps to gain reinforcement or support for the athlete's progress from the coaching staff. In addition, this information, when shared appropriately, allows a continued focus on the behavior change process.

Eating Disorders and Disordered Eating

Involvement in organized sport and general athletic activities offers many positive benefits, both physically and mentally, but the pressure of athletic competition may compound an existing cultural emphasis on thinness. The result is an increased risk for athletes to develop disordered eating patterns and possibly an eating disorder (20, 21). A study evaluating Norwegian athletes showed that 13.5% of the athletes studied had subclinical or clinical eating disorders in comparison with 4.6% of the general population controls (28).

Athletes in many sports face a paradox in that the behavior necessary to achieve a body weight for success in their sport (semistarvation, purging, compulsive exercising) adversely affects health, fuel reserves, physiological and mental functioning, and the ability to train and compete at the level they desire. Reduced carbohydrate intake will affect the body's fuel stores, and a decrease in protein intake may lead to a decrease in lean muscle mass. An overall lack of micronutrients resulting from low energy intake may make growth, repair, and recovery from exercise difficult and put the athlete at increased risk for injury (20, 32).

Eating disorders are traditionally associated with female sports, but disordered eating patterns and eating disorders do occur in male athletes as well, specifically those in sports with an aesthetic component or sports that require making weight or emphasize being small and lean. Men represent 6% to 10% of those with eating disorders (6, 15, 20). In male athletes, 22% of the eating disorders are in those participating in antigravitation sports such as diving, gymnastics, high jumping, and pole vaulting; 9% in aerobic endurance sports; and 5% in ball game sports. In female athletes, 42% of eating disorders are in athletes competing in aesthetic sports, 24% in aerobic endurance sports, 17% in technical sports, and 16% in ball game sports (28). An additional study on the prevalence of eating disorders among males found that 52% of 25 lower weight category collegiate wrestlers and 59 lightweight rowers reported bingeing; 8% of the rowers and 16% of the wrestlers showed pathologic eating disorder index profiles (29).

This particular study is consistent with the remainder of the literature, in which estimates of the prevalence of eating disorders range between 15% and 62% among female athletes; the greatest prevalence is among athletes in aesthetic sports such as ballet, bodybuilding, diving, figure skating, cheerleading, and gymnastics (20).

Eating disorders are classified based on the symptoms they present (32). An eating disorder can be classified as anorexia nervosa, bulimia nervosa, or eating disorder not otherwise specified, but many of those with a diagnosis in one category demonstrate behaviors across the diagnosis continuum. Clinical eating disorders and disordered eating behaviors exist on a·continuum, which makes it important to monitor disordered eating patterns for progression toward eating disorders.

A fine but solid line delineates eating disorders and disordered eating. An eating disorder is a serious mental illness that interferes with an athlete's normal daily activities; disordered eating represents a temporary or mild change in an athlete's eating behaviors. Disordered eating patterns can arise if an athlete is trying to make a weight goal, is under stress, or is intending to change their appearance or performance by making dietary changes. If these patterns are short lived and do not persist, they do not necessarily need to be treated by a psychiatrist or psychologist (although such behaviors should be monitored). Note the behavior, however, because prolonged disordered eating patterns can lead to a diagnosed eating disorder (7, 10).

For people with an eating disorder, the focus on food becomes so strong that the constant sense of stress and anxiety around eating requires professional intervention. Definitions and criteria for common eating disorders are shown in the sidebar. Eating disorders are often the result of an emotional issue or issues. Therefore, appropriate referrals must be made to a medical professional and registered dietitian when working with an athlete who has an eating disorder. Also important is reaching out to more qualified professionals in cases of an eating disorder and lending support to their proposed treatment plan (7, 10).

The complexity, time intensiveness, and expense of managing eating disorders necessitate an interdisciplinary approach. Staff from the following disciplines may be included: medicine, nutrition, mental health, athletic training, and athletics administration. An interdisciplinary approach may make it easier for symptomatic athletes to ask for help and may enhance their potential for full recovery. Establishing educational initiatives for preventing eating disorders is also important.

Diagnostic Criteria for Eating Disorders

The following are modified definitions of eating disorders as specified in *DSM-IV.*

Anorexia Nervosa

Restricting type: The athlete has not regularly engaged in binge eating or purging behavior.

Binge or purge type: The athlete has regularly engaged in binge eating or purging behavior.

- Refusal to maintain body weight at or above a minimally normal weight for height and age (less than 85% of what is expected)
- Intense fear of gaining weight or becoming fat, even though the person is underweight
- Body image disturbances, including a distortion in the way the person experiences body weight or shape, undue influence of body weight or shape on self-evaluation, or denial of the consequences associated with the current low body weight
- In postmenarchal females, amenorrhea (absence of at least three consecutive cycles)

Bulimia Nervosa

Purging type: The athlete has regularly engaged in self-induced vomiting or the misuse of laxatives, diuretics, or enemas.

Nonpurging type: The athlete has used inappropriate compensatory behaviors such as fasting or excessive exercise but has not regularly engaged in self-induced vomiting or the misuse of laxatives, diuretics, or enemas.

- Recurrent episodes of binge eating: (1) eating an amount of food in a discrete period (within any 2-hour period) that is significantly larger than what most people would eat in a similar period and set of circumstances; (2) a sense of a lack of control over eating during the episode
- Recurrent inappropriate compensatory behavior to prevent weight gain (i.e., self-induced vomiting; misuse of laxatives, diuretics, enemas, or other medications; fasting; and excessive exercise)
- Behaviors occurring on average at least two times per week for three months
- Self-evaluation excessively influenced by body shape and weight
- Occurrence of the behavior not exclusively during episodes of anorexia nervosa

Eating Disorder Not Otherwise Specified (EDNOS)

This diagnosis includes disorders of eating that do not meet criteria for any specific eating disorder. Disordered eating patterns are often seen in athletes of all sports as they try to make weight, improve performance, or go through phases of an extreme change in dietary intake and nutrition behavior. EDNOS can look like either anorexia or bulimia or may have the following signs:

- Repeatedly chewing and spitting out, but not swallowing, large amounts of food
- Recurrent episodes of binge eating in the absence of the inappropriate compensatory behaviors that are characteristic of bulimia nervosa (this is categorized as binge eating disorder)

Female Athlete Triad

As mentioned in chapter 1, in 2014 the IOC released an updated consensus statement relating to the female athlete triad and relative energy deficiency in sport (RED-S) (21). The female athlete triad refers to the interrelationship among energy availability, menstrual function, and bone mineral density. Female athletes may be positioned all along a spectrum between health and disease, and those in the danger zone do not exhibit all the clinical conditions at the same time. Low energy availability (with or without eating disorders), amenorrhea, and osteoporosis all pose significant health risks to physically active girls and women. Traditionally, body fat percent has been linked with the female athlete triad, whereas now, low energy availability (the amount of dietary energy remaining after training, metabolic processes, and activities of daily living are accounted for) seems to be the trigger. Some athletes reduce energy availability by increasing energy expenditure more than energy intake; others practice abnormal eating patterns using one or more of the inappropriate compensatory behaviors outlined earlier. Sustained low energy availability can impair both mental and physical health.

The term *RED-S* points to the complexity involved and the fact that male athletes are also affected. The syndrome refers to impaired physiological function including, but not limited to, metabolic rate, menstrual function, bone health, immunity, protein synthesis, and cardiovascular and psychological health caused by relative energy deficiency. The cause of this syndrome is energy deficiency relative to the balance between dietary energy intake and energy expenditure required for health and activities of daily living, growth, and sporting activities. Psychological consequences can either precede RED-S or be the result of RED-S. The clinical phenomenon is not a triad of the three entities of energy availability, menstrual function, and bone health, but rather a syndrome that affects many aspects of physiological function, health, and athletic performance (21); see chapter 1 for more information.

As the number of missed menstrual cycles accumulates secondary to sustained low energy intake, **bone mineral density** (BMD) declines. BMD, the mineral content of bone, is used as a diagnostic criterion for osteopenia and osteoporosis. The loss of BMD may not be fully reversible, and the risk for stress fractures increases.

Being aware of disordered eating patterns and eating disorders among female athletes can help prevent the downward spiral into the triad. The position stand makes several recommendations for screening and diagnosis of the triad:

1. Screening for the triad should occur at the preparticipation exam or the annual health screening exam. Athletes with one component of the triad should be assessed for the others.

2. Athletes with disordered eating should be referred to a mental health practitioner for evaluation, diagnosis, and recommendations for treatment.

3. To diagnose sustained low-energy amenorrhea, other causes must be ruled out. A physical exam by a medical professional and the interpretation of laboratory results will help to rule out other causes of amenorrhea.

4. Finally, athletic administrators and the entire team of professionals working with female athletes should aim for triad prevention through education. Young female athletes often do not see that actions they are taking to enhance performance may cause future problems with bone density and fertility (8).

5. A similar set of tools and protocols has been established for screening and return to play relating to RED-S. All members of an athlete's performance team should be able to identify and properly route the athlete to the right care relating to disordered eating patterns (21).

Professional Applications

Although the process of evaluation and athlete counseling is not likely to change dramatically in the upcoming years, the research on nutrition and supplementation for performance is always changing. In addition, the lists of banned substances change from year to year, as does the list of supplements certified as safe (through groups that test for banned substances). Sport nutritionists must stay current on all this information so that they can answer questions from athletes, coaches, and athletic training staff and be able to make specific, individualized recommendations to athletes. In the

United States, many states require that the person providing medical nutrition therapy or individualized recommendations be a registered and licensed dietitian. Those with sport nutrition certifications, however, can provide general advice to athletes.

Sport nutrition is a field in a constant state of change, and the sport nutritionist must take a comprehensive look at an athlete's lifestyle, medical history, weight history, goals, injury report, lab work, body composition, and training program before helping the athlete develop a plan to achieve their goals. Along with good knowledge of the latest sport science research and its application, the sport nutritionist needs to build good rapport with each athlete, which will let the athlete know they can trust the sport nutritionist and therefore open up. Many clients may have a rational fear of opening up and talking about behavior they are ashamed of (such as binge eating or drinking, overeating, or disordered eating). They also fear that this personal information will be shared with others. Athletes must trust and be comfortable with sport nutritionists to talk about how they feel, exactly what they are eating, how much they are exercising, and what they think about their body. That trust may take some time to build and develops only through conversation.

This book includes many research findings that can be used to fine-tune a nutrition program but that also support some general recommendations that athletes need to be reminded of. The following are 10 general guidelines that will help athletes make wiser food choices:

1. Come back to earth. Choose the least processed forms of food most of the time.

2. Eat a rainbow often. Eat as many colorful fruits, vegetables, and whole grains as you can.

3. When it comes to protein, the fewer legs, the better. Try to choose lean protein sources as often as possible.

4. Eat fats that give something back. Choose a variety of unsaturated fats and essential fatty acids in the diet.

5. Three for three. Eat minimeals consisting of carbohydrate, protein, and fat every 3 hours or at the right time cadence to support your performance goals.

6. Eat breakfast every day. After you wake up, try to eat breakfast as soon as you can.

7. Hydrate. Be sure to meet your hydration needs.

8. Do not waste your workout. Consume a blend of carbohydrate and protein after your training session or competition.

9. Supplement wisely. Check with your dietitian or doctor before starting a new supplement. Also, be aware of the rules and regulations of your sport's governing body when it comes to banned substances.

10. Get back in the kitchen. The more you can prepare your own food, the more control you will have over the nourishment of your body.

Summary Points

- The practice of sport nutrition is somewhere between science and art. Getting athletes to change the way they eat can positively affect their performance, although bringing about behavior change is not always easy.

- Fitness professionals, although they may be knowledgeable about nutrition and performance, should make sure they have the appropriate credentials before providing nutrition information to athletes. Some laws restrict which professionals can provide nutrition counseling.

- When working on a nutrition plan, professionals should take care to keep medical information confidential.

- Always ask athletes' permission before sharing any information with their coach or other members of their team except in the case of a life-threatening condition or eating disorder.

- Building good rapport with athletes is of utmost importance in helping them make changes.

- The steps in creating a nutrition plan include assessment, evaluation, intervention and education, and monitoring and evaluation.

- Using a systematic approach to assessment, evaluation of needs, and intervention and education and then building a deep relationship with the athlete during the monitoring phase not only sets up the nutrition program for success but also may help to change the way that the athlete views nutrition and the way they eat, well beyond their athletic career.

- The sport nutritionist may be on the front line for detecting the RED-S and the female athlete triad of disordered eating, amenorrhea, and osteoporosis (or low bone density signaling a problem in young athletes).

References

Chapter 1

1. Anderson, JW, Konz, EC, Frederich, RC, and Wood, CL. Long-term weight-loss maintenance: A meta-analysis of U.S. studies. *Am J Clin Nutr* 75:579-584, 2001.

2. Antonio, J, Ellerbroek, A, Silver, T, Orris, S, Scheiner, M, Gonzalez, A, and Peacock, CA. A high protein diet (3.4 g/kg/d) combined with a heavy resistance training program improves body composition in healthy trained men and women—a follow-up investigation. *J Int Soc Sports Nutr* 12:39, 2015.

3. Areta, JL, Burke, LM, Camera, DM, West, DWD, Crawshay, S, Moore, DR, Stellingwerff, T, Phillips, S, Hawley, JA, and Coffey, VG. Reduced resting skeletal muscle protein synthesis is rescued by resistance exercise and protein ingestion following short-term energy deficit. *Am J Physiol—Endocrinol Metab* 306:989-997, 2014.

4. Ball, SD, Keller, KR, Moyer-Mileur, LJ, Ding, YW, Donaldson, D, and Jackson, W. Prolongation of satiety after low versus moderately high glycemic index meals in obese adolescents. *Pediatrics* 111:488-494, 2003.

5. Barkeling, B, Rossner, S, and Bjorvell, H. Effects of a high-protein meal (meat) and a high-carbohydrate meal (vegetarian) on satiety measured by automated computerized monitoring of subsequent food intake, motivation to eat and food preferences. *Int J Obes* 14:743-751, 1990.

6. Barrack, MT, Fredericson, M, Tenforde, AS, and Nattiv, A. Evidence of a cumulative effect for risk factors predicting low bone mass among male adolescent athletes. *Br J Sports Med* 51:200-205, 2017.

7. Borsheim, E, Tipton, KD, Wolf, SE, and Wolfe, RR. Essential amino acids and muscle protein recovery from resistance exercise. *Appl J Physiol* 283:E648-657, 2002.

8. Bouche, C, Rizkalla, SW, Luo, J, Vidal, H, Veronese, A, Pacher, N, Fouquet, C, Lang, V, and Slama, G. Five-week, low glycemic index diet increases total fat mass and improves plasma lipid profile in moderately overweight nondiabetic men. *Diabet Care* 25:822-828, 2002.

9. Bray, GA. Afferent signals regulating food intake. *Proceedings of the Nutrition Society*, 59(3):373-384, 2000.

10. Brehm, BJ and D'Alessio, DA. Benefits of high-protein weight loss diets: Enough evidence for practice? *Curr Opin Endocrinol Diabetes, Obes* 15:416-421, 2008.

11. Brown, AF, Welsh, T, Panton, LB, Moffatt, RJ, and Ormsbee, MJ. Higher protein intake improves body composition index in female collegiate dancers. Appl Physiol Nutr Metab, 45(5);547-554, 2020.

12. Brynes, AE, Adamson, J, Dornhorst, A, and Frost, GS. The beneficial effect of a diet with low glycaemic index on 24 h glucose profiles in healthy young people as assessed by continuous glucose monitoring. *Br J Nutr* 93:179-182, 2005.

13. Burke, LM, Close, GL, Lundy, B, Mooses, M, Morton, JP, and Tenforde, AS. Relative energy deficiency in sport in male athletes: A commentary on its presentation among selected groups of male athletes. *Int J Sport Nutr Exerc Metab* 28:364-374, 2018.

14. Campbell, BI, Aguilar, D, Conlin, L, Vargas, A, Schoenfeld, BJ, Corson, A, Gai, C, Best, S, Galvan, E, and Couvillion, K. Effects of high versus low protein intake on body composition and maximal strength in aspiring female physique athletes engaging in an 8-week resistance training program. *Int J Sport Nutr Exerc Metab* 28:580-585, 2018.

15. Campbell, BI, Aguilar, D, and Vargas, A. Effects of a high (2.4 g/kg) vs. low/moderate (1.2 g/kg) protein intake on body composition in aspiring female physique athletes engaging in an 8-week resistance training program. *J Int Soc Sport* 13(Suppl 1):P20, 2016.

16. Cook, CM and Haub, MD. Low Carbohydrate Diets and Performance. *Curr Sport Med Rep* 6:225-229, 2007.

17. Cox, KL, Burke, V, Morton, AR, Beilin, LJ, and Puddey, IB. The independent and combined effects of 16 weeks of vigorous exercise and energy restriction on body mass and composition in free-living overweight men-a randomized controlled trial. *Metabolism* 52:107-115, 2003.

18. Das, SK, Gilhooly, CH, Golden, JK, Pittas, AG, Fuss, PJ, Cheatham, RA, Tyler, S, Tsay, M, McCrory, MA, Lichtenstein, AH, Dallal, GE, Dutta, C, Bhapkar, MV, DeLany, JP, Saltzman, E, and Roberts, SB. Long-term effects of 2 energy-restricted diets differing in glycemic load on dietary adherence, body composition, and metabolism in CALERIE: A 1-y randomized controlled trial. *Am J Clin Nutr* 85:1023-1030, 2007.

19. Demling, RH and Desanti, L. Effect if a hypocaloric diet, increased protein intake and resistance training on lean mass gains and fat mass loss in overweight police officers. *Ann Nutr Metab* 44:21-29, 2000.

20. Dengel, DR, Hagberg, JM, Coon, PJ, Drinkwater, DT, and Goldberg, AP. Effects of weight loss by diet alone or combined with aerobic exercise on body composition in older obese men. *Metabolism* 43:867-871

21. Dengel, DR, Hagberg, JM, Coon, PJ, Drinkwater, DT, and Goldberg, AP. Comparable effects of diet and exercise on body composition and lipoproteins in older men. *Med Sci Sports Exerc* 26:1307-1315

22. DeSouza, MJ, Hontscharuk, R, Olmsted, M, Kerr, G, and Williams, NI. Drive for thinness score is a proxy indicator of energy deficiency in exercising women. *Appetite* 48:359-367, 2007.

23. DeSouza, MJ, Koltun, KJ, Strock, NC, and Williams, NI. Rethinking the concept of an energy availability threshold and its role in the female athlete triad. *Curr Opin Physiol* 10:35-42, 2019.

24. DeSouza, MJ, Williams, NI, Nattiv, A, Joy, E, Misra, M, Loucks, AB, Matheson, G, Olmsted, M, Barrack, M, Mallinson, RJ, Gibbs, JC, Goolsby, M, Nichols,

JF, Drinkwater, B, Sanborn, C, Agostini, R, Otis, CL, Johnson, MD, Hoch, AZ, Alleyne, JMK, Wadsworth, LT, Koehler, K, VanHeest, J, Harvey, P, Kelly, AKW, Fredericson, M, Brooks, GA, O'Donnell, E, Callahan, LR, Putukian, M, Costello, L, Hecht, S, Rauh, MJ, and McComb, J. Misunderstanding the female athlete triad: Refuting the IOC consensus statement on relative energy deficiency in sport (RED-S). *Br J Sports Med* 48:1461-1465, 2014.

25. Drew, MK, Vlahovich, N, Hughes, D, Appaneal, R, Peterson, K, Burke, L, Lundy, B, Toomey, M, Watts, D, Lovell, G, Praet, S, Halson, S, Colbey, C, Manzanero, S, Welvaert, M, West, N, Pyne, DB, and Waddington, G. A multifactorial evaluation of illness risk factors in athletes preparing for the Summer Olympic Games. *J Sci Med Sport* 20:745-750, 2017.

26. Eston, RG, Shephard, S, Kreitzman, S, Coxon, A, Brodie, DA, Lamb, KL, and Baltzopoulos, V. Effect of very low calorie diet on body composition and exercise response in sedentary women. *Eur J Appl Physiol Occup Physiol* 65:452-458, 1992.

27. Forbes, GB. Body fat content influences the body. *Ann N Y Acad Sci* 904:359-365, 2000.

28. Frimel, TN, Sinacore, DR, and Villareal, DT. Exercise attenuates the weight-loss-induced reduction in muscle mass in frail obese older adults. *Med Sci Sports Exerc* 40:1213-1219, 2008.

29. Gordon, CM, Ackerman, KE, Berga, SL, Kaplan, JR, Mastorakos, G, Misra, M, Murad, H, Santoro, NF, and Warren, MP. Functional hypothalamic amenorrhea: An endocrine society clinical practice guideline. *J Clin Endocrinol Metab* 102:1413-1439, 2017.

30. Gornall, J and Villani, RG. Short-term changes in body composition and metabolism with severe dieting and resistance exercise. *Int J Sport Nutr* 6:285-294, 1996.

31. Hackney, AC, Sinning, WE, and Bruot, BC. Reproductive hormonal profiles of endurance-trained and untrained males. *Med Sci Sport Exerc* 20:60-65, 1988.

32. Halton, TL and Hu, FB. The effects of high protein diets on thermogenesis, satiety and weight loss: A critical review. *J Am Coll Nutr* 23:373-385, 2004.

33. Holick, MF, Binkley, NC, Bischoff-Ferrari, HA, Gordon, CM, Hanley, DA, Heaney, RP, Murad, H, and Weaver, CM. Evaluation, treatment, and prevention of vitamin D deficiency: An endocrine society clinical practice guideline. *J Clin Endocrinol Metab* 96:1911-1930, 2011.

34. Horswill, CA, Hickner, RC, Scott, JR, Costill, DL, and Gould, D. Weight loss, dietary carbohydrate modifications, and high intensity, physical performance. *Med Sci Sports Exerc* 22:470-476, 1990.

35. Hunter, GR, Byrne, NM, Sirikul, B, Fernández, JR, Zuckerman, PA, Darnell, BE, and Gower, BA. Resistance training conserves lean body mass and resting energy expenditure following weight loss. *Obesity (Silver Spring)* 16:1045-1051, 2008.

36. Jäger, R, Kerksick, CM, Campbell, BI, Cribb, PJ, Wells, SD, Skwiat, TM, Purpura, M, Ziegenfuss, TM, Ferrando, AA, Arent, SM, Smith-Ryan, A, Stout, JR, Arciero, PJ, Ormsbee, MJ, Taylor, LW, Wilborn, CD, Kalman, DS, Krieder, RB,

Willoughby, DS, Hoffman, JR, Krzykowski, JL, and Antonio, J. International Society of Sports Nutrition Position Stand: Protein and exercise. *J Int Soc Sports Nutr* 14:1-25, 2017.

37. Jeukendrup, A and Gleeson, M. *Sport Nutrition*, 3rd ed. Champaign, IL: Human Kinetics, 193-226, 2019.

38. Johnston, CS, Day, CS, and Swan, PD. Postprandial thermogenesis is increased 100% on a high-protein, low-fat diet versus a high-carbohydrate, low-fat diet in healthy, young women. *J Am Coll Nutr* 21:55-61, 2002.

39. Kraemer, WJ, Ratamess, NA, Volek, JS, Häkkinen, K, Rubin, MR, French, DN, Gomez, AL, McGuigan, MR, Scheett, TP, Newton, RU, Spiering, BA, Izquierdo, M, and Dioguardi, FS. The effects of amino acid supplementation on hormonal responses to resistance training overreaching. *Metabolism* 55:282-291, 2006.

40. Kraemer, WJ, Volek, JS, Clark, KL, Gordon, SE, Incledon, T, Puhl, SM, Triplett-McBride, T, McBride, JM, Putukian, M, and Sebastianelli, WJ. Physiological adaptations to a weight-loss dietary regimen and exercise programs in women. *J Appl Physiol* 83:270-279, 1997.

41. Krotkiewski, M, Landin, K, Mellstrom, D, and Tolli, J. Loss of total body potassium during rapid weight loss does not depend on the decrease of potassium concentration in muscles. Different methods to evaluate body composition during a low energy diet. *Int J Obes Relat Metab Disord* 24:101-107, 2000.

42. Kushner, RF and Doerfler, B. Low-carbohydrate, high-protein diets revisited. *Curr Opin Gastroenterol* 24:198-203, 2008.

43. Lambert, CP, Frank, LL, and Evan, WJ. Macronutrient consideration for the sport of bodybuilding. *Sport Med* 34:317-323, 2004.

44. Latner, JD and Schwartz, M. The effects of a high-carbohydrate, high-protein or balanced lunch upon later food intake and hunger ratings. *Appetite* 33:119-128, 1999.

45. Layman, DK, Boileau, R a, Erickson, DJ, Painter, JE, Shiue, H, Sather, C, and Christou, DD. A reduced ratio of dietary carbohydrate to protein improves body composition and blood lipid profiles during weight loss in adult women. *J Nutr* 133:411-417, 2003.

46. Leaf, A and Antonio, J. The effects of overfeeding on body composition: The role of macronutrient composition—a narrative review. *Int J Exerc Sci* 10:1275-1296, 2017.

47. Livesey, G. A perspective on food energy standards for nutrition labelling. *Br J Nutr* 85:271-287, 2001.

48. Loucks, AB and Thuma, JR. Luteinizing hormone pulsatility is disrupted at a threshold of energy availability in regularly menstruating women. *J Clin Endocrinol Metab* 88:297-311, 2003.

49. McColl, EM, Wheeler, GD, Gomes, P, Bhambhani, Y, and Cumming, DC. The effects of acute exercise on pulsatile release LH release in high-mileage male runners. *Clin Endocrinol (Oxf)* 31:617-621, 1989.

50. Moayyedi, P. The epidemiology of obesity and gastrointestinal and other diseases: An overview. *Dig Dis Sci* 53:2293-2299, 2008.

51. Morton, RW, Murphy, KT, McKellar, SR, Schoenfeld, BJ, Henselmans, M, Helms, E, Aragon, AA, Devries, MC, Banfield, L, Krieger, JW, and Phillips, SM. A systematic review, meta-analysis and meta-regression of the effect of protein supplementation on resistance training-induced gains in muscle mass and strength in healthy adults. *Br J Sports Med* 52:376-384, 2018.

52. Mountjoy, M, Sundgot-Borgen, J, Burke, L, Ackerman, KE, Blauwet, C, Constantini, N, Lebrun, C, Lundy, B, Melin, A, Meyer, N, Sherman, R, Tenforde, AS, Torstveit, MK, and Budgett, R. International Olympic Committee (IOC) Consensus statement on relative energy deficiency in sport (RED-S): 2018 update. *Int J Sport Nutr Exerc Metab* 28:316-331, 2018.

53. Mountjoy, M, Sundgot-Borgen, J, Burke, L, Carter, S, Constantini, N, Lebrun, C, Meyer, N, Sherman, R, Steffen, K, Budgett, R, and Ljungqvist, A. The IOC consensus statement: Beyond the female athlete triad--relative energy deficiency in sport (RED-S). *Br J Sports Med* 48:491-7, 2014.

54. Mourier, A, Bigard, A, de Kerviler, E, Roger, B, Legrand, H, and Guezennec, C. Combined effects of caloric restriction and branched-chain amino acid supplementation on body composition and exercise performance in elite wrestlers. *Int J Sport Nutr* 18:47-55, 1997.

55. Müller, W, Gröschl, W, Müller1, R, and Sudi, K. Underweight in ski jumping: The solution of the problem. *Int J Sports Med* 27:926-934, 2006.

56. National Task Force on the Prevention and Treatment of Obesity and National Institutes of Health. Very low-caloric diets. *J Am Med Assoc* 270:967-974, 1993.

57. Nattiv, A, Loucks, AB, Manore, MM, Sanborn, CF, Sundgot-Borgen, J, and Warren, MP. American College of Sports Medicine position stand. The female athlete triad. *Med Sci Sport Exerc* 39:i-ix, 2007.

58. Nieman, DC, Brock, DW, Butterworth, D, Utter, AC, and Nieman, CC. Reducing diet and/or exercise training decreases the lipid and lipoprotein risk factors of moderately obese women. *J Am Coll Nutr* 21:344-350, 2002.

59. Noble, CA and Kushner, RF. An update on low-carbohydrate, high-protein diets. *Curr Opin Gastroenterol* 22:153-159, 2006.

60. Norris, ML, Harrison, ME, Isserlin, L, Robinson, A, Feder, S, and Sampson, M. Gastrointestinal complications associated with anorexia nervosa: A systematic review. *Int J Eat Disord* 49:216-237, 2016.

61. Papageorgiou, M, Elliott-Sale, KJ, Parsons, A, Tang, JCY, Greeves, JP, Fraser, WD, and Sale, C. Effects of reduced energy availability on bone metabolism in women and men. *Bone* 105:191-199, 2017.

62. Rasmussen, BB, Tipton, KD, Miller, SL, Wolf, SE, and Wolfe, RR. An oral essential amino acid-carbohydrate supplement enhances muscle protein anabolism after resistance exercise. *J Appl Physiol* 88:386-392, 2000.

63. Reaven, GM. Insulin resistance: The link between obesity and cardiovascular disease. *Endocrinol Metab Clin North Am* 37:581-601, 2008.

64. Redman, LM, Heilbronn, LK, Martin, CK, Alfonso, A, Smith, SR, and Ravussin, E. Effect of calorie restriction with or without exercise on body composition and fat distribution. *J Clin Endocrinol Metab* 92:865-872, 2007.

65. Rennie, MJ and Tipton, KD. Protein and amino acid metabolism during and after exercise and the effects of nutrition. *Annu Rev Nutr* 20:457-483, 2006.

66. Rickenlund, A, Eriksson, MJ, and Schenck-Gustafsson, K. and Hirschberg, AL. Amenorrhea in female athletes is associated with endothelial dysfunction and unfavorable lipid profile. *J Adolesc* 22:379-388, 2005.

67. Rodriguez, NNR, Di Marco, N, Langley, S, and DiMarco, NM. American College of Sports Medicine, American Dietetic Association, and Dietitians of Canada joint position statement: Nutrition and athletic performance. *Med Sci Sports Exerc* 41:709-731, 2009.

68. de Rougemont, A, Normand, S, Nazare, JA, Skilton, MR, Sothier, M, Vinoy, S, and Laville, M. Beneficial effects of a 5-week low-glycaemic index regimen on weight control and cardiovascular risk factors in overweight non-diabetic subjects. *Br J Nutr* 98:1288-1298, 2007.

69. Saris, WH, Astrup, A, Prentice, AM, Zunft, HJ, Formiguera, X, Venne, WPV de, Raben, A, Poppitt, SD, Seppelt, B, Johnston, S, Vasilaras, TH, and Keogh, GF. Randomized controlled trial of changes in dietary carbohydrate/fat ratio and simple vs complex carbohydrates on body weight and blood lipids: The CARMEN study. The Carbohydrate Ratio Management in European National diets. *Int J Obes Relat Metab Disord* 24:1310-1318, 2000.

70. Sichieri, R, Moura, AS, Genelhu, V, Hu, F, and Willett, WC. An 18-mo randomized trial of a low-glycemic-index diet and weight change in Brazilian women. *Am J Clin Nutr* 86:707-713, 2007.

71. Skov, AR, Toubro, S, Rønn, B, Holm, L, and Astrup, A. Randomized trial on protein vs carbohydrate in ad libitum fat reduced diet for the treatment of obesity. *Int J Obes Relat Metab Disord* 23:528-536, 1999.

72. Sloth, B, Krog-Mikkelsen, I, Flint, A, Tetens, I, Björck, I, Vinoy, S, Elmstahl, H, Astrup, A, Lang, and V, Raben, A. No difference in body weight decrease between a low-glycemic-index and a high-glycemic-index diet but reduced LDL cholesterol after 10-wk ad libitum intake of the low-glycemic-index diet. *Am J Clin Nutr* 80:337-347, 2004.

73. Stevenson, E, Williams, C, Nute, M, Swaile, P, and Tsui, M. The effect of the glycemic index of an evening meal on the metabolic responses to standard high glycemic index breakfast and subsequent exercise in men. *Int J Sport Nutr Exerc Metab* 15:308-322, 2005.

74. Stiegler, P and Cunliffe, A. The role of diet and exercise for the maintenance of lean body mass and resting metabolic rate during weight loss. *Sports Med* 36:239-262, 2006.

75. Strasser, B, Spreitzer, A, and Haber, P. Fat loss depends on energy deficit only, independently of the method for weight loss. *Ann Nutr Metab* 51:428-432, 2007.

76. Strychar, I. Diet in the management of weight loss. *CMAJ* 174:56-63, 2006.

77. Tappy, L. Thermic effect of food and sympathetic nervous system activity in humans. *Reprod Nutr Dev* 36:391-397, 1996.

78. Tarnopolsky, MA, Zawada, C, Richmond, LB, Carter, S, Shearer, J, Graham, T, and Phillips, SM. Gender differences in carbohydrate loading are related to energy intake. *J Appl Physiol* 91:225-230, 2001.

79. Tipton, KD, Borsheim, E, Wolf, SE, Sanford, AP, and Wolfe, RR. Acute response of net muscle protein balance reflects 24-h balance after exercise and amino acid ingestion. *Am J Physiol—Endocrinol Metab* 284:76-89, 2003.

80. Tipton, KD, Elliott, TA, Cree, MG, Aarsland, AA, Sanford, AP, and Wolfe, RR. Stimulation of net muscle protein synthesis by whey protein ingestion before and after exercise. *Am J Physiol Endocrinol Metab* 292: E71-E76, 2007.

81. Tipton, KD, Elliott, TA, Cree, MG, Wolf, SE, Sanford, AP, and Wolfe, RR. Ingestion of casein and whey proteins result in muscle anabolism after resistance exercise. *Med Sci Sports Exerc* 36:2073-2081, 2004.

82. Tipton, KD, Rasmussen, BB, Miller, SL, Wolf, SE, Owens-Stovall, SK, Petrini, BE, and Wolfe, RR. Timing of amino acid-carbohydrate ingestion alters anabolic response of muscle to resistance exercise. *Am J Physiol—Endocrinol Metab* 281:197-206, 2001.

83. Tsai, AG and Wadden, TA. The evolution of very-low-calorie diets: An update and meta-analysis. *Obesity (Silver Spring)* 14:1283-1293, 2006.

84. Valtuena, S, Blanch, S, Barenys, M, Sola, R, and Salas-Salvado, J. Changes in body composition and resting energy expenditure after rapid weight loss: Is there an energy-metabolism adaptation in obese patients? *Int J Obes Relat Metab Disord* 19:119-125, 1995.

85. Vgontzas, AN. Does obesity play a major role in the pathogenesis of sleep apnoea and its associated manifestations via inflammation, visceral adiposity, and insulin resistance? *Arch Physiol Biochem* 114:211-223, 2008.

86. Vogt, S, Heinrich, L, Schumacher YO, Grosshauser, M, Blum, A, Konig, D, Berg, A, and Schmid, A. Energy intake and energy expenditure of elite cyclists during preseason training. *Int J Sports Med* 26:701-706, 2005.

87. Wadden, TA and Frey, DL. A multicenter evaluation of a proprietary weight loss program for the treatment of marked obesity: A five-year follow-up. *Int J Eat Disord* 22:203-212, 1997.

88. Woods, AL, Garvican-Lewis, LA, Lundy, B, Rice, AJ, and Thompson, KG. New approaches to determine fatigue in elite athletes during intensified training: Resting metabolic rate and pacing profile. *PLoS One* 12:1-17, 2017.

89. World Health Organization. *Obesity: Preventing and managing the global epidemic.* Report of a WHO consultation, 2000.

90. Zahouani, A, Boulier, A, and Hespel, JP. Short- and long-term evolution of body composition in 1,389 obese outpatients following a very low calorie diet (Pro'gram18 VLCD). *Acta Diabetol* 40:149-150, 2003.

Chapter 2

1. Ball, SD, and Altena, TS. Comparison of the BOD POD and dual energy x-ray absorptiometry in men. *Physiol Meas* 25:671-678, 2004.

2. Batsis, JA, Mackenzie, TA, Bartels, SJ, Sahakyan, KR, Somers, VK, and Lopez-Jimenez, F. Diagnostic accuracy of body mass index to identify obesity in older adults: NHANES 1999-2004. *Int J Obes (Lond)* 40:761-767, 2016.

3. Bazzocchi, A, Filonzi, G, Ponti, F, Albisinni, U, Guglielmi, G, and Battista, G. Ultrasound: Which role in body composition? *Eur J Radiol* 85:1469-1480, 2016.

4. Bentzur, KM, Kravitz, L, and Lockner, DW. Evaluation of the BOD POD for estimating percent body fat in collegiate track and field female athletes: A comparison of four methods. *J Strength Cond Res* 22:1985-1991, 2008.

5. Bera, TK. Bioelectrical impedance methods for noninvasive health monitoring: A review. *J Med Eng* 2014:381251, 2014.

6. Berrington de Gonzalez, A, Hartge, P, Cerhan, JR, Flint, AJ, Hannan, L, MacInnis, RJ, Moore, SC, Tobias, GS, Anton-Culver, H, Freeman, LB, Beeson, WL, Clipp, SL, English, DR, Folsom, AR, Freedman, DM, Giles, G, Hakansson, N, Henderson, KD, Hoffman-Bolton, J, Hoppin, JA, Koenig, KL, Lee, IM, Linet, MS, Park, Y, Pocobelli, G, Schatzkin, A, Sesso, HD, Weiderpass, E, Willcox, BJ, Wolk, A, Zeleniuch-Jacquotte, A, Willett, WC, and Thun, MJ. Body-mass index and mortality among 1.46 million white adults. *N Engl J Med* 363:2211-2219, 2010.

7. Bhutani, S, Kahn, E, Tasali, E, and Schoeller, DA. Composition of two-week change in body weight under unrestricted free-living conditions. *Physiol Rep* 5, 2017.

8. Blijdorp, K, van den Heuvel-Eibrink, MM, Pieters, R, Boot, AM, Delhanty, PJ, van der Lely, AJ, and Neggers, SJ. Obesity is underestimated using body mass index and waist-hip ratio in long-term adult survivors of childhood cancer. *PLoS One* 7:e43269, 2012.

9. Carter, MC, Burley, VJ, Nykjaer, C, and Cade, JE. 'My Meal Mate' (MMM): Validation of the diet measures captured on a smartphone application to facilitate weight loss. *Br J Nutr* 109:539-546, 2013.

10. Coughlin, SS, Whitehead, M, Sheats, JQ, Mastromonico, J, Hardy, D, and Smith, SA. Smartphone applications for promoting healthy diet and nutrition: A literature review. *Jacobs J Food Nutr* 2:021, 2015.

11. Ghesmaty Sangachin, M, Cavuoto, LA, and Wang, Y. Use of various obesity measurement and classification methods in occupational safety and health research: A systematic review of the literature. *BMC Obes* 5:28, 2018.

12. Heyward, V and Gibson, AL. *Advaned Fitness Assessment and Exercise Prescription*. Champaign, IL: Human Kinetics, 229-278, 2014.

13. Hollis, JF, Gullion, CM, Stevens, VJ, Brantley, PJ, Appel, LJ, Ard JD, Champagne, CM, Dalcin, A, Erlinger, TP, Funk, K, Laferriere, D, Lin, P, Loria, CM, Samuel-Hodge, C, Vollmer, WM, and Svetkey, LP. Weight loss during the intensive intervention phase of the weight-loss maintenance trial. *Arch Phys Med Rehab* 35:118-126, 2008.

14. Johansson, AG, Forslund, A, Sjodin, A, Mallmin, H, Hambraeus, L, and Ljunghall, S. Determinaton of body composition – A comparison of dual-energy X-ray absorptiometry and hydrodensitometry. *Am J Clin Nutr* 57:323-326, 1993.

15. Lee, SY and Gallagher, D. Assessment methods in human body composition. *Curr Opin Clin Nutr Metab Care* 11:566-572, 2008.

16. Levinson, CA, Fewell, L, and Brosof, LC. My Fitness Pal calorie tracker usage in the eating disorders. *Eat Behav* 27:14-16, 2017.

17. Linardon, J and Messer, M. My fitness pal usage in men: Associations with eating disorder symptoms and psychosocial impairment. *Eat Behav* 33:13-17, 2019.

18. Lowry, DW and Tomiyama, AJ. Air displacement plethysmography versus dual-energy x-ray absorptiometry in underweight, normal-weight, and overweight/obese individuals. *PLoS One* 10:e0115086, 2015.

19. McArdle, WD, Katch, FI, and Katch, VL. *Essentials of Exercise Physiology.* Baltimore: Lippincott, 558-627, 2005.

20. Moon, JR, Tobkin, SE, Costa, PB, Smalls, M, Mieding, WK, O'Kroy, JA, Zoeller, RF, and Stout, JR. Validity of the BOD POD for assessing body composition in athletic high school boys. *J Strength Cond Res* 22:263-268, 2008.

21. Ortiz-Hernández, L, López Olmedo, NP, Genis Gómez, MT, Melchor López, DP, and Valdés Flores, J. Application of body mass index to schoolchildren of Mexico City. *Ann Nutr Metab* 53:205-214, 2008.

22. Pi-Sunyer, X. The medical risks of obesity. *Postgrad Med* 121:21-33, 2009.

23. Pineau, JC, Filliard, JR, and Bocquet, M. Ultrasound techniques applied to body fat measurement in male and female athletes. *Journal of athletic training* 44:142-147, 2009.

24. Romero-Corral, A, Somers, VK, Sierra-Johnson, J, Thomas, RJ, Collazo-Clavell, ML, Korinek J, Allison TG, Batsis JA, Sert-Kuniyoshi FH, and Lopez-Jimenez F. Accuracy of body mass index in diagnosing obesity in the adult general population. *Int J Obes* 32:959-966, 2008.

25. Sergi, G, De Rui, M, Stubbs, B, Veronese, N, and Manzato E. Measurement of lean body mass using bioelectrical impedance analysis: A consideration of the pros and cons. *Aging Clin Exp Res* 29:591-597, 2017.

26. Simpson, CC and Mazzeo, SE. Calorie counting and fitness tracking technology: Associations with eating disorder symptomatology. *Eat Behav* 26:89-92, 2017.

27. Sun, G, French, CR, Martin, GR, Younghusband, B, Green, RC, Xie, Y, Mathews, M, Barron, JR, Fitzpatrick, DG, Gulliver, W, and Zhang, H. Comparison of multifrequency bioelectrical impedance analysis with dual-energy X-ray absorptiometry for assessment of percentage body fat in a large, healthy population. *Am J Clin Nutr* 81:74-78, 2005.

28. Tollosa, DN, Van Camp, J, Huybrechts, I, Huybregts, L, Van Loco, J, De Smet, S, Sterck, E, Rabai, C, Van Hecke, T, Vanhaecke, L, Vossen, E, Peeters, M, and Lachat, C. Validity and reproducibility of a food frequency questionnaire for dietary factors related to colorectal cancer. *Nutrients* 9, 2017.

29. Utter, AC and Hager, ME. Evaluation of ultrasound in assessing body composition of high school wrestlers. *Med Sci Sports Exerc* 40:943-949, 2008.

30. Wagner, DR. Ultrasound as a tool to assess body fat. *J Obes* 2013:280713, 2013.

31. Witt, K and Bush, E. College athletes with an elevated body mass index often have a high upper arm muscle area, but not elevated triceps and subscapular skinfolds. *J Am Diet Assoc* 105:599- 602, 2005.

Chapter 3

1. Ahlborg, BG, Bergström, J, Brohult, J, Ekelund, LG, Hultman, E, and Maschino, G. Human muscle glycogen content and capacity for prolonged exercise after different diets. *Foersvarsmedicin* 3:85-99, 1967.

2. Areta, JL and Hopkins, WG. Skeletal muscle glycogen content at rest and during endurance exercise in humans: A meta-analysis. *Sports Med* 48:2091-2102, 2018.

2a. Atkinson, F.S., K. Foster-Powell, and J.C. Brand-Miller. 2008. International table of glycolic index and glycolic load values: 2008. *Diab Care* 31 (12): 2281-2283.

3. Baar, K and McGee, SL. Optimizing training adaptation by manipulating glycogen. *Euro J Sport Sci* 8, 2008.

4. Balsom, PD, Gaitanos, GC, Soderlund, K, and Ekblom, B. High-intensity exercise and muscle glycogen availability in humans. *Acta Physiol Scand* 165:337-345, 1999.

5. Bartlett, JD, Hawley, JA, and Morton, JP. Carbohydrate availability and exercise training adaptation: Too much of a good thing? *Eur J Sport Sci* 15:3-12, 2015.

6. Bergström J, Hermansen, L, Hultman, E, and Saltin, B. Diet, muscle glycogen and physical performance. *Acta Physiol Scand* 71:140-150, 1967.

7. Biolo, G, Williams, BD, Fleming, RY, and Wolfe, RR. Insulin action on muscle protein kinetics and amino acid transport during recovery after resistance exercise. *Diabetes* 48:949-957, 1999.

8. Burke, LM, Collier, GR, and Hargreaves, M. Glycemic index—a new tool in sport nutrition? *Int J Sport Nutr* 8:401-415, 1998.

9. Burke, LM, Ross, ML, Garvican-Lewis, LA, Welvaert, M, Heikura, IA, Forbes, SG, Mirtschin, JG, Cato, LE, Strobel, N, Sharma, AP, and Hawley, JA. Low carbohydrate, high fat diet impairs exercise economy and negates the performance benefit from intensified training in elite race walkers. *J Physiol* 595:2785-2807, 2017.

10. Carter, JM, Jeukendrup, AE, and Jones, DA. The effect of carbohydrate mouth rinse on 1-h cycle time trial performance. *Med Sci Sports Exerc* 36:2107-2111, 2004.

11. Carter, JM, Jeukendrup, AE, Mann, CH, and Jones, DA. The effect of glucose infusion on glucose kinetics during a 1-h time trial. *Med Sci Sports Exerc* 36:1543-1550, 2004.

12. Casey, A, Short, AH, Curtis, S, and Greenhaff, PL. The effect of glycogen availability on power output and the metabolic response to repeated bouts of maximal, isokinetic exercise in man. *Eur J Appl Physiol Occup Physiol* 72:249-255, 1996.

13. Chambers, ES, Bridge, MW, and Jones, DA. Carbohydrate sensing in the human mouth: Effects on exercise performance and brain activity. *J Physiol* 587:1779-1794, 2009.

14. Coleman, E. Update on carbohydrate: Solid versus liquid. *Int J Sport Nutr* 4:80-88, 1994.

15. Conley, MS and Stone, MH. Carbohydrate ingestion/supplementation or resistance exercise and training. *Sports Med* 21:7-17, 1996.

16. Costill, DL. Carbohydrates for exercise: Dietary demands for optimal performance. *Int J Sports Med* 9:1-18, 1988.

17. Coyle, EF. Substrate utilization during exercise in active people. *Am J Clin Nutr* 61:968S-979S, 1995.

18. Coyle, EF, Coggan, AR, Hemmert, MK, and Ivy, JL. Muscle glycogen utilization during prolonged strenuous exercise when fed carbohydrate. *J Appl Physiol* 61:165-172, 1986.

19. Coyle, EF, Coggan, AR, Hemmert, MK, Lowe, RC, and Walters, TJ. Substrate usage during prolonged exercise following a preexercise meal. *J Appl Physiol* 59:429-433, 1985.

20. Devaki, M, Nirupama, R, and Yajurvedi, HN. Chronic stress-induced oxidative damage and hyperlipidemia are accompanied by atherosclerotic development in rats. *Stress* 16:233-243, 2013.

20a. Diogenes GI Database. 2010. www.diogenes-eu.org/GI-Database/Default.htm.

21. Essen, B and Henriksson, J. Glycogen content of individual muscle fibres in man. *Acta Physiol Scand* 90:645-647, 1974.

22. Fairchild, TJ, Dillon, P, Curtis, C, and Dempsey, AR. Glucose ingestion does not improve maximal isokinetic force. *J Strength Cond Res* 30:194-199, 2016.

23. Foster, C, Costill, DL, and Fink, WJ. Effects of preexercise feedings on endurance performance. *Med Sci Sports* 11:1-5, 1979.

24. Foster-Powell, K, Holt, SH, and Brand-Miller, JC. International table of glycemic index and glycemic load values: 2002. *Am J Clin Nutr* 76:5-56, 2002.

25. Gollnick, PD, Piehl, K, and Saltin, B. Selective glycogen depletion pattern in human muscle fibres after exercise of varying intensity and at varying pedalling rates. *J Physiol* 241:45-57, 1974.

26. Gordon, B, Kohn, LA, Levine, SA, Matton, M, Scriver, WM, and Whiting, WB. Sugar content of the blood following a marathon race with especial reference to the prevention of hypoglycemia: Further observations. *JAMA* 85: 508-509, 1925.

27. Green, KJ, Croaker, SJ, and Rowbottom, DG. Carbohydrate supplementation and exercise-induced changes in T-lymphocyte function. *J Appl Physiol* 95:1216-1223, 2003.

28. Haff, GG, Koch, AJ, Potteiger, JA, Kuphal, KE, Magee, LM, Green, SB, and Jakicic, JJ. Carbohydrate supplementation attenuates muscle glycogen loss during acute bouts of resistance exercise. *Int J Sport Nutr Exerc Metab* 10:326-339, 2000.

29. Haff, GG, Lehmkuhl, MJ, McCoy, LB, and Stone, MH. Carbohydrate supplementation and resistance training. *J Strength Cond Res* 17:187-196, 2003.

30. Haff, GG, Schroeder, CA, Koch, AJ, Kuphal, KE, Comeau, MJ, and Potteiger, JA. The effects of supplemental carbohydrate ingestion on intermittent isokinetic leg exercise. *J Sports Med Phys Fitness* 41:216-222, 2001.

31. Hargreaves, M. Carbohydrate replacement during exercise. In *Nutrition in Sport*. R Maughan, ed. Oxford: Blackwell Science, 112-118, 2000.

32. Hawley, JA, Burke, LM, Phillips, SM, and Spriet, LL. Nutritional modulation of training—induced skeletal muscle adaptations. *J Appl Physiol* 110:834-845, 2011.

33. Hawley, JA, Schabort, EJ, Noakes, TD, and Dennis, SC. Carbohydrate-loading and exercise performance. An update. *Sports Med* 24:73-81, 1997.

33a. Henry, C.J.K., H.J. Lightowler, C.M. Stirk, H. Renton, and S. Hails. 2005. Glycaemic index and glycaemic load values of commercially available products in the UK. *Br J Nutr* 94:922-930.

33b. Herda, T.J., and Cramer, J.T. "Bioenergetics of exercise and training" in *Essentials of strength training and conditioning*, 4th ed. Champaign, IL: Human Kinetics 47; 2016.

34. Hultman, E. Studies on muscle metabolism of glycogen and active phosphate in man with special reference to exercise and diet. *Scand J Clin Lab Invest Suppl* 94:1-63, 1967.

35. Ihalainen, JK, Vuorimaa, T, Puurtinen, R, Hamalainen, I, and Mero, AA. Effects of carbohydrate ingestion on acute leukocyte, cortisol, and interleukin-6 response in high-intensity long-distance running. *J Strength Cond Res* 28:2786-2792, 2014.

36. Institute of Medicine (U.S.). Panel on Macronutrients. and Institute of Medicine (U.S.). Standing Committee on the Scientific Evaluation of Dietary Reference Intakes. *Dietary Reference Intakes for energy, carbohydrate, fiber, fat, fatty acids, cholesterol, protein, and amino acids*. Washington, DC: National Academies Press, 2005.

37. Ivy, JL. Dietary strategies to promote glycogen synthesis after exercise. *Can J Appl Physiol* 26 Suppl:S236-245, 2001.

38. Jenkins, DJ, Wolever, TM, Taylor, RH, Barker, H, Fielden, H, Baldwin, JM, Bowling, AC, Newman, HC, Jenkins, AL, and Goff, DV. Glycemic index of foods: A physiological basis for carbohydrate exchange. *Am J Clin Nutr* 34:362-366, 1981.

39. Jentjens, RL, Moseley, L, Waring, RH, Harding, LK, and Jeukendrup, AE. Oxidation of combined ingestion of glucose and fructose during exercise. *J Appl Physiol* 96:1277-1284, 2004.

40. Jentjens, RL, Venables, MC, and Jeukendrup, AE. Oxidation of exogenous glucose, sucrose, and maltose during prolonged cycling exercise. *J Appl Physiol* 96:1285-1291, 2004.

41. Jeukendrup, AE. Carbohydrate intake during exercise and performance. *Nutrition* 20: 669-677, 2004.

41a. Jeukendrup, A. and Gleeson, M. *Sport Nutrition,* 3rd ed. Champaign, IL: Human Kinetics; 2019.

42. Jeukendrup, AE and Jentjens, R. Oxidation of carbohydrate feedings during prolonged exercise: Current thoughts, guidelines and directions for future research. *Sports Med* 29: 407-424, 2000.

43. Kjaer, M. Hepatic glucose production during exercise. *Adv Exp Med Biol* 441:117-127, 1998.

44. Koh, A, De Vadder, F, Kovatcheva-Datchary, P, and Backhed, F. From dietary fiber to host physiology: Short-chain fatty acids as key bacterial metabolites. *Cell* 165:1332-1345, 2016.

45. Krings, BM, Rountree, JA, McAllister, MJ, Cummings, PM, Peterson, TJ, Fountain, BJ, and Smith, JW. Effects of acute carbohydrate ingestion on anaerobic exercise performance. *J Int Soc Sports Nutr* 13:40, 2016.

46. Kulik, JR, Touchberry, CD, Kawamori, N, Blumert, PA, Crum, AJ, and Haff, GG. Supplemental carbohydrate ingestion does not improve performance of high-intensity resistance exercise. *J Strength Cond Res* 22:1101-1107, 2008.

47. Kumari, M, Grahame-Clarke, C, Shanks, N, Marmot, M, Lightman, S, and Vallance, P. Chronic stress accelerates atherosclerosis in the apolipoprotein E deficient mouse. *Stress* 6:297-299, 2003.

48. Leloir, LF. Two decades of research on the biosynthesis of saccharides. *Science* 172: 1299-1303, 1971.

49. Levine, SA, Gordon, B, and Derick, CL. Some changes in the chemical constituents of the blood following a marathon race with special reference to the development of hypoglycemia. *JAMA* 82:1778-1779, 1924.

50. Long, JE. High fructose corn syrup. In *Alternative Sweeteners*. Nabors, LO, Gelardi RC, eds. New York: Marcel Dekker, 247-258, 1991.

51. Makki, K, Deehan, EC, Walter, J, and Backhed, F. The impact of dietary fiber on gut microbiota in host health and disease. *Cell Host Microbe* 23:705-715, 2018.

52. Marlett, JA, McBurney, MI, Slavin, JL, and American Dietetic A. Position of the American Dietetic Association: Health implications of dietary fiber. *J Am Diet Assoc* 102:993-1000, 2002.

53. Marmy-Conus, N, Fabris, S, Proietto, J, and Hargreaves, M. Preexercise glucose ingestion and glucose kinetics during exercise. *J Appl Physiol* 81:853-857, 1996.

54. Maughan, RJ, Greenhaff, PL, Leiper, JB, Ball, D, Lambert, CP, and Gleeson, M. Diet composition and the performance of high-intensity exercise. *J Sports Sci* 15:265-275, 1997.

55. McAnulty, SR, McAnulty, LS, Nieman, DC, Morrow, JD, Utter, AC, Henson, DA, Dumke, CL, and Vinci, DM. Influence of carbohydrate ingestion on oxidative stress and plasma antioxidant potential following a 3-h run. *Free Radic Res* 37:835-840, 2003.

56. McArdle, WD, Katch, FI, and Katch, VL. *Sports and Exercise Nutrition*. Philadelphia: Lippincott, Williams & Wilkens, 238-241, 2019.

57. Nardone, A, Romano, C, and Schieppati, M. Selective recruitment of high-threshold human motor units during voluntary isotonic lengthening of active muscles. *J Physiol* 409:451-471, 1989.

58. Nehlsen-Cannarella, SL, Fagoaga, OR, Nieman, DC, Henson, DA, Butterworth, DE, Schmitt, RL, Bailey, EM, Warren, BJ, Utter, A, and Davis, JM. Carbohydrate and the cytokine response to 2.5 h of running. *J Appl Physiol* 82:1662-1667, 1997.

59. Randell, RK, Rollo, I, Roberts, TJ, Dalrymple, KJ, Jeukendrup, AE, and Carter, JM. Maximal fat oxidation rates in an athletic population. *Med Sci Sports Exerc* 49:133-140, 2017.

60. Rauch, HG, St Clair Gibson, A, Lambert, EV, and Noakes, TD. A signalling role for muscle glycogen in the regulation of pace during prolonged exercise. *Br J Sports Med* 39:34-38, 2005.

61. Robergs, RA, Pearson, DR, Costill, DL, Fink, WJ, Pascoe, DD, Benedict, MA, Lambert, CP, and Zachwieja, JJ. Muscle glycogenolysis during differing intensities of weight-resistance exercise. *J Appl Physiol* 70:1700-1706, 1991.

62. Rockwell, MS, Rankin, JW, and Dixon, H. Effects of muscle glycogen on performance of repeated sprints and mechanisms of fatigue. *Int J Sport Nutr Exerc Metab* 13:1-14, 2003.

63. Roediger, WE. Utilization of nutrients by isolated epithelial cells of the rat colon. *Gastroenterology* 83:424-429, 1982.

64. Shulman, RG and Rothman, DL. The "glycogen shunt" in exercising muscle: A role for glycogen in muscle energetics and fatigue. *Proc Natl Acad Sci USA* 98:457-461, 2001.

65. Smith, JW, Krings, BM, Shepherd, BD, Waldman, HS, Basham, SA, and McAllister, MJ. Effects of carbohydrate and branched-chain amino acid beverage ingestion during acute upper body resistance exercise on performance and postexercise hormone response. *Appl Physiol Nutr Metab* 43:504-509, 2018.

66. Smith, JW, Pascoe, DD, Passe, DH, Ruby, BC, Stewart, LK, Baker, LB, and Zachwieja, JJ. Curvilinear dose-response relationship of carbohydrate (0-120 g.h(-1)) and performance. *Med Sci Sports Exerc* 45:336-341, 2013.

67. Smith, JW, Zachwieja, JJ, Peronnet, F, Passe, DH, Massicotte, D, Lavoie, C, and Pascoe, DD. Fuel selection and cycling endurance performance with ingestion of [13C]glucose: Evidence for a carbohydrate dose response. *J Appl Physiol* 108:1520-1529, 2010.

68. Spriet, LL. Regulation of fat/carbohydrate interaction in human skeletal muscle during exercise. *Adv Exp Med Biol* 441:249-261, 1998.

69. Tesch, PA, Colliander, EB, and Kaiser, P. Muscle metabolism during intense, heavy-resistance exercise. *Eur J Appl Physiol Occup Physiol* 55:362-366, 1986.

70. Tesch, PA, Ploutz-Snyder, LL, Yström, L, Castro, MJ, and Dudley, GA. Skeletal muscle glycogen loss evoked by resistance exercise. *J Strength Cond Res* 12:67-73, 1998.

71. Thomas, DT, Erdman, KA, and Burke, LM. American College of Sports Medicine Joint Position Statement. Nutrition and athletic performance. *Med Sci Sports Exerc* 48:543-568, 2016.

72. Tipton, KD, Rasmussen, BB, Miller, SL, Wolf, SE, Owens-Stovall, SK, Petrini, BE, and Wolfe, RR. Timing of amino acid-carbohydrate ingestion alters ana-

bolic response of muscle to resistance exercise. *Am J Physiol Endoc Metab* 281: E197-206, 2001.

73. U.S. Department of Agriculture ARS, Beltsville Human Nutrition Research Center, Food Surveys Research Group (Beltsville, MD) and U.S. Department of Health and Human Services, Centers for Disease Control and Prevention, National Center for Health Statistics (Hyattsville, MD). *What we eat in America, NHANES 2015-2016*, individuals 2 years and over (excluding breast-fed children), day 1. www.ars.usda.gov/nea/bhnrc/fsrg, 2016.

74. Van Hall, G. Lactate as a fuel for mitochondrial respiration. *Acta Physiol Scand* 168:643-656, 2000.

75. Wax, B, Brown, SP, Webb, HE, and Kavazis, AN. Effects of carbohydrate supplementation on force output and time to exhaustion during static leg contractions superimposed with electromyostimulation. *J Strength Cond Res* 26:1717-1723, 2012.

76. Wax, B, Kavazis, AN, and Brown, SP. Effects of supplemental carbohydrate ingestion during superimposed electromyostimulation exercise in elite weightlifters. *J Strength Cond Res* 27:3084-3090, 2013.

77. White, JS. Sucrose, HFCS, and fructose: History, manufacture, composition, applications, and production. In *Fructose, High Fructose Corn Syrup, Sucrose and Health*. Rippe, JM, ed. New York: Springer Science+Business Media, 13-34, 2014.

78. Widrick, JJ, Costill, DL, Fink, WJ, Hickey, MS, McConell, GK, and Tanaka, H. Carbohydrate feedings and exercise performance: Effect of initial muscle glycogen concentration. *J Appl Physiol* 74:2998-3005, 1993.

Chapter 4

1. Areta, JL, Burke, LM, Ross, ML, Camera, DM, West, DW, Broad, EM, Jeacocke, NA, Moore, DR, Stellingwerff, T, Phillips, SM, Hawley, JA, and Coffey, VG. Timing and distribution of protein ingestion during prolonged recovery from resistance exercise alters myofibrillar protein synthesis. *J Physiol* 591:2319-2331, 2013.

2. Atherton, PJ, Etheridge, T, Watt, PW, Wilkinson, D, Selby, A, Rankin, D, Smith, K, and Rennie, MJ. Muscle full effect after oral protein: Time-dependent concordance and discordance between human muscle protein synthesis and mTORC1 signaling. *Am J Clin Nutr* 92(5):1080-1088, 2010.

3. Barr, D. *The Anabolic Index: Optimized Nutrition and Supplementation Manual*. Montreal: Lepine, 45-48, 2008.

4. Burd, NA, West, DW, Moore, DR, Atherton, PJ, Staples, AW, Prior, T, Tang, JE, Rennie, MJ, Baker, SK, and Phillips, SM. Enhanced amino acid sensitivity of myofibrillar protein synthesis persists for up to 24 h after resistance exercise in young men. *J Nutr* 141(4):568-573, 2011.

5. Castro, LH, S de Araújo, FH, Olimpio, MY, de B Primo R, Pereira, T, Lopes, LA, S de M Trindade, E, Fernandes, R, and Oesterreich, S. A Comparative meta-analysis of the effect of concentrated, hydrolyzed, and isolated whey protein supplementation on body composition of physical activity practitioners. *Nutrients* 11(9):E2047, 2019.

6. Churchward-Venne, TA, Breen, L, Di Donato, DM, Hector, AJ, Mitchell, CJ, Moore, DR, Stellingwerff, T, Breuille, D, Offord, EA, Baker, SK, and Phillips, SM. Leucine supplementation of a low-protein mixed macronutrient beverage enhances myofibrillar protein synthesis in young men: A double-blind, randomized trial. *Am J Clin Nutr* 99(2):276-286, 2014.

7. Cotter, JA and Barr, D. Dietary protein efficacy: Dose and peri-exercise timing. In *Dietary Protein and Resistance Exercise*. Lowery, JM, Antonio, J, eds. Boca Raton: CRC Press 69-94, 2012.

8. Elliot, TA, Cree, MG, Sanford, AP, Wolfe, RR, and Tipton, KD. Milk ingestion stimulates net muscle protein synthesis following resistance exercise. *Med Sci Sports Exerc* 38:667-674, 2006.

9. Farup, J, Rahbek, SK, Storm, AC, Klitgaard, S, Jørgensen, H, Bibby, BM, Serena, A, and Vissing, K. Effect of degree of hydrolysis of whey protein on in vivo plasma amino acid appearance in humans. *Springerplus* 5:382, 2016.

10. Fürst, P and Stehle, P. What are the essential elements needed for the determination of amino acid requirements in humans? *J Nutr* 134(6 Suppl):1558S-1565S, 2004.

11. Hamilton-Reeves, JM, Vazquez, G, Duval, SJ, Phipps, WR, Kurzer, MS, and Messina, MJ. Clinical studies show no effects of soy protein or isoflavones on reproductive hormones in men: Results of a meta-analysis. *Fertil Steril* 94(3):997-1007, 2010.

12. Hulmi JJ, Lockwood CM, and Stout JR. Effect of protein/essential amino acids and resistance training on skeletal muscle hypertrophy: A case for whey protein. *Nutr Metab (Lond)* 7:51, 2010.

13. Jäger, R, Kerksick, CM, Campbell, BI, Cribb, PJ, Wells, SD, Skwiat, TM, Purpura, M, Ziegenfuss, TN, Ferrando, AA, Arent, SM, Smith-Ryan, AE, Stout, JR, Arciero, PJ, Ormsbee, MJ, Taylor, LW, Wilborn, CD, Kalman, DS, Kreider, RB, and Willoughby, DS, Hoffman, JR, Krzykowski, JL, and Antonio, J. International Society of Sports Nutrition Position Stand: Protein and exercise. *J Int Soc Sports Nutr* 14:20, 2017.

14. Kerksick, CM, Arent, S, Schoenfeld, BJ, Stout, JR, Campbell, B, Wilborn, CD, Taylor, L, Kalman, D, Smith-Ryan, AE, Kreider, RB, Willoughby, D, Arciero, PJ, VanDusseldorp, TA, Ormsbee, MJ, Wildman, R, Greenwood, M, Ziegenfuss, TN, Aragon, AA, and Antonio, J. International society of sports nutrition position stand: Nutrient timing. *J Int Soc Sports Nutr* 14:33, 2017.

15. Lemon, PW, Tarnopolsky, MA, MacDougall, JD, and Atkinson, SA. Protein requirements and muscle mass/strength changes during intensive training in novice bodybuilders. *J Appl Physiol (1985)* 73(2):767-775, 1992.

16. Lockwood, CM, Roberts, MD, Dalbo, VJ, Smith-Ryan, AE, Kendall, KL, Moon, JR, and Stout, JR. Effects of hydrolyzed whey versus other whey protein supplements on the physiological response to 8 weeks of resistance exercise in college-aged males. *J Am Coll Nutr* 36:16-27, 2017.

17. Lugo, JP, Saiyed, ZM, Lau, FC, Molina, JP, Pakdaman, MN, Shamie, AN, and Udani, JK. Undenatured type II collagen (UC-II®) for joint support: A random-

ized, double-blind, placebo-controlled study in healthy volunteers. *J Int Soc Sports Nutr* 10(1):48, 2013.

18. Marinangeli, C and House, JD. Potential impact of the digestible indispensable amino acid score as a measure of protein quality on dietary regulations and health. *Nutr Rev* 75(8):658-667, 2017.

19. Marsh, KA, Munn, EA, and Baines, SK. Protein and vegetarian diets. *Med J Aust* 199(S4):S7-S10, 2013.

20. Messina, M, Lynch, H, Dickinson, JM, and Reed, KE. No difference between the effects of supplementing with soy protein versus animal protein on gains in muscle mass and strength in response to resistance exercise. *Int J Sport Nutr Exerc Metab* 28(6):674-685, 2018.

21. Mettler, S, Mitchell, N, and Tipton, KD. Increased protein intake reduces lean body mass loss during weight loss in athletes. *Med Sci Sports Exerc* 42(2):326-337, 2010.

22. Moore, DR, Tang, JE, Burd, NA, Rerecich, T, Tarnopolsky, MA, and Phillips, SM. Differential stimulation of myofibrillar and sarcoplasmic protein synthesis with protein ingestion at rest and after resistance exercise. *J Physiol* 587(Pt 4):897-904, 2009.

23. Moore, DR, Robinson, MJ, Fry, JL, Tang, JE, Glover, EI, Wilkinson, SB, Prior, T, Tarnopolsky, MA, and Phillips, SM. Ingested protein dose response of muscle and albumin protein synthesis after resistance exercise in young men. *Am J Clin Nutr* 89(1):161-168, 2009.

24. Moore DR. Maximizing post-exercise anabolism: The case for relative protein intakes. *Front Nutr* 6:147, 2019.

25. Morifuji, M, Ishizaka, M, Baba, S, Fukuda, K, Matsumoto, H, Koga, J, Kanegae, M, and Higuchi, M. Comparison of different sources and degrees of hydrolysis of dietary protein: Effect on plasma amino acids, dipeptides, and insulin responses in human subjects. *J Agric Food Chem* 58:8788-8797, 2010.

26. Morton, RW, Murphy, KT, McKellar, SR, Schoenfeld, BJ, Henselmans, M, Helms, E, Aragon, AA, Devries, MC, Banfield, L, Krieger, JW, and Phillips, SM. A systematic review, meta-analysis and meta-regression of the effect of protein supplementation on resistance training-induced gains in muscle mass and strength in healthy adults. *Br J Sports Med* 52:376-384, 2018.

27. Murphy, CH, Hector, AJ, and Phillips, SM. Considerations for protein intake in managing weight loss in athletes. *Eur J Sport Sci* 15:21-28, 2015.

28. Res, PT, Groen, B, Pennings, B, Beelen, M, Wallis, GA, Gijsen, AP, Senden, JM, and Van Loon, LJ. Protein ingestion before sleep improves postexercise overnight recovery. *Med Sci Sports Exerc* 44(8):1560-1569, 2012.

29. Shimomura, Y, Yamamoto, Y, Bajotto, G, Sato, J, Murakami, T, Shimomura, N, Kobayashi, H, and Mawatari, K. Nutraceutical effects of branched-chain amino acids on skeletal muscle. *J Nutr* 136(2):529S-532S, 2006.

30. Snijders, T, Res, PT, Smeets, JS, van Vliet, S, van Kranenburg, J, Maase, K, Kies, AK, Verdijk, LB, and van Loon, LJ. Protein ingestion before sleep increases

muscle mass and strength gains during prolonged resistance-type exercise training in healthy young men. *J Nutr* 145:1178-1184, 2015.

31. Spano, M, Basic nutrition factors in health. In *Essentials of Strength Training and Conditioning*. 4th ed. Haff, GG, Triplett, TN, eds. Champaign, IL: Human Kinetics, 175-199, 2016.

32. Thomas, DT, Erdman, KA, and Burke, LM. American College of Sports Medicine joint position statement. Nutrition and athletic performance. *Med Sci Sports Exerc* 48(3):543-568, 2016.

33. Trommelen, J, Holwerda, AM, Kouw, IW, Langer, H, Halson, SL, Rollo, I, Verdijk, LB, and Van Loon, LJ. Resistance exercise augments postprandial overnight muscle protein synthesis rates. *Med Sci Sports Exerc* 48:2517-2525, 2016.

34. Trommelen, J, and van Loon, LJ. Pre-sleep protein ingestion to improve the skeletal muscle adaptive response to exercise training. *Nutrients* 8(12):E763, 2016.

35. Trumbo, P, Schlicker, S, Yates, AA, and Poos, M. Food and Nutrition Board of the Institute of Medicine, National Academies. Dietary Reference Intakes for energy, carbohydrate, fiber, fat, fatty acids, cholesterol, protein and amino acids. *J Am Diet Assoc* 102(11):1621-1630, 2002.

36. Van Huis, A, Klunder, H, Itterbeeck, JV, Mertens, E, Halloran, A, Muir, G, and Vantomme, P. *Edible Insects: Future Prospects for Food and Feed Security*. Food and Agriculture Organization of the United Nations: Rome, Italy, 2013.

37. van Vliet, S, Shy, EL, Abou Sawan, S, Beals, JW, West, DW, Skinner, SK, Ulanov, AV, Li, Z, Paluska, SA, Parsons, CM, Moore, DR, and Burd, NA. Consumption of whole eggs promotes greater stimulation of postexercise muscle protein synthesis than consumption of isonitrogenous amounts of egg whites in young men. *Am J Clin Nutr* 106(6):1401-1412, 2017.

38. van Vliet, SV, Beals, JW, Martinez, IG, Skinner, SK, and Burd, NA. Achieving optimal post-exercise muscle protein remodeling in physically active adults through whole food consumption. *Nutrients* 10(2): E224, 2018.

39. Vangsoe, MT, Joergensen, MS, Heckmann, LL, and Hansen, M. Effects of insect protein supplementation during resistance training on changes in muscle mass and strength in young men. *Nutrients* 10(3)E335, 2018.

40. Vangsoe, MT, Thogersen, R, Bertram, HC, Heckmann, LL, and Hansen, M. Ingestion of insect protein isolate enhances blood amino acid concentrations similar to soy protein in a human trial. *Nutrients* 10(10): E1357, 2018.

41. Witard, OC, Jackman, SR, Breen, L, Smith, K, Selby, A, and Tipton, KD. Myofibrillar muscle protein synthesis rates subsequent to a meal in response to increasing doses of whey protein at rest and after resistance exercise. *Am J Clin Nutr* 99(1):86-95, 2014.

42. Wolfe, RR, Cifelli, AM, Kostas, G, and Kim, IY. Optimizing protein intake in adults: Interpretation and application of the recommended dietary allowance compared with the acceptable macronutrient distribution range. *Adv Nutr* 8(2):266-275, 2017.

43. Yetley, EA, MacFarlane, AJ, Greene-Finestone, LS, Garza, C, Ard, JD, Atkinson, SA, Bier, DM, Carriquiry, AL, Harlan, WR, Hattis, D, King, JC, Krewski, D, O'Connor, DL, Prentice, RL, Rodricks, JV, and Wells, GA. Options for basing dietary reference intakes (DRIs) on chronic disease endpoints: Report from a joint US-Canadian-sponsored working group. *Am J Clin Nutr* 105(1):249S-285S, 2017.

44. Yi, L, Lakemond, CMM, Sagis, LMC, Eisner-Schadler, V, van Huis, A, and van Boekel, MAJS. Extraction and characterisation of protein fractions from five insect species. *Food Chem* 141:3341-3348, 2013.

Chapter 5

1. Ahrén, B, Mari, A, Fyfe, CL, Tsofliou, F, Sneddon, AA, Wahle, KW, Winzell, MS, Pacini G, and Williams, L. Effects of conjugated linoleic acid plus n-3 polyunsaturated fatty acids on insulin secretion and estimated insulin sensitivity in men. *Eur J Clin Nutr* 63(6):778-786, 2009.

2. Andersson, A, Sjodin, A, Hedman, A, Olsson, R, and Vessby, B. Fatty acid profile of skeletal muscle phospholipids in trained and untrained young men. *Am J Physiol Endocrinol Metab* 279(4):E744-E751, 2000.

3. Aoyama, T, Nosaka, N, and Kasai, M. Research on the nutritional characteristics of medium-chain fatty acids. *J Med Investig* 54(3-4):385-388, 2007.

4. Archer, S, Green, D, Chamberlain, M, Dyer, A, and Liu, K. Association of dietary fish and n-3 fatty acid intake with hemostatic factors in the coronary artery risk development in young adults (CARDIA) study. *Arterioscler, Thromb Vasc Biol* 18:1119-1123, 1998.

5. Arterburn, LM, Hall, EB, and Oken, H. Distribution, interconversion, and dose response of n-3 fatty acids in humans. *Am J Clin Nutr* 83(6 Suppl):1467S-1476S, 2006.

6. Bastard, J, Maachi, M, Lagathu, C, Kim, M, Caron, M, Vidal, H, Capeau, J, and Feve, B. Recent advances in the relationship between obesity, inflammation, and insulin resistance. *Eur Cytokine Network* 17(1):4-12, 2006.

7. Boudreau, MD, Chanmugam, PS, Hart, SB, Lee, SH, and Hwang, DH. Lack of dose response by dietary n-3 fatty acids at a constant ratio of n-3 to n-6 fatty acids in suppressing eicosanoid biosynthesis from arachidonic acid. *Am J Clin Nutr* 54(1):111-117, 1991.

8. Breslow, J. n-3 fatty acids and cardiovascular disease. *Am J Clin Nutr* 83(6 Suppl): 1477S-1482S, 2006.

9. Brooks, GA. Importance of the "crossover" concept in exercise metabolism. *Clin Exper Pharm Physiol* 24(11):889-895, 1997.

10. Browning, L. n-3 Polyunsaturated fatty acids, inflammation and obesity-related disease. *Proc Nutr Soc* 62(2):447-453, 2003.

11. Bueno, NB, de Melo, IS, de Oliveira, SL, and da Rocha Ataide, T. Very-low carbohydrate ketogenic diet v. Low- fat diet for long-term weight loss: A meta-analysis of randomised controlled trials. *Brit J Nutr* 110(07):1178-1187, 2013.

12. Burke, L. Re-examining high-fat diets for sports performance: Did we call the 'nail in the coffin' too soon? *Sports Med* 45 Suppl 1:S33-49, 2015.

13. Burke, L, Ross, M, Garvican-Lewis, L, Welavaert, M, Heikura, I, Forbes, S, Mirtschin, J, Cato, L, Strobel, N, Sharma, A, and Hawley, J. Low carbohydrate, high fat diet impairs exercise economy and negates the performance benefit from intensified training in elite race walkers. *J Physiol* 595(9):2785-2807, 2017.

14. Calabrese, C, Myer, S, Munson, S, Turet, P, and Birdsall, T. A cross-over study of the effect of a single oral feeding of medium chain triglyceride oil vs. canola oil on post-ingestion plasma triglyceride levels in healthy men. *Alt Med Rev* 4(1): 23-28, 1999.

15. Calder, P. n-3 polyunsaturated fatty acids, inflammation, and inflammatory diseases. *Am J Clin Nutr* 83(6 Suppl):1505S-1519S, 2006.

16. Cannon, J, Fiatarone, M, Meydani, M, Gong, J, Scott, L, Blumberg, J, and Evans, W. Aging and dietary modulation of elastase and interleukin-1 beta secretion. *Am J Physiol* 268(1 Pt 2):R208-213, 1995.

17. Childs, C, Romeu-Nadal, M, Burdge, G, and Calder, P. Gender differences in the n-3 fatty acid content of tissues. *Proc Nutr Soc* 67(1):19-27, 2008.

18. Curtis, C, Hughes, C, Flannery, C, Little, C, Harwood, J, and Caterson, B. n-3 fatty acids specifically modulate catabolic factors involved in articular cartilage degradation. *J Biol Chem* 275(2):721-724, 2000.

19. Delarue, J, Matzinger, O, Binnert, C, Schneiter, P, Chiolero, R, and Tappy L. Fish oil prevents the adrenal activation elicited by mental stress in healthy men. *Diab Metab* 29(3):289-295, 2003.

20. Dorgan, J, Judd, J, Longcope, C, Brown, C, Schatzkin, A, Clevidence, B, Campbell, W, Nair, P, Franz, C, Kahle, L, and Taylor, P. Effects of dietary fat and fiber on plasma and urine androgens and estrogens in men: A controlled feeding study. *Am J Clin Nutr* 64(6): 850-855, 1996.

21. Dowden, A. Bulletproof coffee: Plenty of bull. And fat too. New York: American Council on Science and Health, acsh.org/news/2019/06//08/bulletproof-coffee-plenty-bull-and-fat-too-14079. Accessed November 20, 2019.

22. Ehringer, W, Belcher, D, Wassall, S, and Stillwell, W. A comparison of the effects of linolenic (18:3 omega 3) and docosahexaenoic (22:6 omega 3) acids on phospholipid bilayers. *Chem Physics Lipids* 54(2):79-88, 1990.

23. Endres, S, Ghorbani, R, Kelley, V, Georgilis, K, Lonnemann, G, van der Meer, J, Cannon, J, Rogers, T, Klempner, M, and Weber, P. The effect of dietary supplementation with n-3 polyunsaturated fatty acids on the synthesis of interleukin-1 and tumor necrosis factor by mononuclear cells. *New Eng J Med* 320(5):265-271, 1989.

24. Fernandes, G, Lawrence, R, and Sun, D. Protective role of n-3 lipids and soy protein in osteoporosis. *Prostaglandins, Leukot Essent Fatty Acids* 68(6):361-372, 2003.

25. Fleming, J, Sharman, M, Avery, N, Love, D, Gomez, A, Scheett, T, Kraemer, W, and Volek, J. Endurance capacity and high-intensity exercise performance responses to a high fat diet. *Int J Sport NutrExerc Metab* 13(4):466-478, 2003.

26. Flickinger, B, and Matsuo, N. Nutritional characteristics of DAG oil. *Lipids* 38(2):129-132, 2003.

27. Graham, T, Hibbett, E, and Sathasivam, P. Metabolic and exercise endurance effects of coffee and caffeine ingestion. *J Appl Physiol* 85(3):883-889, 1998.

28. Greene, D, Varley, B, Hartwig, T, Chapman, P, and Rigney, M. A low-carbohydrate ketogenic diet reduces body mass without compromising performance in powerlifting and Olympic weightlifting athletes. *J Str Cond Res* 32(12):3373-3382, 2018.

29. Hamalainen, E, Adlercreutz, H, Puska, P, and Pietinen, P. Decrease of serum total and free testosterone during a low-fat high-fibre diet. *J Steroid Biochem* 18(3):369-370, 1983.

30. Hargreaves, M, Hawley, J, and Jeukendrup, A. Pre-exercise carbohydrate and fat ingestion: Effects on metabolism and performance. *J Sports Sci Med* 22:31-38, 2004.

31. Harris, M, Putman, R, Ruffner, K, Slack, G, Vansickle, A, Mendel, R, and Lowery, L. The effects of gender on psychometric and epinephrine responses to pre-exercise coffee. Proceedings of the Sixteenth International Society of Sports Nutrition (ISSN) Conference and Expo, Las Vegas, Nevada. *J Int Soc Sports Nutr* 16. In press, 2019.

32. Harvey, C, Schofield, G, and Williden, M. The use of nutritional supplements to induce ketosis and reduce symptoms associated with keto-induction: A narrative review. *PeerJ* 6: e4488, 2018.

33. Haveman L, West, S, Goedecke, J, MacDonald, I, Saint Clair Gibson, A, Noakes, T, and Lambert. E. Fat adaptation followed by carbohydrate loading compromises high-intensity sprint performance. *J Appl Physiol (1985)*. 100(1):194-202, 2006.

34. Hawley, J, Dennis, S, Lindsay, F, and Noakes, T. Nutritional practices of athletes: Are they sub-optimal? *J Sports Sci Med* 13:S75-S81, 1995.

35. Helge, J, Wu, B, Willer, M, Daugaard, J, Storlien, L, and Kiens, B. Training affects muscle phospholipid fatty acid composition in humans. *J Appl Physiol* 90(2):670-677, 2001.

36. Hoffman, D, Theuer, R, Castañeda, Y, Wheaton, D, Bosworth, R, O'Connor, A, Morale, S, Wiedemann, L, and Birch, E. Maturation of visual acuity is accelerated in breast-fed term infants fed baby food containing DHA-enriched egg yolk. *J Nutr* 134(9):2307-2313, 2004.

37. Horowitz, J, Mora-Rodriguez, R, Byerley, L, and Coyle, E. Pre-exercise medium-chain triglyceride ingestion does not alter muscle glycogen use during exercise. *J Appl Physiol* 88(1):219-225, 2000.

38. Horvath, P, Eagen, C, Fisher, N, Leddy, J, and Pendergast, D. The effects of varying dietary fat on performance and metabolism in trained male and female runners. *J Am Coll Nutr* 19(1):52-60, 2000.

39. Innis, S. Dietary omega 3 fatty acids and the developing brain. *Brain Research* 1237:35-43, 2008.

40. Hultin, G. Coconut oil controversy: Updates in research. *Today's Dietitian* 17(2).

41. Institute of Medicine. *Dietary Reference Intakes for energy, carbohydrate, fiber, fat, fatty acids, cholesterol, protein, and amino acids.* Washington, DC: National Academies Press, 2005 (Update 2018).

42. Jeukendrup, A. Periodized nutrition for athletes. *Sports Med* 47 (Suppl) 10:51-63, 2017.

43. Jeukendrup, A, Thielen, J, Wagenmakers, A, Brouns, F, and Saris, W. Effect of medium-chain triacylglycerol and carbohydrate ingestion during exercise on substrate utilization and subsequent cycling performance. *Am J Clinical Nutr* 67(3):397-404, 1998.

44. Kapoor, R, and Huang Y. Gamma linolenic acid: An anti-inflammatory omega-6 fatty acid. *Curr Pharm Biotech* 7(6):531-534, 2006.

45. Klein, S, Coyle, E, and Wolfe, R. Fat metabolism during low-intensity exercise in endurance-trained and untrained men. *Am J Physiol* 267(6) Pt 1:E934-940, 1994.

46. Kremer, J, Jubiz, W, Michalek, A, Rynes, R, Bartholomew, L, Bigaouette, J, Timchalk, M, Beeler, D, and Lininger, L. Fish-oil fatty acid supplementation in active rheumatoid arthritis: A double-blinded, controlled, crossover study. *Ann Int Med* 106:497-503, 1987.

47. Lenn, J, Uhl, T, Mattacola, C, Boissonneault, G, Yates, J, Ibrahim, W, and Bruckner, G. The effects of fish oil and isoflavones on delayed onset muscle soreness. *Med Sci Sports Exerc* 34(10):1605-1613, 2002.

48. Lindgren, B, Ruokonen, E, Magnusson-Borg, K, and Takala, J. Nitrogen sparing effect of structured triglycerides containing both medium-and long-chain fatty acids in critically ill patients; a double blind randomized controlled trial. *Clin Nutr* 20(1):43-48. 2001.

49. Logan, A. Neurobehavioral aspects of omega-3 fatty acids: Possible mechanisms and therapeutic value in major depression. *Alt Med Review* 8(4):410-425, 2003.

50. Lowery, L. Effects of conjugated linoleic acid on body composition and strength in novice male bodybuilders. In *International Conference on Weight Lifting and Strength Training Conference Book*. Hakkinen, K, ed. Lahti, Finland: Gummerus, 241-242. 1999.

51. Lowery, L. Dietary fat and sports nutrition: A primer. *J Sports Sci Med* 3:106-117, 2004.

52. Mann, N, Johnson, L, Warrick, G, and Sinclair, A. The arachidonic acid content of the Australian diet is lower than previously estimated. *J Nutr* 125(10):2528-2535, 1995.

53. Ma, S and Suzuki, K. Keto-adaptation and endurance exercise capacity, fatigue recovery, and exercise-induced muscle and organ damage prevention: A narrative review. *Sports (Basel)* 13:7(2), 2019.

54. Mathews, E, and Wagner, D. Prevalence of overweight and obesity in collegiate American football players, by position. *J Am Coll Health* 57(1):33-38, 2008.

55. McDonald, B. The Canadian experience: Why Canada decided against an upper limit for cholesterol. *J Am Coll Nutr* 23(6 Suppl):616S-620S, 2004.

56. McSwiney, F, Wardrop, B, Hyde, P, LaFountain, R, Volek, J, and Doyle, L. Keto-adaptation enhances exercise performance and body composition responses to training in endurance athletes. *Metabolism* 81:25-34, 2018.

57. Mensink, R. Effects of stearic acid on plasma lipid and lipoproteins in humans. *Lipids* 40(12):1201-1205, 2005.

58. Meyer, B, Mann, N, Lewis, J, Milligan, G, Sinclair, A, and Howe, P. Dietary intakes and food sources of omega-6 and omega-3 polyunsaturated fatty acids. *Lipids* 38(4):391-398, 2003.

59. Mickleborough, T, Murray, R, Ionescu, A, and Lindley, M. Fish oil supplementation reduces severity of exercise-induced bronchoconstriction in elite athletes. *Am J Respir Crit Care Med* 168(10):1181-1189, 2003.

60. Morcos, N and Camilo K. Acute and chronic toxicity study of fish oil and garlic combination. *Int J Vit Nutr Res* 71(5):306-312, 2001.

61. Muskiet, F, Fokkema, M, Schaafsma, A, Boersma, E, and Crawford, M. Is docosahexaenoic acid (DHA) essential? Lessons from DHA status regulation, our ancient diet, epidemiology and randomized controlled trials. *J Nutr* 134(1):183-186, 2004.

62. Paoli, A. Ketogenic diet for obesity: Friend or foe? *Int J Envir Res Public Health* 11(2):2092-107, 2014.

63. Pariza, M, Park, Y, and Cook, M. The biologically active isomers of conjugated linoleic acid. *Prog Lipid Res* 40:283-298, 2001.

64. Park, Y, Albright, K, Liu, W, Storkson, J, Cook, M, and Pariza M. Effect of conjugated linoleic acid on body composition in mice. *Lipids* 32(8):853-858, 1997.

65. Perez-Jimenez, F, Lopez-Miranda, J, and Mata, P. Protective effect of dietary monounsaturated fat on arteriosclerosis: Beyond cholesterol. *Atheroscler* 163(2):385-398, 2002.

66. Phillips, T, Childs, A, Dreon, D, Phinney, S, and Leeuwenburgh, C. A dietary supplement attenuates IL-6 and CRP after eccentric exercise in untrained males. *Med Sci Sports Exerc* 35(12):2032-2037, 2003.

67. Piper, S, Röhm, K, Boldt, J, Odermatt, B, Maleck, W, and Suttner, S. Hepatocellular integrity in patients requiring parenteral nutrition: Comparison of structured MCT/LCT vs. a standard MCT/LCT emulsion and a LCT emulsion. *Eur J Anaesthesiol* 25(7):557-565, 2008.

68. Powers, M, Goggin, C, Kirk, S, Smith, R, Slotta, A, Betro, A, Santana, K, Hubbell, A, Cox, A, Dreger, K, and Lowery, L. Via® instant coffee enhances explosive bench press performance. *Ann Nutr Metab* 63(Suppl 1):566, 2013.

69. Raatz, S, Bibus, D, Thomas, W, and Kris-Etherton, P. Total fat intake modifies plasma fatty acid composition in humans. *J Nutr* 131(2):231-234, 2001.

70. Rasmussen, O, Thomsen, C, Hansen, K, Vesterlund, M, Winther, E, and Hermansen, K. Favourable effect of olive oil in patients with non-insulin-dependent diabetes. The effect on blood pressure, blood glucose and lipid levels of a high-fat diet rich in monounsaturated fat compared with a carbohydrate-rich diet. *Ugeskr Laeger* 157(8): 1028-1032, 1995.

71. Rawson, E, Branch, J, and Stephenson T. *Nutrition for Health, Fitness and Sport*. New York: McGraw-Hill, 177-185, 2020.

72. Reed, M, Cheng, R, Simmonds, M, Richmond, W, and James, V. Dietary lipids: An additional regulator of plasma levels of sex hormone binding globulin. *J Clin Endocrinol Metab* 64(5):1083-1085, 1987.

73. Richter, W. Long-chain omega-3 fatty acids from fish reduce sudden cardiac death in patients with coronary heart disease. *Eur J Med Res* 8(8):332-336, 2003.

74. Riechman, S, Andrews, R, Maclean, D, and Sheather, S. Statins and dietary and serum cholesterol are associated with increased lean mass following resistance training. *J Gerontol: Biol Sci Med Sci* 62(10):1164-1171, 2007.

75. Sidossis, L, Gastaldelli, A, Klein, S, and Wolfe R. Regulation of plasma fatty acid oxidation during low- and high-intensity exercise. *Am J Physiol* 272(6) Pt 1:E1065-1070, 1997.

76. Sidossis L and Wolfe, R. Glucose and insulin-induced inhibition of fatty acid oxidation: The glucose-fatty acid cycle reversed. *Am J Physiol* 270(4 Pt 1):E733-8, 1996.

77. Simopoulos, A. The importance of the ratio of omega-6/omega-3 essential fatty acids. *Biomed Pharmacother* 56(8):365-379, 2002.

78. Simopoulos, A. Omega-3 fatty acids and athletics. *Curr Sports Med Rep* 6(4):230-236, 2007.

79. Smith, B, Feucht, A, Slack, G, Rogers, J, LaRock, F, Mendel R, and Lowery, L Coffee but not anticipation of coffee alters the outcome of explosive bench pressing. *FASEB J* 30:898.10, 2016.

80. Stellingwerff T, Spriet, L, Watt, M, Kimber, N, Hargreaves, M, Hawley J, and Burke, L. Decreased PDH activation and glycogenolysis during exercise following fat adaptation with carbohydrate restoration. *Am J Physiol Endocrinol Metab* 290(2):E380-8, 2006.

81. Stepto, N. Effect of short-term fat adaptation on high intensity training. *Med Sci Sports Exerc* 34:449-455, 2002.

82. Strzelczyk A. Intravenous initiation and maintenance of ketogenic diet: Proof of concept in super-refractory status epilepticus. *Seizure* 22(7):581-3, 2013.

83. Stubbs, B, Koutnik, A, Poff, A, Ford, K, and D'Agostino, D. Commentary: Ketone diester ingestion impairs time-trial performance in professional cyclists. *Front Physiol* 9:279, 2018.

84. Su, H, Bernardo, L, Mirmiran, M, Ma, X, Nathanielsz, P, and Brenna, J. Dietary 18:3n-3 and 22:6n-3 as sources of 22:6n-3 accretion in neonatal baboon brain and associated organs. *Lipids* 34 Suppl: S347-S350, 1999.

85. Su, K, Huang, S, Chiu, C, and Shen, W. Omega-3 fatty acids in major depressive disorder. A preliminary double-blind, placebo-controlled trial. *Eur Neuropsychopharmacol* 13(4):267-271, 2003.

86. Takeuchi, H, Sekine, S, Kojima, K, and Aoyama, T. The application of medium-chain fatty acids: Edible oil with a suppressing effect on body fat accumulation. *Asia Pacif J Clin Nutr* 17 Suppl 1:320-323, 2008.

87. Terpstra, A. Effect of conjugated linoleic acid on body composition and plasma lipids in humans: An overview of the literature. *Am J Clin Nutr* 79(3):352-361, 2004.

88. Thomsen, C, Rasmussen, O, Hansen, K, Vesterlund, M, and Hermansen, K. Comparison of the effects on the diurnal blood pressure, glucose, and lipid

levels of a diet rich in monounsaturated fatty acids with a diet rich in polyunsaturated fatty acids in type 2 diabetic subjects. *Diab Med 12*(7):600-606, 1995.

89. U.S. Department of Health and Human Services and U.S. Department of Agriculture. *Dietary Guidelines for Americans.* Washington, DC: U.S. Government Printing Office, 2017.

90. van Loon, L, Koopman, R, Manders, R, van der Weegen, W, van Kranenburg, G, and Keizer, H. Intramyocellular lipid content in type 2 diabetes patients compared with overweight sedentary men and highly trained endurance athletes. *Am J Physiol: Endocrinol Metab* 287(3):E558-E565, 2004.

91. Van Zant, R, Conway, J, and Seale, J. A moderate carbohydrate and fat diet does not impair strength performance in moderately trained males. *J Sports Med Phys Fit* 42(1): 31-37, 2002.

92. Vargas, S, Romance, R, Petro, J, Bonilla, D, Galancho, I, Espinar, S, Kreider, R, and Benitez-Porres, J. Efficacy of ketogenic diet on body composition during resistance training in trained men: A randomized controlled trial. *J Int Soc Sports Nutr* 15(1):31, 2018.

93. Venkatraman, J, Leddy, J, and Pendergast, D. Dietary fats and immune status in athletes: Clinical implications. *Med Sci Sports Exerc* 32(7 Suppl):S389-S395, 2000.

94. Venkatraman, J, Feng, X, and Pendergast, D. Effects of dietary fat and endurance exercise on plasma cortisol, prostaglandin E2, interferon-gamma and lipid peroxides in runners. *J Am Coll Nutr* 20(5) (Oct):529-536, 2001.

95. Vistisen, B, Nybo, L, Xu, X, Høy, C, and Kiens, B. Minor amounts of plasma medium-chain fatty acids and no improved time trial performance after consuming lipids. *J Appl Physiol* 95(6):2434-2443, 2003.

96. Vogt, M, Puntschart, A, Howald, H, Mueller, B, Mannhart, C, Gfeller-Tuescher, L, Mullis, P, and Hoppeler, H. Effects of dietary fat on muscle substrates, metabolism, and performance in athletes. *Med Sci Sports Exerc* 35(6):952-960, 2003.

97. Wang, Y and Jones, P. Conjugated linoleic acid and obesity control: Efficacy and mechanisms. *Int J Obes Rel Metab Disord* 28(8):941-955, 2004.

98. Weisinger, H, Vingrys, A, and Sinclair, A. The effect of docosahexaenoic acid on the electroretinogram of the guinea pig. *Lipids* 31(1):65-70, 1996.

99. Whigham, L, Watras, A, and Schoeller, D. Efficacy of conjugated linoleic acid for reducing fat mass: A meta-analysis in humans. *Am J Clin Nutr* 85(5):1203-1211, 2007.

100. Zderic, T, Davidson, C, Schenk, S, Byerley, L, and Coyle E. High-fat diet elevates resting intramuscular triglyceride concentration and whole body lipolysis during exercise. *Am J Physiol: Endocrinol Metab* 286(2):E217-E225, 2004.

Chapter 6

1. Almond, CS, Shin, AY, Fortescue, EB, Mannix, RC, Wypij, D, Binstadt, BA, Duncan, CN, Olson, DP, Salerno, AE, Newburger, JW, and Greenes, DS. Hyponatremia among runners in the Boston Marathon. *N Engl J Med* 352:1550-1556, 2005.

2. American College of Sports Medicine, Sawka, MN, Burke, LM, Eichner, ER, Maughan, RJ, Montain, SJ, and Stachenfeld, NS. American College of Sports Medicine position stand. Exercise and fluid replacement. *Med Sci Sports Exerc* 39:377-390, 2007.

3. Armstrong, LE, Maresh, CM, Castellani, JW, Bergeron, MF, Kenefick, RW, LaGasse, KE, and Riebe, D. Urinary indices of hydration status. *Int J Sport Nutr* 4:265-279, 1994.

4. Beetham, R. Biochemical investigation of suspected rhabdomyolysis. *Ann Clin Biochem* 37 (Pt 5):581-587, 2000.

5. Bergeron, MF, McKeag, DB, Casa, DJ, Clarkson, PM, Dick, RW, Eichner, ER, Horswill, CA, Luke, AC, Mueller, F, Munce, TA, Roberts, WO, and Rowland, TW. Youth football: Heat stress and injury risk. *Med Sci Sports Exerc* 37:1421-1430, 2005.

6. Blatteis, CM. Age-dependent changes in temperature regulation—a mini review. *Gerontology* 58:289-295, 2012.

7. Cairns, RS and Hew-Butler, T. Proof of concept: Hypovolemic hyponatremia may precede and augment creatine kinase elevations during an ultramarathon. *Eur J Appl Physiol* 116:647-655, 2016.

8. Campbell, WW and Geik, RA. Nutritional considerations for the older athlete. *Nutrition* 20:603-608, 2004.

9. Cheuvront, SN, Carter, R,3rd, Montain, SJ, and Sawka, MN. Daily body mass variability and stability in active men undergoing exercise-heat stress. *Int J Sport Nutr Exerc Metab* 14:532-540, 2004.

10. Committee on Military Nutrition Research, Food and Nutrition Board. *Fluid replacement and heat stress.* Institute of Medicine, Washington, DC. 1994.

11. Council on Sports Medicine and Fitness and Council on School Health, Bergeron, MF, Devore, C, Rice, SG, and American Academy of Pediatrics. Policy statement—climatic heat stress and exercising children and adolescents. *Pediatrics* 128:e741-7, 2011.

12. Darrow, DC and Yannet, H. The changes in the distribution of body water accompanying increase and decrease in extracellular electrolyte. *J Clin Invest* 14:266-275, 1935.

13. Devlin, LH, Fraser, SF, Barras, NS, and Hawley, JA. Moderate levels of hypo-hydration impairs bowling accuracy but not bowling velocity in skilled cricket players. *J Sci Med Sport* 4:179-187, 2001.

13a. Dunford, M. *Fundamentals of Sport and Exercise Nutrition.* Champaign, IL: Human Kinetics, 114, 2010.

13b. Dunford, M. *Exercise Nutrition,* 2nd Ed. Champaign, IL: Human Kinetics, 33, 2009.

14. Dunford, M, and Doyle, JA. *Nutrition for Sport and Exercise.* Belmont, CA; Thompson Higher Education, 240-276, 2008.

15. Edwards, AM, Mann, ME, Marfell-Jones, MJ, Rankin, DM, Noakes, TD, and Shillington, DP. Influence of moderate dehydration on soccer performance:

Physiological responses to 45 min of outdoor match-play and the immediate subsequent performance of sport-specific and mental concentration tests. *Br J Sports Med* 41:385-391, 2007.

16. Epstein, M, and Hollenberg, NK. Age as a determinant of renal sodium conservation in normal man. *J Lab Clin Med* 87:411-417, 1976.

17. Evetovich, TK, Boyd, JC, Drake, SM, Eschbach, LC, Magal, M, Soukup, JT, Webster, MJ, Whitehead, MT, and Weir, JP. Effect of moderate dehydration on torque, electromyography, and mechanomyography. *Muscle Nerve* 26:225-231, 2002.

18. Falk, B, Bar-Or, O, and MacDougall, JD. Thermoregulatory responses of pre-, mid-, and late-pubertal boys to exercise in dry heat. *Med Sci Sports Exerc* 24:688-694, 1992.

19. Fortney, SM, Wenger, CB, Bove, JR, and Nadel, ER. Effect of hyperosmolality on control of blood flow and sweating. *J Appl Physiol Respir Environ Exerc Physiol* 57:1688-1695, 1984.

20. Frontera-Cantero, JE, Rivera-Brown, AM, Cabrera-Dávila, Y, Berríos, LE, González, J, and Ramírez-Marrero, F. Fluid and sweat electrolyte loss in heat-acclimatized pre and post menarcheal girl athletes. *Med Sci Sports Exerc* 38:S111-S112, 2006.

21. Ganio, MS, Wingo, JE, Carrolll, CE, Thomas, MK, and Cureton, KJ. Fluid ingestion attenuates the decline in $\dot{V}O_2$peak associated with cardiovascular drift. *Med Sci Sports Exerc* 38:901-909, 2006.

22. Godek, SF, Bartolozzi, AR, Burkholder, R, Sugarman, E, and Peduzzi, C. Sweat rates and fluid turnover in professional football players: A comparison of National Football League linemen and backs. *J Athl Train* 43:184-189, 2008.

23. Goulet, EDB and Hoffman, MD. Impact of ad libitum versus programmed drinking on endurance performance: A systematic review with meta-analysis. *Sports Med* 49:221-232, 2019.

24. Gowans, EM and Fraser, CG. Despite correlation, random spot and 24-h urine specimens are not interchangeable. *Clin Chem* 33:1080-1081, 1987.

25. Hayes, LD and Morse, CI. The effects of progressive dehydration on strength and power: Is there a dose response? *Eur J Appl Physiol* 108:701-707, 2010.

26. Hew-Butler, T, Almond, C, Ayus, JC, Dugas, J, Meeuwisse, W, Noakes, T, Reid, S, Siegel, A, Speedy, D, Stuempfle, K, Verbalis, J, and Weschler, L. Consensus statement of the 1st International Exercise-Associated Hyponatremia Consensus Development Conference. *Clin J Sport Med* 15:208-13, 2005.

27. Hew-Butler, T, Dugas, JP, Noakes, TD, and Verbalis, JG. Changes in plasma arginine vasopressin concentrations in cyclists participating in a 109-km cycle race. *Br J Sports Med* 44:594-597, 2010.

28. Hew-Butler, T, Loi, V, Pani, A, and Rosner, MH. Exercise-associated hyponatremia: 2017 update. *Front Med (Lausanne)* 4:21, 2017.

29. Horswill, CA, Passe, DH, Stofan, JR, Horn, MK, and Murray, R. Adequacy of fluid ingestion in adolescents and adults during moderate-intensity exercise. *Pedi Exerc Sci* 17:41-50, 2005.

30. Inbar, O, Morris, N, Epstein, Y, and Gass, G. Comparison of thermoregulatory responses to exercise in dry heat among prepubertal boys, young adults and older males. *Exp Physiol* 89:691-700, 2004.

31. Institute of Medicine, Food and Nutrition Board. *Dietary reference intakes for water, potassium, chloride, and sodium.* 2005.

32. Jeukendrup, AE, Jentjens, RL, and Moseley, L. Nutritional considerations in triathlon. *Sports Med* 35:163-181, 2005.

33. Judelson, DA, Maresh, CM, Anderson, JM, Armstrong, LE, Casa, DJ, Kraemer, WJ, and Volek, JS. Hydration and muscular performance: Does fluid balance affect strength, power and high-intensity endurance? *Sports Med* 37:907-921, 2007.

34. Judelson, DA, Maresh, CM, Farrell, MJ, Yamamoto, LM, Armstrong, LE, Kraemer, WJ, Volek, JS, Spiering, BA, Casa, DJ, and Anderson, JM. Effect of hydration state on strength, power, and resistance exercise performance. *Med Sci Sports Exerc* 39:1817-1824, 2007.

35. Judelson, DA, Maresh, CM, Yamamoto, LM, Farrell, MJ, Armstrong, LE, Kraemer, WJ, Volek, JS, Spiering, BA, Casa, DJ, and Anderson, JM. Effect of hydration state on resistance exercise-induced endocrine markers of anabolism, catabolism, and metabolism. *J Appl Physiol* 105:816-824, 2008.

36. Katch, VL, McArdle, WD, Katch, FI, and McArdle, WD. *Essentials of Exercise Physiology.* Philadelphia: Wolters Kluwer/Lippincott Williams & Wilkins Health, 513-520, 2011.

37. Kenney, WL, Tankersley, CG, Newswanger, DL, Hyde, DE, Puhl, SM, and Turner, NL. Age and hypohydration independently influence the peripheral vascular response to heat stress. *J Appl Physiol* 68:1902-1908, 1990.

38. Kiningham, RB and Gorenflo, DW. Weight loss methods of high school wrestlers. *Med Sci Sports Exerc* 33:810-813, 2001.

39. Kirchengast, S and Gartner, M. Changes in fat distribution (WHR) and body weight across the menstrual cycle. *Coll Antropol* 26 Suppl:47-57, 2002.

40. Laursen, PB, Suriano, R, Quod, MJ, Lee, H, Abbiss, CR, Nosaka, K, Martin, DT, and Bishop, D. Core temperature and hydration status during an Ironman triathlon. *Br J Sports Med* 40:320-5, 2006.

41. Maughan, RJ and Noakes, TD. Fluid replacement and exercise stress. A brief review of studies on fluid replacement and some guidelines for the athlete. *Sports Med* 12:16-31, 1991.

42. Maughan, RJ and Shirreffs, SM. Development of individual hydration strategies for athletes. *Int J Sport Nutr Exerc Metab* 18:457-472, 2008.

43. Maughan, RJ, Watson, P, Cordery, PAA, Walsh, NP, Oliver, SJ, Dolci, A, Rodriguez-Sanchez, N, and Galloway, SDR. Sucrose and sodium but not caffeine content influence the retention of beverages in humans under euhydrated conditions. *Int J Sport Nutr Exerc Metab* 29:51-60, 2019.

44. Meyer, F, and Bar-Or, O. Fluid and electrolyte loss during exercise. The paediatric angle. *Sports Med* 18:4-9, 1994.

45. Montain, S. Strategies to prevent hyponatremia during prolonged exercise. *Current Sports Med Rep* 7:S28-S35, 2008.

46. Morley, JE. Dehydration, hypernatremia, and hyponatremia. *Clin Geriatr Med* 31:389-399, 2015.

47. Munoz, CX, McKenzie, AL, and Armstrong, LE. Optimal hydration biomarkers: Consideration of daily activities. *Obes Facts* 7 Suppl 2:13-18, 2014.

48. Noakes, T and IMMDA. Fluid replacement during marathon running. *Clin J Sport Med* 13:309-318, 2003.

49. Noonan, B, Mack, G, and Stachenfeld, N. The effects of hockey protective equipment on high-intensity intermittent exercise. *Med Sci Sports Exerc* 39:1327-1335, 2007.

50. Nuccio, RP, Barnes, KA, Carter, JM, and Baker, LB. Fluid balance in team sport athletes and the effect of hypohydration on cognitive, technical, and physical performance. *Sports Med* 47:1951-1982, 2017.

51. Olsson, KE and Saltin, B. Variation in total body water with muscle glycogen changes in man. *Acta Physiol Scand* 80:11-18, 1970.

52. Petrie, HJ, Stover, EA, and Horswill, CA. Nutritional concerns for the child and adolescent competitor. *Nutrition* 20:620-631, 2004.

53. Ray, ML, Bryan, MW, Ruden, TM, Baier, SM, Sharp, RL, and King, DS. Effect of sodium in a rehydration beverage when consumed as a fluid or meal. *J Appl Physiol* 85:1329-1336, 1998.

54. Reaburn, P. Nutrition and the ageing athlete. In *Clinical Sports Nutrition*. Burke, L, Deakin, V, eds. Melbourne: McGraw-Hill, 602-639, 2000.

55. Riddell, MC, Bar-Or, O, Wilk, B, Parolin, ML, and Heigenhauser, GJ. Substrate utilization during exercise with glucose and glucose plus fructose ingestion in boys ages 10-14 yr. *J Appl Physiol* 90:903-911, 2001.

56. Rivera-Brown, AM, Rowland, TW, Ramirez-Marrero, FA, Santacana, G, and Vann, A. Exercise tolerance in a hot and humid climate in heat-acclimatized girls and women. *Int J Sports Med* 27:943-950, 2006.

57. Rolls, BJ, and Phillips, PA. Aging and disturbances of thirst and fluid balance. *Nutr Rev* 48:137-144, 1990.

58. Rosenbloom, CA, and Dunaway, A. Nutrition recommendations for masters athletes. *Clin Sports Med* 26:91-100, 2007.

59. Rosenfeld, R, Livne, D, Nevo, O, Dayan, L, Milloul, V, Lavi, S, and Jacob, G. Hormonal and volume dysregulation in women with premenstrual syndrome. *Hypertension* 51:1225-1230, 2008.

60. Rowland, T. Thermoregulation during exercise in the heat in children: Old concepts revisited. *J Appl Physiol* 105:718-724, 2008.

61. Rowland, T, Hagenbuch, S, Pober, D, and Garrison, A. Exercise tolerance and thermoregulatory responses during cycling in boys and men. *Med Sci Sports Exerc* 40:282-287, 2008.

62. Rowland, T. Fluid replacement requirements for child athletes. *Sports Med* 41:279-288, 2011.

63. Sawka, MN, Wenger, CB, and Pandolf, KB. Thermoregulatory responses to acute exercise-heat stress and heat acclimation. In *Handbook of Physiology*, section 4: Environmental Physiology. Blatteis, CM, Fregly, MJ, eds. New York: Oxford University Press for the American Physiological Society, 94-114, 1996.

64. Seifert, J, Harmon, J, and DeClercq, P. Protein added to a sports drink improves fluid retention. *Int J Sport Nutr Exerc Metab* 16:420-429, 2006.

65. Siegel, AJ, Verbalis, JG, Clement, S, Mendelson, JH, Mello, NK, Adner, M, Shirey, T, Glowacki, J, Lee-Lewandrowski, E, and Lewandrowski, KB. Hyponatremia in marathon runners due to inappropriate arginine vasopressin secretion. *Am J Med* 120:461.e11-461.e17, 2007.

66. Soto-Quijano, DA. The competitive senior athlete. *Phys Med Rehabil Clin N Am* 28:767-776, 2017.

67. Speedy, DB, Noakes, TD, and Schneider, C. Exercise-associated hyponatremia: A review. *Emerg Med (Fremantle)* 13:17-27, 2001.

68. Tarnopolsky, MA. Nutritional consideration in the aging athlete. *Clin J Sport Med* 18:531-538, 2008.

69. White, M, Berning, JR, and Kendig, A. *Nutrition guide.* United States Anti-Doping Association, 2019.

70. Wilk, B, Yuxiu, H, and Bar-Or, O. Effect of body hypohydration on aerobic performance of boys who exercise in the heat. *Med Sci Sports Exerc* 34:5, 2002.

71. Wilk, B, Rivera-Brown, AM, and Bar-Or, O. Voluntary drinking and hydration in non-acclimatized girls exercising in the heat. *Eur J Appl Physiol* 101:727-734, 2007.

72. Yamamoto, LM, Judelson, DA, Farrell, MJ, Lee, EC, Armstrong, LE, Casa, DJ, Kraemer, WJ, Volek, JS, and Maresh, CM. Effects of hydration state and resistance exercise on markers of muscle damage. *J Strength Cond Res* 22:1387-1393, 2008.

73. Yoshida, T, Takanishi, T, Nakai, S, Yorimoto, A, and Morimoto, T. The critical level of water deficit causing a decrease in human exercise performance: A practical field study. *Eur J Appl Physiol* 87:529-534, 2002.

Chapter 7

1. Aguilo, A, Tauler, P, Sureda, A, Cases, N, Tur, J, and Pons, A. Antioxidant diet supplementation enhances aerobic performance in amateur sportsmen. *J Sports Sci* 25:1203-1210, 2007.

2. Antoniak, AE, and Greig CA. The effect of combined resistance exercise training and vitamin D_3 supplementation on musculoskeletal health and function in older adults: A systematic review and meta-analysis. *BMJ Open* 7(7):e014619, 2017.

3. Backx, E, van der Avoort, C, Tieland, M, Maase, K, Kies, A, van Loon, L, de Groot, L, and Mensink, M. Seasonal variation in vitamin D status in elite athletes: A longitudinal study. *Int J Sport Nutr Exerc Metab* 27:6-10, 2017.

4. Bailey, DM, Lawrenson, L, McEneny, J, Young, IS, James, PE, Jackson, SK, Henry, RR, Mathieu-Costello, O, McCord, JM, and Richardson, RS. Electron

paramagnetic spectroscopic evidence of exercise-induced free radical accumulation in human skeletal muscle. *Free Radic Res* 41:182-190, 2007.

5. Bailey, DM, Williams, C, Betts, JA, Thompson, D, and Hurst TL. Oxidative stress, inflammation and recovery of muscle function after damaging exercise: Effect of 6-week mixed antioxidant supplementation. *Eur J Appl Physiol* 111:925-936, 2011.

6. Barker, T, Henriksen, VT, Martins, TB, Hill, HR, Kjeldsberg, CR, Schneider, ED, Dixon, BM, and Weaver, LK. Higher serum 25-hydroxyvitamin D concentrations associate with a faster recovery of skeletal muscle strength after muscular injury. *Nutrients* 5:1253-1275, 2013.

7. Barker, T, Schneider, ED, Dixon, BM, Henriksen, VT, and Weaver, LK. Supplemental vitamin D enhances the recovery in peak isometric force shortly after intense exercise. *Nutr Metab (Lond)* 10(1):69, 2013.

8. Beals, KA and Manore, MM. Nutritional status of female athletes with subclinical eating disorders. *J Am Diet Assoc* 98:419-425, 1998.

9. Belko, AZ, Obarzanek, E, Roach, R, Rotter, M, Urban, G, Weinberg, S, and Roe, DA. Effects of aerobic exercise and weight loss on riboflavin requirements of moderately obese, marginally deficient young women. *Am J Clin Nutr* 40:553-561, 1984.

10. Belko, AZ, Meredith, MP, Kalkwarf, HJ, Obarzanek, E, Weinberg, S, Roach, R, McKeon, G, and Roe, DA. Effects of exercise on riboflavin requirements: Biological validation in weight reducing women. *Am J Clin Nutr* 41:270-277, 1985.

11. Benson, J, Gillen, DM, Bourdet, K, and Loosli, AR. Inadequate nutrition and chronic calorie restriction in adolescent ballerinas. *Phys Sports Med* 13:79-90, 1985.

12. Beshgetoor, D, and Nichols, JF. Dietary intake and supplement use in female master cyclists and runners. *Int J Sport Nutr Exerc Metab* 13:166-172, 2003.

13. Bischoff-Ferrari, HA, Dietrich, T, Orav, EJ, Hu, FB, Zhang, Y, Karlson, EW, and Dawson-Hughes, B. Higher 25-hydroxyvitamin D concentrations are associated with better lower-extremity function in both active and inactive persons aged > or =60 y. *Am J Clin Nutr* 80:752-758, 2004.

14. Bjørnsen, T, Salvesen, S, Berntsen, S, Hetlelid, KJ, Stea, TH, Lohne-Seiler, H, Rohde, G, Haraldstad, K, Raastad, T, Køpp, U, Haugeberg, G, Mansoor, MA, Bastani, NE, Blomhoff, R, Stølevik, SB, Seynnes, OR, and Paulsen, G. Vitamin C and E supplementation blunts increases in total lean body mass in elderly men after strength training. *Scand J Med Sci Sports* 26:755-763, 2016.

15. Brady, PS, Brady, LJ, and Ullrey, DE. Selenium, vitamin E and the response to swimming stress in the rat. *J Nutr* 109:1103-1109, 1979.

16. Bredle, DL, Stager, JM, Brechue, WF, and Farber, MO. Phosphate supplementation, cardiovascular function, and exercise performance in humans. *J Appl Physiol* 65:1821-1826, 1988.

17. Brilla, LR and Haley, TF. Effect of magnesium supplementation on strength training in humans. *J Am Coll Nutr* 11:326-329, 1992.

18. Brownlie, T, 4th, Utermohlen, V, Hinton, PS, and Haas, JD. Tissue iron deficiency without anemia impairs adaptation in endurance capacity after aerobic training in previously untrained women. *Am J Clin Nutr* 79:437-443, 2004.

19. Brun, JF, Dieu-Cambrezy, C, Charpiat, A, Fons, C, Fedou, C, Micallef, JP, Fussellier, M, Bardet, L, and Orsetti, A. Serum zinc in highly trained adolescent gymnasts. *Biol Trace Elem Res* 47:273-278, 1995.

20. Brutsaert, TD, Hernandez-Cordero, S, Rivera, J, Viola, T, Hughes, G, and Haas, JD. Iron supplementation improves progressive fatigue resistance during dynamic knee extensor exercise in iron-depleted, nonanemic women. *Am J Clin Nutr* 77:441-448, 2003.

21. Bryant, RJ, Ryder, J, Martino, P, Kim, J, and Craig, BW. Effects of vitamin E and C supplementation either alone or in combination on exercise-induced lipid peroxidation in trained cyclists. *J Strength Cond Res* 17:792-800, 2003.

22. Cannell, JJ, Hollis, BW, Sorenson, MB, Taft, TN, and Anderson, JJ. Athletic performance and vitamin D. *Med Sci Sports Exerc* 41:1102-1110, 2009.

23. Ceglia, L, Niramitmahapanya, S, da Silva Morais, M, Rivas, DA, Harris, SS, Bischoff-Ferrari, H, Fielding, RA, and Dawson-Hughes, B. A randomized study on the effect of vitamin D_3 supplementation on skeletal muscle morphology and vitamin D receptor concentration in older women. *J Clin Endocrinol Metab* 98:E1927-1935, 2013.

24. Ciocoiu, M, Badescu, M, and Paduraru, I. Protecting antioxidative effects of vitamins E and C in experimental physical stress. *J Physiol Biochem* 63:187-194, 2007.

25. Clénin, G, Cordes, M, Huber, A, Schumacher, YO, Noack, P, Scales, J, and Kriemler, S. Iron deficiency in sports—definition, influence on performance and therapy. *Swiss Med Wkly* 145:w14196, 2015.

26. Close, GL, Ashton, T, Cable, T, Doran, D, Holloway, C, McArdle, F, and MacLaren, DP. Ascorbic acid supplementation does not attenuate post-exercise muscle soreness following muscle-damaging exercise but may delay the recovery process. *Br J Nutr* 95:976-981, 2006.

27. Close, GL, Leckey, J, Patterson, M, Bradley, W, Owens, DJ, Fraser, WD, and Morton, JP. The effects of vitamin D(3) supplementation on serum total 25[OH] D concentration and physical performance: A randomised dose-response study. *Br J Sports Med* 47:692-696, 2013.

28. Close, GL and Jackson, MJ. Antioxidants and exercise: A tale of the complexities of relating signalling processes to physiological function? *J Physiol* 592:1721-1722, 2014.

29. Cohen, JL, Potosnak, L, Frank, O, and Baker, H. A nutritional and hematological assessment of elite ballet dancers. *Phys Sports Med* 13:43-54, 1985.

30. Collings, R, Harvey, LJ, Hooper, L, Hurst, R, Brown, TJ, Ansett, J, King, M, and Fairweather-Tait, SJ. The absorption of iron from whole diets: A systematic review. *Am J Clin Nutr* 98:65-81, 2013.

31. Deuster, PA, Kyle, SB, Moser, PB, Vigersky, RA, Singh, A, and Schoomaker, EB. Nutritional survey of highly trained women runners. *Am J Clin Nutr* 44:954-962, 1986.

32. Deuster, PA, Dolev, E, Kyle, SB, Anderson, RA, and Schoomaker, EB. Magnesium homeostasis during high-intensity anaerobic exercise in men. *J Appl Physiol* 62:545-550, 1987.

33. Deuster, PA, and Cooper, JA. Choline. In *Sports Nutrition: Vitamins and Minerals.* 2nd ed. Driskell, JA, Wolinsky, I, eds. Boca Raton, FL: CRC Press, 139-162, 2006.

34. Dillard, CJ, Litov, RE, Savin, WM, Dumelin, EE, and Tappel, AL. Effects of exercise, vitamin E, and ozone on pulmonary function and lipid peroxidation. *J Appl Physiol Respir Environ Exerc Physiol* 45:927-932, 1978.

35. Donato, AJ, Uberoi, A, Bailey, DM, Wray, DW, and Richardson, RS. Exercise-induced brachial artery vasodilation: Effects of antioxidants and exercise training in elderly men. *Am J Physiol Heart Circ Physiol* 298:H671-H678, 2010.

36. Doyle, MR, Webster, MJ, and Erdmann, LD. Allithiamine ingestion does not enhance isokinetic parameters of muscle performance. *Int J Sport Nutr* 7:39-47, 1997.

37. Dressendorfer, RH, and Sockolov, R. Hypozincemia in runners. *Phys Sports Med* 8:97-100, 1980.

38. Dutra, MT, Alex, S, Silva, AF, Brown, LE, and Bottaro, M. Antioxidant supplementation impairs changes in body composition induced by strength training in young women. *Int J Exerc Sci* 12:287-296, 2019.

39. Economos, CD, Bortz, SS, and Nelson, ME. Nutritional practices of elite athletes. Practical recommendations. *Sports Med (Auckland, NZ)* 16:381-399, 1993.

40. Edgerton, VR, Ohira, Y, Hettiarachchi, J, Senewiratne, B, Gardner, GW, and Barnard, RJ. Elevation of hemoglobin and work tolerance in iron-deficient subjects. *J Nutr Sci Vitaminol* 27:77-86, 1981.

41. EFSA Panel on Dietetic Products, Nutrition and Allergies. Scientific opinion paper on tolerable upper limit level of vitamin D. *EFSA J* 10:2813, 2012.

42. EFSA Panel on Dietetic Products, Nutrition and Allergies. Scientific opinion paper on dietary reference values for vitamin D. *EFSA J* 14:4547, 2016.

43. Evans, GW. The effect of chromium picolinate on insulin-controlled parameters in humans. *Int J Biosci Med Res* 11:163-180, 1989.

44. Faber, M and Benade, AJ. Mineral and vitamin intake in field athletes (discus-, hammer-, javelin-throwers and shot-putters). *Int J Sports Med* 12:324-327, 1991.

45. Farrokhyar, F, Sivakumar, G, Savage, K, Koziarz, A, Jamshidi, S, Ayeni, OR, Peterson, D, and Bhandari, M. Effects of vitamin D supplementation on serum 25-hydroxyvitamin D concentrations and physical performance in athletes: A systematic review and meta-analysis of randomized controlled trials. *Sports Med* 47:2323-2339, 2017.

46. Filaire, E and Lac, G. Nutritional status and body composition of juvenile elite female gymnasts. *J Sports Med Phys Fitness* 42:65-70, 2002.

47. Fischer, CP, Hiscock, NJ, Basu, S, Vessby, B, Kallner, A, Sjöberg, LB, Febbraio, MA, and Pedersen BK. Vitamin E isoform-specific inhibition of the

exercise-induced heat shock protein 72 expression in humans. *J Appl Physiol* 100:1679-1687, 2006.

48. Fletcher, RH and Fairfield, KM. Vitamins for chronic disease prevention in adults. Clinical applications. *J Am Med Assoc* 287:3127-3129, 2002.

49. Fogelholm, GM, Himberg, JJ, Alopaeus, K, Gref, GC, Laakso, JT, Lehto, JJ, and Mussalo-Rauhamaa, H. Dietary and biochemical indices of nutritional status in male athletes and controls. *J Am Coll Nutr* 11:181-191, 1992.

50. Fogelholm, M, Ruokonen, I, Laakso, JT, Vuorimaa, T, and Himberg JJ. Lack of association between indices of vitamin B_1, B_2, and B_6 status and exercise-induced blood lactate in young adults. *Int J Sport Nutr* 3:165-176, 1993.

51. Gaeini, AA, Rahnama, N, and Hamedinia MR. Effects of vitamin E supplementation on oxidative stress at rest and after exercise to exhaustion in athletic students. *J Sports Med Phys Fitness* 46:458-461, 2006.

52. Galbo, H, Holst, JJ, Christensen, NJ, and Hilsted, J. Glucagon and plasma catecholamines during beta-receptor blockade in exercising man. *J Appl Physiol* 40:855-863, 1976.

53. Gallagher, JC. Vitamin D and falls—the dosage conundrum. *Nat Rev Endocrinol* 12:680-684, 2016.

54. Gardner, GW, Edgerton, VR, Senewiratne, B, Barnard, RJ, and Ohira, Y. Physical work capacity and metabolic stress in subjects with iron deficiency anemia. *Am J Clin Nutr* 30: 910-917, 1997.

55. Garthe, I and Maughan, RJ. Athletes and supplements: Prevalence and perspectives. *Int J Sport Nutr Exerc Metab* 28:126-138, 2018.

56. Gey, GO, Cooper, KH, and Bottenberg, RA. Effect of ascorbic acid on endurance performance and athletic injury. *JAMA* 211:105, 1970.

57. Girgis, CM, Clifton-Bligh, RJ, Hamrick, MW, Holick, MF, and Gunton JE. The roles of vitamin D in skeletal muscle: Form, function, and metabolism. *Endocr Rev* 34:33-83, 2013.

58. Girgis, CM, Clifton-Bligh, RJ, Turner, N, Lau, SL, and Gunton, JE. Effects of vitamin D in skeletal muscle: Falls, strength, athletic performance and insulin sensitivity. *Clin Endocrinol* 80:169-181, 2014.

59. Golf, SW, Bohmer, D, and Nowacki, PE. Is magnesium a limiting factor in competitive exercise? A summary of relevant scientific data. In *Magnesium*. Golf, S, Dralle, D, and Vecchiet, L, eds. London: John Libbey, 209-220, 1993.

60. Gomez-Cabrera, MC, Domenech, E, Romagnoli, M, Arduini, A, Borras, C, Pallardo, FV, Sastre, J, and Viña, J. Oral administration of vitamin C decreases muscle mitochondrial biogenesis and hampers training-induced adaptations in endurance performance. *Am J Clin Nutr* 87:142-149. 2008.

61. Guilland, JC, Penaranda, T, Gallet, C, Boggio, V, Fuchs, F, and Klepping, J. Vitamin status of young athletes including the effects of supplementation. *Med Science Sports Exerc* 21:441-449, 1989.

62. Haas, JD and Brownlie 4th, T. Iron deficiency and reduced work capacity: A critical review of the research to determine a causal relationship. *J Nutr* 131:676S, 688S; discussion 688S-690S, 2001.

63. Haub, MD, Loest, HB, and Hubach, KL. Assessment of vitamin status of athletes. In *Nutritional Status of Athletes*. 2nd ed. Driskell, JA, Wolinsky, I, eds. Boca Raton, FL: CRC Press, 290-310, 2011.

64. Haymes, EM. Iron. In *Sports Nutrition*. 2nd ed. Driskell, JA. Wolinsky, I, eds. Boca Raton, FL: CRC Press, 203-216, 2006.

65. Heath, EM. Niacin. In *Sports Nutrition*. 2nd ed. Driskell, JA, Wolinsky, I, eds. Boca Raton, FL: CRC Press, 69-80, 2006.

66. Herrmann, M, Obeid, R, Scharhag, J, Kindermann, W, and Herrmann, W. Altered vitamin B_{12} status in recreational endurance athletes. *Int J Sport Nutr Exerc Metabol* 15:433-441, 2005.

67. Hickson, JF, Jr., Schrader, J, and Trischler, LC. Dietary intakes of female basketball and gymnastics athletes. *J Am Diet Assoc* 86:251-253, 1986.

68. Hinton, PS, Giordano, C, Brownlie, T, and Haas JD. Iron supplementation improves endurance after training in iron-depleted, nonanemic women. *J Appl Physiol* 88:1103-1111, 2000.

69. Hinton, PS and Sinclair, LM. Iron supplementation maintains ventilatory threshold and improves energetic efficiency in iron-deficient nonanemic athletes. *Eur J Clin Nutr* 61:30-39, 2007.

70. Holick, MF, Binkley, NC, Bischoff-Ferrari, HA, Gordon, CM, Hanley, DA, Heaney, RP, Murad, MH, and Weaver, CM; Endocrine Society. Evaluation, treatment, and prevention of vitamin D deficiency: An Endocrine Society clinical practice guideline. *J Clin Endocrinol Metab* 96:1911-1930, 2011.

71. Holick, MF. The vitamin D deficiency pandemic: Approaches for diagnosis, treatment and prevention. *Rev Endocr Metab Disor* 18:153-165, 2017.

72. Hoogendijk, WJ, Lips, P, Dik, MG, Deeg, DJ, Beekman, AT, and Penninx, BW. Depression is associated with decreased 25-hydroxyvitamin D and increased parathyroid hormone levels in older adults. *Arch Gen Psychiatry* 65:508-512, 2008.

73. Institute of Medicine, Food and Nutrition Board. *Dietary Reference Intakes for calcium, phosphorus, magnesium, vitamin D, and fluoride*. Washington, DC: National Academies Press, 1997.

74. Institute of Medicine, Food and Nutrition Board. *Dietary References Intakes for thiamin, riboflavin, niacin, vitamin B_{12}, folate, pantothenic acid, biotin, and choline*. Washington, DC: National Academies Press, 1998.

75. Institute of Medicine, Food and Nutrition Board. *Dietary Reference Intakes for vitamin C, vitamin E, selenium, and carotenoids*. Washington, DC: National Academies Press, 2000.

76. Institute of Medicine, Food and Nutrition Board. *Dietary Reference Intakes for vitamin A, vitamin K, arsenic, boron, chromium, copper, iodine, iron, manganese, molybdenum, nickel, silicon, vanadium, and zinc*. Washington, DC: National Academies Press, 2001.

77. Institute of Medicine, Food and Nutrition Board. *Dietary Reference Intakes: Applications in dietary planning*. Washington, DC: National Academies Press, 2003.

78. Institute of Medicine. *Dietary Reference Intakes: The essential guide to nutrient requirements.* Washington, DC: National Academies Press, 2006.

79. Institute of Medicine, Food and Nutrition Board. *Dietary Reference Intakes for calcium and vitamin D.* Washington, DC: National Academies Press, 2011.

80. Isaacson, A, and Sandow, A. Effects of zinc on responses of skeletal muscle. *J Gen Physiol* 46:655-677, 1963.

81. Johnston, CS, Swan, PD, and Corte, C. Substrate utilization and work efficiency during submaximal exercise in vitamin C depleted-repleted adults. *Int J Vitamin Nutr Res* 69:41-44, 1999.

82. Keith, RE, O'Keeffe, KA, Alt, LA, and Young, KL. Dietary status of trained female cyclists. *J Am Dietet Assoc* 89:1620-1623, 1989.

83. Keith, RE and Alt, LA. Riboflavin status of female athletes consuming normal diets. *Nutr Res* 11:727-734, 1991.

84. Keith, RE. Ascorbic acid. In *Sports Nutrition.* 2nd ed. Driskell, JA, Wolinsky, I, eds. Boca Raton, FL: CRC Press, 29-46, 2006.

85. Keys, A, Henschel, AF, Michelsen, O, and Brozek, JM. The performance of normal young men on controlled thiamin intakes. *J Nutr* 26:399-415, 1943.

86. Keren, G and Epstein, Y. The effect of high dosage vitamin C intake on aerobic and anaerobic capacity. *J Sports Med Phys Fitness* 20:145-148, 1980.

87. Khaled, S, Brun, JF, Micallel, JP, Bardet, L, Cassanas, G, Monnier, JF, and Orsetti, A. Serum zinc and blood rheology in sportsmen (football players). *Clin Hemorheol Microcirc* 17:47-58, 1997.

88. Khaled, S, Brun, JF, Cassanas, G, Bardet, L, and Orsetti, A. Effects of zinc supplementation on blood rheology during exercise. *Clin Hemorheol Microcirc* 20:1-10, 1999.

89. Khassaf, M, McArdle, A, Esanu, C, Vasilaki, A, McArdle, F, Griffiths, RD, Brodie, DA, and Jackson, MJ. Effect of vitamin C supplements on antioxidant defence and stress proteins in human lymphocytes and skeletal muscle. *J Physiol* 549:645-652, 2003.

90. Kirchner, EM, Lewis, RD, and O'Connor, PJ. Bone mineral density and dietary intake of female college gymnasts. *Med Sci Sports Exerc* 27:543-549, 1995.

91. Knez, WL, Jenkins, DG, and Coombes, JS. Oxidative stress in half and full Ironman triathletes. *Med Sci Sports Exerc* 39:283-288, 2007.

92. Kreider, RB, Miller, GW, Williams, MH, Somma, CT, and Nasser, TA. Effects of phosphate loading on oxygen uptake, ventilatory anaerobic threshold, and run performance. *Med Sci Sports Exerc* 22:250-256, 1990.

93. Krotkiewski, M, Gudmundsson, M, Backstrom, P, and Mandroukas, K. Zinc and muscle strength and endurance. *Acta Physiol Scand* 116:309-311, 1982.

94. Książek A, Zagrodna A, and Słowińska-Lisowska M. Vitamin D, skeletal muscle function and athletic performance in athletes—a narrative review. *Nutrients* 11(8):1800, 2019.

95. Lamprecht, M, Hofmann, P, Greilberger, JF, and Schwaberger, G. Increased lipid peroxidation in trained men after 2 weeks of antioxidant supplementation. *Int J Sport Nutr Exerc Metab* 19:385-399, 2009.

96. Larson-Meyer, DE, Woolf, K, and Burke, L. Assessment of nutrient status in athletes and the need for supplementation. *Int J Sport Nutr Exerc Metab* 28:139-158, 2018.

97. Lawrence, JD, Bower, RC, Riehl, WP, and Smith, JL. Effects of alpha-tocopherol acetate on the swimming endurance of trained swimmers. *Am J Clin Nutr* 28:205-208, 1975.

98. Leklem, JE. Vitamin B$_6$: A status report. *J Nutr* 120(Suppl 11):1503-1507, 1990.

99. Lemmel, G. Vitamin C deficiency and general capacity for work. *Munchener Medizinische Wochenschrift* 85:1381, 1938.

100. Loosli, AR, Benson, Gillen, DM, and Bourdet, K. Nutritional habits and knowledge in competitive adolescent female gymnasts. *Phys Sports Med* 14:118-121, 1986.

101. Loosli, AR and Benson, J. Nutritional intake in adolescent athletes. *Pediatr Clin N Am* 37:1143-1152, 1990.

102. Lukaski, HC, Hoverson, BS, Gallagher, SK, and Bolonchuk, WW. Physical training and copper, iron, and zinc status of swimmers. *Am J Clin Nutr* 51:1093-1099, 1990.

103. Lukaski, HC, Hall, CB, and Siders, WA. Altered metabolic response of iron-deficient women during graded, maximal exercise. *Eur J Appl Physiol Occup Physiol* 63:140-145, 1991.

104. Lukaski, H. Chromium as a supplement. *Ann Rev Nutr* 19:279-302, 1999.

105. Lukaski, HC and Nielsen, FH. Dietary magnesium depletion affects metabolic responses during submaximal exercise in postmenopausal women. *J Nutr* 132:930-935, 2002.

106. Lukaski, H. Vitamin and mineral status: Effects on physical performance. *Nutrition* 20: 632-644, 2004.

107. Lukaski, HC. Low dietary zinc decreases erythrocyte carbonic anhydrase activities and impairs cardiorespiratory function in men during exercise. *Am J Clin Nutr* 81:1045-1051, 2005.

108. Lukaski, HC. Zinc. In *Sports Nutrition*. 2nd ed. Driskell, JA, Wolinsky, I, eds. Boca Raton, FL: CRC Press, 217-234, 2006.

109. Lukaski, HC and Scrimgeour, AG. Assessment of mineral status in athletes. In *Nutritional Assessment of Athletes*. 2nd ed. Driskell, JA, Wolinsky, I, eds. Boca Raton, FL: CRC Press, 311-340, 2011.

110. Lukaski, HC. Effects of chromium(III) as a nutritional supplement. In *The Nutritional Biochemistry of Chromium(III)*. 2nd ed. Vincent, JB, ed. Amsterdam: Elsevier, 61-78, 2019.

111. Magkos, F and Yannakoulis, M. Methodology of dietary assessment in athletes: Concepts and pitfalls. *Curr Opin Clin Nutr Metabol Care* 6:539-549, 2003.

112. Manore, MM. Effect of physical activity on thiamine, riboflavin, and vitamin B$_6$ requirements. *Am J Clin Nutr* 72(2 Suppl): 598S-606S, 2000.

113. Matter, M, Stittfall, T, Graves, J, Myburgh, K, Adams, B, Jacobs, P, and Noakes, TD. The effect of iron and folate therapy on maximal exercise performance

in female marathon runners with iron and folate deficiency. *Clin Sci* 72:415-422, 1987.

114. Maughan, RJ and Burke LM. *Nutrition for Athletes—a Practical Guide for Eating for Health and Performance*. Lausanne, Switzerland: IOC Medical Commission on Sports Nutrition, 2012.

115. McClung, J.P. Marchitelli, LJ, Friedl, KE, and Young, AJ. Prevalence of iron deficiency and iron deficiency anemia among three populations of female military personnel in the US army. *J Am Coll Nutr* 25:64-69, 2006.

116. Montoye, HJ, Spata, PJ, Pinckney, V, and Barron, L. Effects of vitamin B_{12} supplementation on physical fitness and growth of young boys. *J Appl Physiol* 7:589-592, 1955.

117. Moreira-Pfrimer, LD, Pedrosa, MA, Teixeira, L, and Lazaretti-Castro, M. Treatment of vitamin D deficiency increases lower limb muscle strength in institutionalized older people independently of regular physical activity: A randomized double-blind controlled trial. *Ann Nutr Metab* 54:291-300, 2009.

118. Morrison, D, Hughes, J, Della Gatta, PA, Mason, S, Lamon, S, Russell, AP, and Wadley GD. Vitamin C and E supplementation prevents some of the cellular adaptations to endurance-training in humans. *Free Radic Biol Med* 89:852-862, 2015.

119. Murray, R, Bartoli, WP, Eddy, DE, and Horn, MK. Physiological and performance responses to nicotinic-acid ingestion during exercise. *Med Sci Sports Exerc* 27:1057-1062, 1995.

120. National Academies of Science, Engineering and Medicine. *Dietary Reference Intakes for sodium and potassium*. Washington, DC: National Academies Press, 2019.

121. Niekamp, RA and Baer, JT. In-season dietary adequacy of trained male cross-country runners. *Int J Sport Nutr* 5:45-55, 1995.

122. Nielsen, FH and Lukaski, HC. Update on the relationship between magnesium and exercise. *Mag Res* 19:180-189, 2006.

123. Nieman, DC, Henson, DA, McAnulty, SR, McAnulty, LS, Morrow, JD, Ahmed, A, and Heward, CB. Vitamin E and immunity after the Kona Triathlon World Championship. *Med Sci Sports Exerc* 36:1328-1335, 2004.

124. Owens, DJ, Sharples, AP, Polydorou, I, Alwan, N, Donovan, T, Tang, J, Fraser, WD, Cooper, RG, Morton, JP, Stewart, C, and Close, GL. A systems-based investigation into vitamin D and skeletal muscle repair, regeneration, and hypertrophy. *Am J Physiol Endocrinol Metab* 309:E1019-E1031, 2015.

125. Owens, DJ, Tang, JC, Bradley, WJ, Sparks, AS, Fraser, WD, Morton, JP, and Close GL. Efficacy of high-dose vitamin D supplements for elite athletes. *Med Sci Sports Exerc* 49:349-356, 2017.

126. Owens, DJ, Allison, R, and Close, GL. Vitamin D and the athlete: Current perspectives and new challenges. *Sports Med* 48(Suppl 1):3-16, 2018.

127. Paschalis, V, Theodorou, AA, Kyparos, A, Dipla, K, Zafeiridis, A, Panayiotou, G, Vrabas, IS, and Nikolaidis, MG. Low vitamin C values are linked with decreased

physical performance and increased oxidative stress: Reversal by vitamin C supplementation. *Eur J Nutr* 55:45-53, 2016.

128. Pasricha, SR, Low, M, Thompson, J, Farrell, A, and De-Regil, LM. Iron supplementation benefits physical performance in women of reproductive age: A systematic review and meta-analysis. *J Nutr* 144:906-914, 2014.

129. Paulsen, G, Cumming, KT, Holden, G, Hallén, J, Rønnestad, BR, Sveen, O, Skaug, A, Paur, I, Bastani, NE, Østgaard, HN, Buer, C, Midttun, M, Freuchen, F, Wiig, H, Ulseth, ET, Garthe, I, Blomhoff, R, Benestad, HB, and Raastad, T. Vitamin C and E supplementation hampers cellular adaptation to endurance training in humans: A double-blind, randomised, controlled trial. *J Physiol* 592:1887-1901, 2014.

130. Paulsen, G, Hamarsland, H, Cumming, KT, Johansen, RE, Hulmi, JJ, Børsheim, E, Wiig, H, Garthe, I, and Raastad T. Vitamin C and E supplementation alters protein signalling after a strength training session, but not muscle growth during 10 weeks of training. *J Physiol* 592:5391-5408, 2014.

131. Peeling, P, Dawson, B, Goodman, C, Landers, G, and Trinder, D. Athletic induced iron deficiency: New insights into the role of inflammation, cytokines and hormones. *Eur J Appl Physiol* 103:381-391, 2008.

132. Peeling, P, Dawson, B, Goodman, C, Landers, G, Wiegerinck, ET, Swinkels, DW, and Trinder, D. Effects of exercise on hepcidin response and iron metabolism during recovery. *Int J Sport Nutr Exerc Metab* 19:583-597, 2009.

133. Pernow, B and Saltin, B. Availability of substrates and capacity for prolonged heavy exercise in man. *J Appl Physiol* 31:416-422, 1971.

134. Peternelj, TT and Coombes, JS. Antioxidant supplementation during exercise training: Beneficial or detrimental? *Sports Med* 41:1043-1069, 2011.

135. Peters, AJ, Dressendorfer, RH, Rimar, J, and Keen, CL. Diet of endurance runners competing in a 20-day road race. *Phys Sports Med* 14:63-70, 1986.

136. Pfeifer, M, Begerow, B, and Minne, HW. Vitamin D and muscle function. *Osteoporosis Int* 13:187-194, 2002.

137. Pfeiffer, CM and Looker, AC. Laboratory methodologies for indicators of iron status: Strengths, limitations, and analytical challenges. *Am J Clin Nutr* 106(Suppl 6):1606S-1614S, 2017.

138. Plotnikoff, GA and Quigley, JM. Prevalence of severe hypovitaminosis D in patients with persistent, nonspecific musculoskeletal pain. *Mayo Clinic Proc* 78:1463-1470, 2003.

139. Pompano, LM and Haas, JD. Increasing iron status through dietary supplementation in iron-depleted, sedentary women increases endurance performance at both near-maximal and submaximal exercise intensities. *J Nutr* 149:231-239, 2019.

140. Radak, Z, Zhao, Z, Koltai, E, Ohno, H, and Atalay, M. Oxygen consumption and usage during physical exercise: The balance between oxidative stress and ROS-dependent adaptive signaling. *Antioxid. Redox Signal* 18:1208-1246, 2013.

141. Read, MH and McGuffin, SL. The effect of B-complex supplementation on endurance performance. *J Sports Med Phys Fitness* 23:178-184, 1983.

142. Richardson, JH and Drake PD. The effects of zinc on fatigue of striated muscle. *J Sports Med Phys Fitness* 19:133-134, 1979.

143. Richardson, RS, Donato, AJ, Uberoi, A, Wray, DW, Lawrenson, L, Nishiyama, S, and Bailey, DM. Exercise-induced brachial artery vasodilation: Role of free radicals. *Am J Physiol Heart Circ Physiol* 292:H1516-H522, 2007.

144. Ristow, M, Zarse, K, Oberbach, A, Klöting, N, Birringer, M, Kiehntopf, M, Stumvoll, M, Kahn, CR, and Blüher, M. Antioxidants prevent health-promoting effects of physical exercise in humans. *Proc Natl Acad Sci USA* 106:8665-8670, 2009.

145. Rokitzki, L, Logemann, E, Huber, G, Keck, E, and Keul, J. Alpha-tocopherol supplementation in racing cyclists during extreme endurance training. *Int J Sport Nutr* 4:253-264, 1994.

146. Rowland, TW, Deisroth, MB, Green, GM, and Kelleher, GF. The effect of iron therapy on the exercise capacity of nonanemic iron-deficient adolescent runners. *Am J Dis Child* 142:165-169, 1988.

147. Sanders, KM, Stuart, AL, Williamson, EJ, Simpson, JA, Kotowicz, MA, Young, D, and Nicholson, GC. Annual high-dose oral vitamin D and falls and fractures in older women: A randomized controlled trial. *JAMA* 303:1815-1822, 2010.

148. Schoene, RB, Escourrou, P, Robertson, HT, Nilson, KL, Parsons, JL, and Smith, NJ. Iron repletion decreases maximal exercise lactate concentrations in female athletes with minimal iron-deficiency anemia. *J Lab Clin Med* 102:306-312, 1983.

149. Sharman, IM, Down, MG, and Sen, RN. The effects of vitamin E and training on physiological function and athletic performance in adolescent swimmers. *Brit J Nutr* 26:265-276, 1971.

150. Sharman, IM, Down, MG, and Norgan, NG. The effects of vitamin E on physiological function and athletic performance of trained swimmers. *J Sports Med Phys Fitness* 16:215-225, 1976.

151. Shephard, RJ, Campbell, R, Pimm, R, Stuart, D, and Wright, GR. Vitamin E, exercise, and the recovery from physical activity. *Eur J Appl Physiol Occup Physiol* 33:119-126, 1974.

152. Short, SH and Short, WR. Four-year study of university athletes' dietary intake. *J Am Dietet Assoc* 82:632-645, 1983.

153. Sim, M, Garvican-Lewis, LA, Cox, GR, Govus, A, McKay, AKA, Stellingwerff, T, and Peeling, P. Iron considerations for the athlete: A narrative review. *Eur J Appl Physiol* 119:1463-1478, 2019.

154. Simon-Schnass, I and Pabst, H. Influence of vitamin E on physical performance. *Int J Vitamin Nutr Res* 58: 49-54, 1988.

155. Singh, A, Deuster, PA, and Moser, PB. Zinc and copper status in women by physical activity and menstrual status. *J Sports Med Phys Fitness* 30:29-36, 1990.

156. Singh, A, Moses, FM, and Deuster, PA. Chronic multivitamin-mineral supplementation does not enhance physical performance. *Med Sci Sports Exerc* 24:726-732, 1992.

157. Smith, LM, Gallagher, JC, and Suiter C. Medium doses of daily vitamin D decrease falls and higher doses of daily vitamin D3 increase falls: A randomized clinical trial. *J Steroid Biochem Mol Biol* 173:317-322, 2017.

158. Soric, M, Misigoj-Durakovic, M, and Pedisic, Z. Dietary intake and body composition of prepubescent female aesthetic athletes. *Int J Sport Nutr Exerc Metab* 18:343-354, 2008.

159. Speich, M, Pineau, A, and Ballereau, F. Minerals, trace elements and related biological variables in athletes and during physical activity. *Clin Chim Acta* 312:1-11, 2001.

160. Stacewicz-Sapuntzakis, M and Borthakur, G. Vitamin A. In *Sports Nutrition*. 2nd ed. Driskell, JA, Wolinsky, I, eds. Boca Raton, FL: CRC Press, 163-174, 2006.

161. Steen, SN and McKinney, S. Nutritional assessment of college wrestlers. *Phys Sports Med* 14:101-116, 1986.

162. Steen, SN, Mayer, K, Brownell, KD, and Wadden, TA. Dietary intake of female collegiate heavyweight rowers. *Int J Sport Nutr* 5:225-231, 1995.

163. Stofan, JR, Zachwieja, JJ, Horswill, CA, Murray, R, Anderson, SA, and Eichner, ER. Sweat and sodium losses in NCAA football players: A precursor to heat cramps? *Int J Sport Nutr Exerc Metabol* 15:641-652, 2005.

164. Suboticanec, K, Stavljenic, A, Schalch, W, and Buzina, R. Effects of pyridoxine and riboflavin supplementation on physical fitness in young adolescents. *Int J Vitamin Nutr Res* 60:81-88, 1990.

165. Telford, RD, Catchpole, EA, Deakin, V, Hahn, AG, and Plank, AW. The effect of 7 to 8 months of vitamin/mineral supplementation on athletic performance. *Int J Sport Nutr* 2:135-153, 1992.

166. Teixeira, VH, Valente, HF, Casal, SI, Marques, AF, and Moreira PA. Antioxidants do not prevent postexercise peroxidation and may delay muscle recovery. *Med Sci Sports Exerc* 41:1752-1760, 2009.

167. Thomas, DT, Erdman, KA, and Burke, LM. American College of Sports Medicine Joint Position Statement. Nutrition and Athletic Performance. *Med Sci Sports Exerc* 48:543-568, 2016.

168. Tin-May-Than, Ma-Win-May, Khin-Sann-Aung, and M. Mya-Tu. The effect of vitamin B_{12} on physical performance capacity. *Br J Nutr* 40:269-273, 1978.

169. van der Beek, EJ, van Dokkum, W, Schrijver, J, Wesstra, A, Kistemaker, C, and Hermus, RJ. Controlled vitamin C restriction and physical performance in volunteers. *J Am Coll Nutr* 9:332-339, 1990.

170. van der Beek, EJ, van Dokkum, W, Wedel, M, Schrijver, J, and van den Berg, H. Thiamin, riboflavin and vitamin B_6: Impact of restricted intake on physical performance in man. *J Am Coll Nutr* 13:629-640, 1994.

171. Van Loan, MD., Sutherland, B, Lowe, NM, Turnlund, JR, and King, JC. The effects of zinc depletion on peak force and total work of knee and shoulder extensor and flexor muscles. *Int J Sport Nutr* 9:125-135, 1999.

172. Vincent, JB. The potential value and toxicity of chromium picolinate as a nutritional supplement, weight loss agent and muscle development agent. *Sports Med* 33:213-30, 2003.

173. Virk, RS, Dunton, NJ, Young, JC, and Leklem, JE. Effect of vitamin B$_6$ supplementation on fuels, catecholamines, and amino acids during exercise in men. *Med Sci Sports Exerc* 31:400-408, 1999.

174. Volek, JS, Silvestre, R, Kirwan, JP, Sharman, MJ, Judelson, DA, Spiering, BA, Vingren, JL, Maresh, CM, Vanheest, JL, and Kraemer, WJ. Effects of chromium supplementation on glycogen synthesis after high-intensity exercise. *Med Sci Sports Exerc* 38:2102-2109, 2006.

175. Volpe, SL. Micronutrient requirements for athletes. *Clin Sports Med* 26:119-130, 2007.

176. Wald, G, Brougha, L, and Johnson, R. Experimental human vitamin A deficiency and ability to perform muscular exercise. *Am J Physiol* 137:551-554, 1942.

177. Watt, T, Romet, TT, McFarlane, I, McGuey, D, Allen, C, and Goode, RC. Letter: Vitamin E and oxygen consumption. *Lancet* 2(7876): 354-355, 1974.

178. Webster, MJ. Physiological and performance responses to supplementation with thiamin and pantothenic acid derivatives. *Eur J Appl Physiol Occup Physiol* 77:486-491, 1998.

179. Weight, LM, Myburgh, KH, and Noakes, TD. Vitamin and mineral supplementation: Effect on the running performance of trained athletes. *Am J Clin Nutr* 47:192-195, 1998.

180. Welch, PK, Zager, KA, Endres, J, and Poon, SW. Nutrition education, body composition and dietary intake of female college athletes. *Phys Sports Med* 15:63-74, 1987.

181. Williams, MH. Dietary supplements and sports performance: Introduction and vitamins. *J Int Soc Sports Nutr* 1:1-6, 2004.

182. Williams, MH. Dietary supplements and sports performance: Minerals. *J Int Soc Sports Nutr* 2:43-49, 2005.

183. Wood, B, Gijsbers, A, Goode, A, Davis, S, Mulholland, J, and Breen, K. 1980. A study of partial thiamin restriction in human volunteers. *Am J Clin Nutr* 33:848-861, 1980.

184. Woolf, K and Manore, MM. B-vitamins and exercise: Does exercise alter requirements? *Int J Sport Nutr Exerc Metab* 16:453-484, 2006.

185. Wray, DW, Nishiyama, SK, Harris, RA, Zhao, J, McDaniel, J, Fjeldstad, AS, Witman, MA, Ives, SJ, Barrett-O'Keefe, Z, and Richardson, RS. Acute reversal of endothelial dysfunction in the elderly after antioxidant consumption. *Hypertension* 59:818-824, 2012.

186. Zhu, K, Austin, N, Devine, A, Bruce, D, and Prince, RL. A randomized controlled trial of the effects of vitamin D on muscle strength and mobility in older women with vitamin D insufficiency. *J Am Geriatr Soc* 58:2063-2068, 2010.

187. Ziegler, PJ, Nelson, JA, and Jonnalagadda, SS. Nutritional and physiological status of U.S. national figure skaters. *Int J Sport Nutr* 9:345-360, 1999.

188. Zürcher, SJ, Quadri, A, Huber, A, Thomas, L, Close, GL, Brunner, S, Noack, P, Gojanovic, B, and Kriemler, S. Predictive factors for vitamin D concentrations in Swiss athletes: A cross-sectional study. *Sports Med Int Open* 2:E148-E156, 2018.

Chapter 8

1. Balsom, PD, Soderlund, K, and Ekblom, B. Creatine in humans with special reference to creatine supplementation. *Sports Med* 18(4):268-280, 1994.

2. Besset, A, Bonardet, A, Rondouin, G, Descomps, B, and Passouant, P. Increase in sleep related GH and Prl secretion after chronic arginine aspartate administration in man. *Acta Endocrinologica (Copenhagen)* 99:18-23, 1982.

3. Biolo, G, Maggi, SP, Williams, BD, Tipton, KD, and Wolfe, RR. Increased rates of muscle protein turnover and amino acid transport after resistance exercise in humans. *Am J Physiol* 268(3Pt1):E514-E20, 1995.

4. Biolo, G, Tipton, KD, Klein, S, and Wolfe, RR. An abundant supply of amino acids enhances the metabolic effect of exercise on muscle protein. *Am J Physiol* 273(1Pt1):E122-E129, 1997.

5. Boirie, Y, Dangin, M, Gachon, P, Vasson, MP, Maubois, JL, and Beaufrere, B. Slow and fast dietary proteins differently modulate postprandial protein accretion. *P Natl Acad Sci USA* 94(26):14930-14935, 1997.

6. Branch, JD. Effect of creatine supplementation on body composition and performance: A meta-analysis. *Int J Sport Nutr Exe* 13(2):198-226, 2003.

7. Brose, A, Parise, G, and Tarnopolsky, MA. Creatine supplementation enhances isometric strength and body composition improvements following strength exercise training in older adults. *J Gerontol A Biol Sci Med Sci* 58(1):B11-B19, 2003.

8. Brown, GA, Vukovich, MD, Martini, ER, Kohut, ML, Franke, WD, Jackson, DA, and King, DS. Endocrine responses to chronic androstenedione intake in 30- to 56-year-old men. *J Clin Endocrinol Metab* 85: 4074-4080, 2000.

9. Brown, GA, Vukovich, MD, Sharp, RL, Reifenrath, TA, Parsons, KA, and King, DS. Effect of oral DHEA on serum testosterone and adaptations to resistance training in young men. *J Appl Physiol* 87:2274-2283, 1999.

10. Buford, TW, Kreider, RB, Stout, JR, Greenwood, M, Campbell, B, Spano, M, Ziegenfuss T, Lopez, H, Landis, J, Antonio, J. International society of sports nutrition position stand: Creatine supplementation and exercise. *J Int Soc Sports Nutr* 4:6, 2007.

11. Campbell, B, Kreider, RB, Ziegenfuss, T, La Bounty, P, Roberts, M, Burke, D, Landis, J, Lopez, H, and Antonio, J. International society of sports nutrition position stand: Protein and exercise. *J Int Soc Sports Nutr* 4:8, 2007.

12. Campbell, B, Roberts, M., Kerksick, C, Wilborn, C, Marcello, B, Taylor, L, Nassar, E, Leutholtz, B, Bowden, R, Rasmussen, C, Greenwood, M, and Kreider, R. Pharmacokinetics, safety, and effects on exercise performance of l-arginine alpha-ketoglutarate in trained adult men. *Nutrition* 22:872-881, 2006.

13. Candow, DG, Chilibeck, PD, Burke, DG, Davison, KS, and Smith-Palmer, T. Effect of glutamine supplementation combined with resistance training in young adults. *Eur J Appl Physiol* 86:142-149, 2001.

14. Castell, LM and Newsholme, EA. The effects of oral glutamine supplementation on athletes after prolonged, exhaustive exercise. *Nutrition* 13(7-8):738-742, 1997.

15. Chrusch, MJ, Chilibeck, PD, Chad, KE, Davison, KS, and Burke, DG. Creatine supplementation combined with resistance training in older men. *Med Sci Sports Exerc* 33(12):2111-2117, 2001.

16. Clarkson, PM. Nutritional ergogenic aids: Caffeine. *Int J Sport Nutr* 3:103-111, 1993.

17. Costill, DL, Dalsky, GP, and Fink, WJ. Effects of caffeine ingestion on metabolism and exercise performance. *Med Sci Sports* 10:155-158, 1978.

18. Cribb, PJ, Williams, AD, Carey, MF, and Hayes, A. The effect of whey isolate and resistance training on strength, body composition, and plasma glutamine. *Int J Sport Nutr Exerc Metab* 16(5):494-509, 2006.

19. Dangin, M, Boirie, Y, Garcia-Rodenas, C, Gachon, P, Fauquant, J, Callier, P, Ballevre, O, and Beaufrere, B. The digestion rate of protein is an independent regulating factor of postprandial protein retention. *Am J Physiol Endocrinol Metab* 280(2):E340-348, 2001.

20. Demling, RH and DeSanti, L. Effect of a hypocaloric diet, increased protein intake and resistance training on lean mass gains and fat mass loss in overweight police officers. *Ann Nutr Metab* 44(1):21-29, 2000.

21. Driskell, J and Wolinsky, I. *Energy-Yielding Macronutrients and Energy Metabolism in Sports Nutrition*. Boca Raton, FL: CRC Press, 201, 2000.

22. Dunnett, M and Harris, RC. Influence of oral beta-alanine and L-histidine supplementation on the carnosine content of the gluteus medius. *Equine Vet J* 30:499-504, 1999.

23. Earnest, CP, Snell, PG, Rodriguez, R, Almada, AL, and Mitchell, TL. The effect of creatine monohydrate ingestion on anaerobic power indices, muscular strength and body composition. *Acta Physiol Scand* 153(2):207-209, 1995.

24. Eckerson, JM, Stout, JR, Moore, GA, Stone, NJ, Nishimura, K, and Tamura, K. Effect of two and five days of creatine loading on anaerobic working capacity in women. *J Strength Cond Res* 18:168-173, 2004.

25. Elam, RP, Hardin, DH, Sutton, RA, and Hagen, L. Effects of arginine and ornithine on strength, lean body mass and urinary hydroxyproline in adult males. *J Sport Med Phys Fit* 29:52-56, 1989.

26. Esmarck, B, Andersen, JL, Olsen, S, Richter, EA, Mizuno, M, and Kjaer, M. Timing of postexercise protein intake is important for muscle hypertrophy with resistance training in elderly humans. *J Physiol* 535(Pt1):301-311, 2001.

27. Falkoll, P, Sharp, R, Baier, S, Levenhagen, D, Carr, C, and Nissen, S. Effect of beta-hydroxy-beta-methylbutyrate, arginine, and lysine supplementation on strength, functionality, body composition, and protein metabolism in elderly women. *Nutrition* 20(5):445-451, 2004.

28. Forslund, AH, El-Khoury, AE, Olsson, RM, Sjodin, AM, Hambraeus, L, and Young, VR. Effect of protein intake and physical activity on 24-h pattern and rate of macronutrient utilization. *Am J Physiol Endocrinol Metab* 276(5Pt1):E964-E976, 1999.

29. Friedman, JE and Lemon, PW. Effect of chronic endurance exercise on retention of dietary protein. *Int J Sports Med* 10(2):118-123, 1989.

30. Gallagher, PM, Carrithers, JA, Godard, MP, Schulze, KE, and Trappe, SW. Beta-hydroxy-beta-methylbutyrate ingestion, part I: Effects on strength and fat free mass. *Med Sci Sports Exerc* 32(12):2109-2115, 2000a.

31. Gallagher, PM, Carrithers, JA, Godard, MP, Schulze, KE, and Trappe, SW. Beta-hydroxy-beta-methylbutyrate ingestion, part II: Effects on hematology, hepatic and renal function. *Med Sci Sports Exerc* 32(12):2116-2119, 2000b.

32. Gonzalez, AM, Walsh, AL, Ratamess, NA, Kang, J, and Hoffman, JR. Effect of a pre-workout energy supplement on acute multi-joint resistance exercise. *J Sport Sci Med* 10: 261-266, 2011.

33. Graham, TE and Spriet, LL. Performance and metabolic responses to a high caffeine dose during prolonged exercise. *J Appl Physiol* 71:2292-2298, 1991.

34. Greenwood, M, Farris, J, Kreider, R, Greenwood, L, and Byars, A. Creatine supplementation patterns and perceived effects in select Division I collegiate athletes. *Clin J Sport Med* 10(3):191-194, 2000.

35. Greenwood, M, Kalman, DS, and Antonio, J. *Nutritional Supplements in Sports and Exercise.* New York: Humana Press, 201, 2008.

36. Greenwood, M, Kreider, RB, Melton, C, Rasmussen, C, Lancaster, S, Cantler, E, Milnor, P, and Almada. A. Creatine supplementation during college football training does not increase the incidence of cramping or injury. *Mol Cell Biochem* 244:83-88, 2003.

37. Harris, RC, Hill, CA, Kim, HJ, Boobis, L, Sale, C., Harris, DB, and Wise, JA. Beta-alanine supplementation for 10 weeks significantly increased muscle carnosine levels. *FASEB J* 19:A1125, 2005.

38. Harris, RC, Tallon, MJ, Dunnett, M, Boobis, L, Coakley, J, Kim, HJ, Fallowfield, JL, Hill, CA, Sale, C, and Wise, JA. The absorption of orally supplied β-alanine and its effect on muscle carnosine synthesis in human vastus lateralis. *Amino Acids* 30(3):279-289, 2006.

39. Heymsfield, SB, Arteaga, C, McManus, C, Smith, J, and Moffitt, S. Measurement of muscle mass in humans: Validity of the 24-hour urinary creatinine method. *Am J Clin Nutr* 37(3):478-494, 1983.

40. Hirvonen, J, Rehunen, S, Rusko, H, and Harkonen, M. Breakdown of high-energy phosphate compounds and lactate accumulation during short supra-maximal exercise. *Eur J Appl Physiol* 56(3):253-259, 1987.

41. Hoffman, JR, Cooper, J, Wendell, M, Im, J, and Kang, J. Effects of b-hydroxy-b-methylbutyrate on power performance and indices of muscle damage and stress during high intensity training. *J Strength Cond Res* 18(94):745-752, 2004.

42. Hoffman, JR, Ratamess, NA, Faigenbaum, AD, Ross, R, Kang, J, Stout, JR, and Wise, JA. Short duration beta-alanine supplementation increases training volume and reduces subject feelings of fatigue in college football players. *Nutr Res* 28(1):31-35, 2008a.

43. Hoffman, J, Ratamess, N, Kang, J, Mangine, G, Faigenbaum, A, and Stout, J. Effect of creatine and beta-alanine supplementation on performance and endocrine responses in strength/power athletes. *Int J Sport Nutr Exerc Metab* 16(4):430-446, 2006.

44. Hoffman, J, Ratamess, NA, Ross, R, Kang, J, Magrelli, J, Neese, K, Faigenbaum, AD, and Wise, JA. Beta-alanine and the hormonal response to exercise. *Int J Sports Med 29*(12):952-958, 2008b.

45. Hoffman, JR, and Stout, JR. Performance enhancing supplements. In *Essentials of Strength Training and Conditioning*. Baechle, TR, Earle, RW, eds. Champaign, IL: Human Kinetics, 180, 2008.

46. Jackman, SR, Wiltard, OC, Philp, A, Wallis, GA, Baar, K, and Tipton, KD. Branched-chain amino acid ingestion stimulates muscle myofibrillar protein synthesis following resistance exercise in humans. *Front Physiol* 8:390, 2017.

47. Jagim, AR, Harty, PS, and Camic, CL. Common Ingredient Profiles of Multi-Ingredient Pre-Workout Supplements. *Nutrients* 11(2):E254, 2019.

48. Jones, AM, Atter, T, and Georg, KP. Oral creatine supplementation improves multiple sprint performance in elite ice-hockey players. *J Sport Med Phys Fit* 39(3):189-196, 1999.

49. Joyner, MJ. Over-the-counter supplements and strength training. *Exerc Sport Sci Rev* 28:2-3, 2000.

50. Kendrick, IP, Harris, RC, Kim, HJ, Kim, CK, Dang, VH, Lam, TQ, Bui, TT, Smith, M, and Wise, JA. The effects of 10 weeks of resistance training combined with beta-alanine supplementation on whole body strength, force production, muscular endurance and body composition. *Amino Acids* 34(4):547-554, 2008.

51. Kendall, KL, Moon, JR, Fairman, CM, Spradley, BD, Tai, CY, Falcone, PH, Carson, LR, Mosman, MM, Joy, JM, Kim, MP, Serrano, ER, and Esposito, EN. Ingesting a preworkout supplement containing caffeine, creatine, beta-alanine, amino acids, and B vitamins for 28 days is both safe and efficacious in recreationally active men. *Nutr Res* 34:442-449, 2014.

52. Kerksick, CM, Rasmussen, CJ, Lancaster, SL, Magu, B, Smith, P, Melton, C, Greenwood, M, Almada, AL, Earnest, CP, and Kreider, RB. The effects of protein and amino acid supplementation on performance and training adaptations during ten weeks of resistance training. *J Strength Cond Res* 20(3):643-653, 2006.

53. King, DS, Sharp, RL, Vukovich, MD, Brown, GA, Reifenrath, TA, Uhl, NL, and Parsons, KA. Effect of oral androstenedione on serum testosterone and adaptations to resistance training in young men: A randomized controlled trial. *JAMA* 281:2020-2028, 1999.

54. Kirksey, KB, Stone, MH, Warren, BJ, Johnson, RL, Stone, M, Haff, GG, Williams, FE, and Proulx, C. The effects of 6 weeks of creatine monohydrate supplementation on performance measures and body composition in collegiate track and field athletes. *J Strength Cond Res* 13:148, 1999.

55. Knitter, AE, Panton, L, Rathmacher, JA, Petersen, A, and Sharp, R. Effects of beta-hydroxy-beta-methylbutyrate on muscle damage after a prolonged run. *J Appl Physiol* 89(4):1340-1344, 2000.

56. Kouw, IW, Holwerda, AM, Trommelen, J, Kramer, IF, Bastiaanse, J, Halson, SL, Wodzig, WK, Verdijk, LB, and van Loon, LJ. Protein ingestion before sleep increases overnight muscle protein synthesis rates in healthy older men: A randomized controlled trial. *J Nutr* 147(12):2252-2261, 2017.

57. Kreider, RB. Effects of creatine supplementation on performance and training adaptations. *Mol Cell Biochem* 244(1-2):89-94, 2003a.

58. Kreider, RB. Species-specific responses to creatine supplementation. *Am J Physiol* 285(4):R725-R726, 2003b.

59. Kreider, RB, Ferreira, M, Wilson, M, and Almada, AL. Effects of calcium beta-hydroxy-beta-methylbutyrate (HMB) supplementation during resistance-training on markers of catabolism, body composition and strength. *Int J Sports Med* 20(8):503-9, 1999.

60. Kreider, RB, Ferreira, M, Wilson, M, Grindstaff, P, Plisk, S, Reinardy, J, Cantler, E, and Almada, AL. Effects of creatine supplementation on body composition, strength, and sprint performance. *Med Sci Sports Exerc* 30(1):73-82, 1998.

61. Kreider, RB, Klesges, R, Harmon, K, Grindstaff, P, Ramsey, L, Bullen, D, Wood, L, Li Y, and Almada, A. Effects of ingesting supplements designed to promote lean tissue accretion on body composition during resistance training. *Int J Sport Nutr* 6(3):234-246, 1996.

62. Kreider, RB, Leutholtz, BC, and Greenwood, M. Creatine. In *Nutritional Ergogenic Aids*. Wolinsky, I, Driskel, J, eds. Boca Raton, FL: CRC Press, 81-104, 2004.

63. Kreider, RB, Melton, C, Rasmussen, CJ, Greenwood, M, Lancaster, S, Cantler, EC, Milnor, P, and Almada, AL. Long-term creatine supplementation does not significantly affect clinical markers of health in athletes. *Mol Cell Biochem* 244:95-104, 2003.

64. Lamont, LS, Patel, DG, and Kalhan, SC. Leucine kinetics in endurance-trained humans. *J Appl Physiol* 69(1):1-6, 1990.

65. Lemon, PW. Protein and amino acid needs of the strength athlete. *Int J Sport Nutr* 1(2):127-145, 1991.

66. Lemon, PW. Effects of exercise on dietary protein requirements. *Int J Sport Nutr* 8(4):426-447, 1998.

67. Lemon, PW, Tarnopolsky, MA, MacDougall, JD, and Atkinson, SA. Protein requirements and muscle mass/strength changes during intensive training in novice bodybuilders. *J Appl Physiol* 73(2):767-775, 1992.

68. Meredith, CN, Zackin MJ, Frontera WR, and Evans WJ. Dietary protein requirements and body protein metabolism in endurance-trained men. *J Appl Physiol* 66(6):2850-2856, 1989.

69. Mero, AA, Keskinen, KL, Malvela, MT, and Sallinen, JM. Combined creatine and sodium bicarbonate supplementation enhances interval swimming. *J Strength Cond Res* 18(2):306-310, 2004.

70. Mujika, I, Padilla, S, Ibanez, J, Izquierdo, M, and Gorostiaga, E. 2000. Creatine supplementation and sprint performance in soccer players. *Med Sci Sports Exerc* 32(2):518-525, 2000.

71. Nissen, S, Faidley, TD, Zimmerman, DR, Izard, R, and Fisher, CT. Colostral milk fat percentage and pig performance are enhanced by feeding the leucine metabolite beta-hydroxy-beta-methyl butyrate to sows. *J Anim Sci* 72(9):2331-2337, 1994.

72. Nissen, SL and Sharp, RL. Effect of dietary supplements on lean mass and strength gains with resistance exercise: A meta-analysis. *J Appl Physiol* 94:651-659, 2003.

73. Nissen, S, Sharp, R, Ray, M, Rathmacher, JA, Rice, D, Fuller, Jr. JC, Connelly, AS, and Abumrad, N. Effect of leucine metabolite beta-hydroxy-beta-methylbutyrate on muscle metabolism during resistance-exercise training. *J Appl Physiol* 81(5):2095-2104, 1996.

74. Noonan, D, Berg, K, Latin, RW, Wagner, JC, and Reimers, K. Effects of varying dosages of oral creatine relative to fat free body mass on strength and body composition. *J Strength Cond Res* 12:104, 1998.

75. O'Connor, DM, and Crowe, MJ. Effects of beta-hydroxy-beta-methylbuterate and creatine monohydrate supplementation on the aerobic and anaerobic capacity of highly trained athletes. *J Sport Med Phys Fit* 43:64-68, 2003.

76. Ormsbee, MJ, Mandler, WK, Thomas, DD, Ward, EG, Kinsey, AW, Simonavice, E, Panton, LB, and Kim, JS. The effects of six weeks of supplementation with multi-ingredient performance supplements and resistance training on anabolic hormones, body composition, strength, and power in resistance-trained men. *J Int Soc Sports Nutr* 9:49, 2012.

77. Ormsbee, MJ, Thomas, DD, Mandler, WK, Ward, EG, Kinsey, AW, Panton, LB, Scheett, TP, Hooshmand, S, Simonavice, E, and Kim, JS. The effects of pre- and post-exercise consumption of multi-ingredient performance supplements on cardiovascular health and body fat in trained men after six weeks of resistance training: A stratified, randomized, double-blind study. *Nutr Metab* 10:39, 2013.

78. Ostojic, SM. Creatine supplementation in young soccer players. *Int J Sport Nutr Exerc Metab* 14(1):95-103, 2004.

79. Peeters, B, Lantz, C, and Mayhew, J. Effects of oral creatine monohydrate and creatine phosphate supplementation on maximal strength indices, body composition, and blood pressure. *J Strength Cond Res* 13:3, 1999.

80. Peterson, AL, Qureshi, MA, Ferket, PR, and Fuller, Jr. JC. Enhancement of cellular and humoral immunity in young broilers by the dietary supplementation of beta-hydroxy-beta-methylbutyrate. *Immunopharmacol Immunotoxicol* 21(2):307-330, 1999a.

81. Peterson, AL, Qureshi MA, Ferket PR, and Fuller Jr. JC. In vitro exposure with beta-hydroxy-beta-methylbutyrate enhances chicken macrophage growth and function. *Vet Immunol Immunopathol* 67(1):67-78, 1999b.

82. Phillips, SM, Atkinson, SA, Tarnopolsky, MA, and MacDougall, JD. Gender differences in leucine kinetics and nitrogen balance in endurance athletes. *J Appl Physiol* 75(5):2134-2141, 1993.

83. Phillips, SM, Tipton, KD, Aarsland, A, Wolf, SE, and Wolfe, RR. Mixed muscle protein synthesis and breakdown after resistance exercise in humans. *Am J Physiol* 273(1Pt1):E99-E107, 1997.

84. Phillips, S, Tipton, K, Ferrando, A, and Wolfe, R. Resistance training reduces the acute exercise-induced increase in muscle protein turnover. *Am J Physiol* 276(1Pt1):E118-E124, 1999.

85. Preen, D, Dawson, B, Goodman, C, Lawrence, S, Beilby, J, and Ching, S. Effect of creatine loading on long-term sprint exercise performance and metabolism. *Med Sci Sports Exerc* 33(5):814-821, 2001.

86. Rasmussen, BB, Volpi, E, Gore, DC, and Wolfe, RR. Androstenedione does not stimulate muscle protein anabolism in young healthy men. *J Clin Endocrinol Metab* 85:55-59, 2000.

87. Rawson, E and Persky, AM. Mechanisms of muscular adaptations to creatine supplementation: Review article. *Int J Sports Med* 8(2):43-53, 2007.

88. Rennie, MJ, Wackerhage, H, Spangenburg, EE, and Booth, FW. Control of the size of the human muscle mass. *Annu Rev Physiol* 66:799-828, 2004.

89. Rohle, D, Wilborn, C, Taylor, L, Mulligan, C, Kreider, R, and Willoughby, D. Effects of eight weeks of an alleged aromatase inhibiting nutritional supplement 6-OXO (androst-4-ene-3,6,17-trione) on serum hormone profiles and clinical safety markers in resistance-trained, eugonadal males. *J Int Soc Sports Nutr* 19(4):13, 2007.

90. Sale, C, Hill, CA, Ponte, J, and Harris, RC. B-alanine supplementation improves isometric endurance of the knee extensor muscles. *J Int Soc Sports Nutr* 9:26, 2012.

91. Shimomura, Y, Inaguma, A, Watanabe, S, Yamamoto, Y, Muramatsu, Y, Bajotto, G, Sato, J, Shimomura, N, Kobayashi, H, and Mawatari, K. Branched-chain amino acid supplementation before squat exercise and delayed-onset muscle soreness. *Int J Sport Nutr Exerc Metab* 20(3):236-244, 2010.

92. Skare, OC, Skadberg, and Wisnes, AR. 2001. Creatine supplementation improves sprint performance in male sprinters. *Scand J Med Sci Sports* 11(2):96-102.

93. Slater, G, Jenkins, D, Logan, P, Lee, H, Vukovich, M, Rathmacher, JA, and Hahn, AG. Beta-hydroxy-beta-methylbutyrate (HMB) supplementation does not affect changes in strength or body composition during resistance training in trained men. *Int J Sport Nutr Exerc Metab* 11(3):384-396, 2001.

94. Smith, AE, Fukuda, DH, Kendall, KL, and Stout, JR. The effects of a pre-workout supplement containing caffeine, creatine, and amino acids during three weeks of high-intensity exercise on aerobic and anaerobic performance. *J Int Soc Sports Nutr* 7:10, 2010.

95. Spillane, M, Schwarz, N, Leddy, S, Correa, T, Minter, M, Longoria, V, and Willoughby DS. Effects of 28 days of resistance exercise while consuming commercially available pre- and post-workout supplements, NO-Shotgun(R) and NO-Synthesize(R) on body composition, muscle strength and mass, markers of protein synthesis, and clinical safety markers in males. *Nutr Metab* 8:78, 2011.

96. Spradley, BD, Crowley, KR, Tai, CY, Kendall, KL, Fukuda, DH, Esposito, EN, Moon, SE, and Moon, JR. Ingesting a pre-workout supplement containing caffeine, B-vitamins, amino acids, creatine, and beta-alanine before exercise delays fatigue while improving reaction time and muscular endurance. *Nutr Metab* 9:28, 2012.

97. Stone, MH, Sanborn, K., Smith, LL, O'Bryant, HS, Hoke, T, Utter, AC, Johnson, RL, Boros, R, Hruby, J, Pierce KC, Stone, ME, and Garner, B. Effects

of in-season (5 weeks) creatine and pyruvate supplementation on anaerobic performance and body composition in American football players. *Int J Sport Nutr* 9(2):146-165, 1999.

98. Stout, JR, Cramer, JT, Mielke, M, O'Kroy, J, Torok, DJ, and Zoeller, RF. Effects of twenty-eight days of beta-alanine and creatine monohydrate supplementation on the physical working capacity at neuromuscular fatigue threshold. *J Strength Cond Res* 20(4):928-931, 2006.

99. Stout, J, Eckerson, J, Ebersole, K, Moore, G, Perry, S, Housh, T, Bull, A, Cramer, J, and Batheja, A. Effect of creatine loading on neuromuscular fatigue threshold. *J Appl Physiol* 88(1):109-112, 2000.

100. Stout, JR, Eckerson, J, and Noonan, D. Effects of 8 weeks of creatine supplementation on exercise performance and fat-free weight in football players during training. *Nutr Res* 19:217, 1999.

101. Stout, JR, Graves, BS, Smith, AE, Hartman, MJ, Cramer, JT, Beck, TW, and Harris, RC. The effect of beta-alanine supplementation on neuromuscular fatigue in elderly (55-92 years): A double-blind randomized study. *J Int Soc Sports Nutr* 5:21, 2008.

102. Tarnopolsky, M. Protein requirements for endurance athletes. *Nutrition* 20(78):662-668, 2004.

103. Tarnopolsky, MA, Atkinson, SA, MacDougall, JD, Chesley, A, Phillips, S, and Schwarcz, HP. Evaluation of protein requirements for trained strength athletes. *J Appl Physiol* 73(5):1986-1995, 1992.

104. Tarnopolsky, MA. and MacLennan DP. Creatine monohydrate supplementation enhances high-intensity exercise performance in males and females. *Int J Sport Nutr Exerc Metab* 10(4):452-463, 2000.

105. Teixeira, FJ, Matias, CN, Monteiro, CP, Valamatos, MJ, Reis, JF, Tavares, F, Batista, A, Domingos, C, Alves, F, Sardinha, LB, and Phillips, SM. Leucine metabolites do not enhance training-induced performance or muscle thickness. *Med Sci Sports Exerc* 51(1):56-64, 2019.

106. Theodorou, AS, Cooke, CB, King, RF, Hood, C, Denison, T, Wainwright, B, and Havenetidis, K. The effect of longer-term creatine supplementation on elite swimming performance after an acute creatine loading. *J Sports Sci* 17(11):853-859, 1999.

107. Tipton, KD, Elliot, TA, Cree, MG, Wolf, SE, Sanford, AP, and Wolf, RR. Ingestion of casein and whey proteins result in muscle anabolism after resistance exercise. *Med Sci Sports Exerc* 36(12):2073-2081, 2004.

108. Tipton, KD, Ferrando AA, Phillips SM, Doyle, Jr. D, and Wolfe, RR. Postexercise net protein synthesis in human muscle from orally administered amino acids. *Am J Physiol* 276(4Pt1):E628-E634, 1999.

109. Vandenberghe, K, Goris, M, Van Hecke, P, Van Leemputte, M, Vangerven, L, and Hespel, P. Long-term creatine intake is beneficial to muscle performance during resistance training. *J Appl Physiol* 83(6):2055-2063, 1997.

110. van Gammeren, D, Falk, D, and Antonio, J. Effects of norandrostenedione and norandrostenediol in resistance-trained men. *Nutrition* 18:734-737, 2002.

111. Van Koevering, MT, Dolezal, HG, Gill, DR, Owens, FN, Strasia, CA, Buchanan, DS, Lake, R, and Nissen, S. Effects of beta-hydroxy-beta-methyl butyrate on performance and carcass quality of feedlot steers. *J Anim Sci* 72(8):1927-1935, 1994.

112. van Loon, LJ, Oosterlaar, AM, Hartgens, F, Hesselink, MK, Snow, RJ, and Wagenmakers, AJ. Effects of creatine loading and prolonged creatine supplementation on body composition, fuel selection, sprint and endurance performance in humans. *Clin Sci* 104(2):153-162, 2003.

113. van Someren, KA, Edwards, AJ, and Howatson, G. The effects of HMB supplementation on indices of exercise induced muscle damage in man. *Med Sci Sports Exerc* 35(5):270, 2003.

114. van Someren, KA, Edwards, AJ, and Howatson, G. Supplementation with beta-hydroxy-beta-methylbutyrate (HMB) and alpha-ketoisocaproic acid (KIC) reduces signs and symptoms of exercise-induced muscle damage in man. *Int J Sport Nutr Exerc Metab* 15(4):413-424, 2005.

115. Villareal, DT, and Holloszy, JO. DHEA enhances effects of weight training on muscle mass and strength in elderly women and men. *Am J Physiol Endocrinol Metab* 291:E1003-1008, 2006.

116. Volek, JS, Duncan, ND, Mazzetti, SA, Staron, RS, Putukian, M, Gomez, AL, Pearson, DR, Fink, WJ, and Kraemer, WJ. Performance and muscle fiber adaptations to creatine supplementation and heavy resistance training. *Med Sci Sports Exerc* 3(8):1147-1156, 1999.

117. Volek, JS, Kraemer, WJ, Bush, JA, Boetes, M, Incledon, T, Clark, KL, and Lynch, JM. Creatine supplementation enhances muscular performance during high-intensity resistance exercise. *J Am Diet Assoc* 97(7):765-770, 1997.

118. Vukovich, MD, Stubbs, NB, and Bohlken, RM. Body composition in 70-year-old adults responds to dietary beta-hydroxy-beta-methylbutyrate similarly to that of young adults. *J Nutr* 131(7):2049-2052, 2001.

119. Wagenmakers, AJ. Tracers to investigate protein and amino acid metabolism in human subjects. *P Nutr Soc* 58(4):987-1000, 1999.

120. Wallace, MB, Lim, J, Cutler, A, and Bucci, L. Effects of dehydroepiandrosterone vs androstenedione supplementation in men. *Med Sci Sports Exerc* 31:1788-1792, 1999.

121. Walsh, AL, Gonzalez, AM, Ratamess, NA, Kang, J, and Hoffman, JR. Improved time to exhaustion following ingestion of the energy drink Amino Impact. *J Int Soc Sports Nutr* 7:14, 2010.

122. Wang, CC, Yang, MT, Lu, KH, and Chan, KH. The effects of creatine supplementation on explosive performance and optimal individual postactivation potentiation time. *Nutrients* 8(3):143, 2016.

123. Wang, CC, Lin, SC, Hsu, SC, Yang, MT, and Chan, KH. The effects of creatine supplementation on muscle strength and optimal individual post-activation potentiation time of the upper body in canoeists. *Nutrients* 9(11):1169, 2017.

124. Welbourne, TC. Increased plasma bicarbonate and growth hormone after an oral glutamine load. *Am J Clin Nutr* 61:1058-1061, 1995.

125. Willoughby, DS, and Rosene, J. Effects of oral creatine and resistance training on myosin heavy chain expression. *Med Sci Sports Exerc* 33(10):1674-1681, 2001.

126. Willoughby, DS, Stout, JR, and Wilborn, CD. Effects of resistance training and protein plus amino acid supplementation on muscle anabolism, mass, and strength. *Amino Acids* 32(4):467-477, 2007.

127. Willoughby, DS, Wilborn, C., Taylor, L., and Campbell, B. Eight weeks of aromatase inhibition using the nutritional supplement Novedex XT: Effects in young, eugonadal men. *Int J Sport Nutr Exerc Metab* 17:92-108, 2007.

128. Wiroth, JB, Bermon, S, Andrei, S, Dalloz, E, Hebuterne, X, and Dolisi, C. Effects of oral creatine supplementation on maximal pedalling performance in older adults. *Eur J Appl Physiol* 84(6):533-539, 2001.

129. Zoeller, RF, Stout, JR, O'Kroy, JA, Torok, DJ, and Mielke, M. Effects of 28 days of beta-alanine and creatine monohydrate supplementation on aerobic power, ventilatory and lactate thresholds, and time to exhaustion. *Amino Acids* 33(3):505-510, 2007.

Chapter 9

1. American College of Sports Medicine, American Dietetic Association, and Dietitians of Canada. Joint position statement: Nutrition and athletic performance. *Med Sci Sports Exerc* 48(3):543-568, 2016.

2. Astorino, TA and Roberson, DW. Efficacy of acute caffeine ingestion for short-term high-intensity exercise performance: A systematic review. *J Strength Cond Res* 24(1):257-265, 2010.

3. Aulin, KP, Soderlund, K, and Hultman, F. Muscle glycogen resynthesis rate in humans after supplementation of drinks containing carbohydrates with low and high molecular masses. *Eur J of Appl Physiol* 81:346-351, 2000.

4. Baker, LB, Munce, TA, and Kenney, WL. Sex differences in voluntary fluid intake by older adults during exercise. *Med Sci Sports Exerc* 37:789-796, 2005.

5. Banister, EW, Allen, ME, Mekjavic, IB, Singh, AK, Legge, B, and Mutch, BJC. The time course of ammonia and lactate accumulation in blood during bicycle exercise. *Eur J Appl Physiol* 51:195-202, 1983.

6. Bassit, RA, Sawada, LA, Bacarau, RFP, Navarro, F, and Costa Rosa, LFBP. The effect of BCAA supplementation upon the immune response of triathletes. *Med Sci Sports Exerc* 32:1214-1219, 2000.

7. Bell, DG and McLellan, TM. Effect of repeated caffeine ingestion on repeated exhaustive exercise aerobic endurance. *Med Sci Sports Exerc* 35(8):1348-1354, 2003.

8. Berardi, JM, Price, TB, Noreen, EE, Lemon, PW. Postexercise muscle glycogen recovery enhanced with a carbohydrate-protein supplement. *Med Sci Sports Exerc* 38(60):1106-1113, 2006.

9. Bernadot, D. *Advanced Sports Nutrition*. Champaign, IL: Human Kinetics, 1-341, 2006.

10. Betts, JA, Williams, C, Boobis, L, and Tsintzas, K. Increased carbohydrate oxidation after ingesting carbohydrate with added protein. *Med Sci Sports Exerc* 40(5):903-912, 2008.

11. Blomstrand, E, Celsing, E, and Newsholme, EA. Changes in plasma concentrations of aromatic and branched-chain amino acids during sustained exercise in man and their possible role in fatigue. *Acta Physiol* 133(1):115-121, 1988.

12. Blomstrand, E, Hassmen, P, Ek, S, Ekblom, B, and Newsholme, EA. Influence of ingesting a solution of branched-chain amino acids on perceived exertion during exercise. *Acta Physiol* 159(1):41-49, 1997.

13. Blomstrand, E, Hassmen, P, Ekblom, B, and Newsholme, EA. Administration of branched-chain amino acids during sustained exercise; effect on performance and on plasma concentration of some amino acids. *Eur J Appl Physiol* 63:83-88, 1991.

14. Brouns, F. Heat-sweat-dehydration-rehydration: A praxis oriented approach. *J Sports Sci* 9:143-152, 1991.

15. Burke, L. Caffeine and sports performance. *Appl Physiol Nutr Metab* 33(6):1319-34, 2008.

16. Butterfield, GE and Calloway, DH. Physical activity improves protein utilization in young men. *Brit J Nutr* 51:171-184, 1984.

17. Carr, AJ, Hopkins WG, and Gore, CJ. Effects of acute alkalosis and acidosis on performance: A meta-analysis. *Sports Med* 41(10):801-814, 2011.

18. Carli, G, Bonifazi, M, Lodi, L, Lupo, C, Martelli, G, and Viti, A. Changes in the exercise-induced hormone response to branched chain amino acid administration. *Eur J Appl Physiol Occup Physiol* 64:272-277, 1992.

19. Castell, LM. Glutamine supplementation in vitro and vivo, in exercise and in immunodepression. *Sports Med* 33:323-345, 2003.

20. Costill, DL, Dalsky, GP, and Fink, WJ. Effects of caffeine ingestion on metabolism and exercise performance. *Med Sci Sports* 10:155-158, 1978.

21. Coombes, JS and McNaughton, LR. Effects of branched-chain amino acid supplementation on serum creatine kinase and lactate dehydrogenase after prolonged exercise. *J Sport Med Phys Fit* 40:240-246, 2000.

22. Cureton, KJ, Warren, GL, Millard-Stafford, ML, Wingo, JE, Trilk, J, and Buyckx, J. Caffeinated sports drink: Ergogenic effects and possible mechanisms. *Int J Sport Nutr Exerc Metab* 17:35-55, 2007.

23. Currell, K and Jeukendrup, AE. Superior aerobic endurance performance with ingestion of multiple transportable carbohydrates. *Med Sci Sports Exerc* 40(2):275-281, 2008.

24. Demura, S, Yamada, T, and Terasawa, N. Effect of coffee ingestion on physiological responses and ratings of perceived exertion during submaximal aerobic endurance exercise. *Percept Mot Ski* 105(3 Pt 2):1109-1116, 2007.

25. Doherty, M and Smith, PM. Effects of caffeine ingestion on exercise testing: A meta-analysis. *Int J Sport Nutr Exerc Metab* 14(6):626-646, 2004.

26. Dunford, M. *Sports Nutrition: A Practice Manual for Professionals*. 4th ed. American Dietetic Association. Chicago, IL, 445-459, 2006.

27. Fredholm, B, Battig, K, Holmen, J, Nehlig, A, and Zvartau, EE. Actions of caffeine in the brain with special reference to factors that contribute to its widespread use. *Pharmacol Rev* 51(1):83-133, 1999.

28. Gleeson, M. Interrelationship between physical activity and branched-chain amino acids. *J Nutr* 135:1591S-1595S, 2005.

29. Gleeson, M. Dosing and efficacy of glutamine supplementation in human exercise and sport training. *J Nutr* 138:2045-2049, 2008.

30. Goodpaster, BH, Costill, DL, Fink, WJ, Trappe, TA, Jozi, AC, Starling, RD, and Trappe, SW. The effects of pre-exercise starch ingestion on aerobic endurance performance. *Int J Sports Med* 17(5):366-372, 1996.

31. Graham, TE. Caffeine and exercise: Metabolism, aerobic endurance and performance. *Sports Med* 31:785-807, 2001

32. Graham, TE and Spriet, LL. Caffeine and exercise performance. *Gatorade Sports Science Exchange* 9(1):1-5, 1996.

33. Green, MS, Corona, BT, Doyle, JA, and Ingalls, CP. Carbohydrate-protein drinks do not enhance recovery from exercise-induced muscle injury. *Int J Sport Nutr Exerc Metab* 18: 1-18, 2008.

34. Greer, BK, Woodard, JL, White, JP, Arguello, EM, and Haymes, EM. Branched-chain amino acid supplementation and indicators of muscle damage after aerobic endurance exercise. *Int J Sport Nutr Exerc Metab* 17:595-607, 2007.

35. Halton, TL and Hu, FB. The effects of high protein diets on thermogenesis, satiety and weight loss: A critical review. *J Am Coll Nutr* 23(5):373-385, 2004.

36. Hargreaves, M. Muscle glycogen and metabolic regulation. *P Nutr Soc* 63(2):217-220, 2004.

37. Hassmen, P, Blomstrand, E, Ekblom, B, and Newsholme, EA. Branched-chain amino acid supplementation during 30-km competitive run: Mood and cognitive performance. *Nutr J* 10(5):405-410, 1994.

38. Hawley, JA and Reilly, T. Fatigue revisited. *J Sports Sci* 15:245-246, 1997.

39. Hearris, MA, Hammond, KM, Fell, JM, and Morton, JP. Regulation of muscle glycogen metabolism during exercise: Implications for endurance performance and training adaptations. *Nutrients* 10(3):298, 2018.

40. Heibel, AB, Perim, PHL, Oliveira, LF, McNaughton, LR, and Saunders, B. Time to optimize supplementation: Modifying factors influencing the individual responses to extracellular buffering agents. *Front Nutr* 5:35, 2018.

41. Hobson, RM, Harris, RC, Martin, D, Smith, P, Macklin, B, Elliot-Sale, KJ, and Sale, C. Effect of sodium bicarbonate supplementation on 2000-m rowing performance. *Int J Sports Phyiol Perform* 9:139-144, 2014.

42. Hoffman, JR, Kang, J, Ratamess, NA, Jennings, PF, Mangine, GT, and Faigenbaum, AD. Effect of nutritionally enriched coffee consumption on aerobic and anaerobic exercise performance. *J Strength Cond Res* 21(2):456-459, 2007.

43. Jafari, H, Barrett, R, and Emhoff, CW. Effects of branched-chain amino acid supplementation on exercise performance and recovery in highly endurance-trained athletes. *FASEB J* 30:1 lb683, 2016.

44. Jentjens, RL, Achten, J, and Jeukendrup, AE. High oxidation rates from combined carbohydrates ingested during exercise. *Med Sci Sports Exerc* 36:1551-1558, 2004.

45. Jeukendrup, A and Gleeson, M. *Sports Nutrition: An Introduction to Energy Production and Performance.* Champaign, IL: Human Kinetics, 204-205, 2004.

46. Johannsen, NM and Sharp, RL. Effect of preexercise ingestion of modified cornstarch on substrate oxidation during aerobic endurance exercise. *Int J Sport Nutr Exerc Metab* 17(3):232-243, 2007.

47. Jozsi, AC, Trappe, TA, Starling, RD, Goodpaster, BH, Trappe, SW, Fink, WJ, and Costill, DL. The influence of starch structure on glycogen resynthesis and subsequent cycling performance. *Int J Sports Med* 17(5):373-378, 1996.

48. Kiens, B, Raben, AB, Valeur, AK, and Richter, EA. Benefit of dietary simple carbohydrates on the early post-exercise muscle glycogen repletion in male athletes. *Med Sci Sports Exerc* 22:S88, 1990.

49. Killer, SC, Blannin, AK, and Jeukendrup, AE. No evidence of dehydration with moderate daily coffee intake: A counterbalanced cross-over study in a free-living population. *PLoS One* 9(1):e84154, 2014.

50. Knuiman P, Hopman, MTE, Verbruggen, C, and Mensink, M. Protein and the adaptive response with endurance training: Wishful thinking or a competitive edge? *Front Physiol* 2018;9:598, 2018.

51. Koopman, R, Pannemans, DLE, Jeukendrup, AE, Gijsen, AP, Senden, JMG, Halliday, D, Saris, WH, van Loon, LJ, and Wagenmakers, AJ. Combined ingestion of protein and carbohydrate improves protein balance during ultra-aerobic endurance exercise. *Am J Physiol Endoc M* 287:E712-E720, 2004.

52. Lamont, LS, McCullough, AJ, and Kalhan, SC. Comparison of leucine kinetics in aerobic endurance-trained and sedentary humans. *J Appl Physiol* 86:320-325, 1999.

53. Latner, JD and Schwartz, M. The effects of a high-carbohydrate, high-protein or balanced lunch upon later food intake and hunger ratings. *Appetite* 33(1):119-128, 1999.

54. Leiper, JB, Aulin, KP, and Soderlund, K. Improved gastric emptying rate in humans of a unique glucose polymer with gel-forming properties. *Scand J Gastroenterol* 35:1143-1149, 2000.

55. Lemon, PW. Effects of exercise on dietary protein requirements. *Int J Sport Nutr* 8:426-447, 1998.

56. Lemon, PW and Proctor, DN. Protein intake and athletic performance. *Sports Med* 12: 313-325, 1991.

57. Luden, ND, Saunders, MJ, and Todd, MK. Postexercise carbohydrate-protein-antioxidant ingestion decreases plasma creatine kinase and muscle soreness. *Int J Sport Nutr Exerc Metab* 17:109-123, 2007.

58. Maughan, RJ. Fluid and electrolyte loss and replacement in exercise. *J Sports Sci* 9:117-142, 1991.

59. Maughan, RJ and Murray, R. Gastric emptying and intestinal absorption of fluids, carbohydrates, and electrolytes. In *Sports Drinks: Basic Science and Practical Aspects*. New York: CRC Press, 1-279, 2001.

60. McLellan, TM, Bell, GD, and Kamimori, GH. Caffeine improves physical performance during 24 h of active wakefulness. *Aerosp Med Hum Perform* 75(8):666-672, 2004.

61. McNaughton, LR, Siegler, J, and Midgley, A. Ergogenic effects of sodium bicarbonate. *Curr Sports Med Rep* 7:230-236, 2008.

62. Millard-Stafford, ML, Cureton, KJ, Wingo, JE, Trilk, J, Warren, GJ, and Buyckx, M. Hydration during exercise in warm, humid conditions: Effect of a caffeinated sports drink. *Int J Sport Nutr Exerc Metab* 17:163-177, 2007.

63. Morgan, RM, Patterson, MJ, and Nimmo, MA. Acute effects of dehydration on sweat composition in men during prolonged exercise in the heat. *Acta Physiol* 182(1):37-43, 2004.

64. Murray, R and Kenney, WL. Sodium balance and exercise. *Curr Sport Med Rep* 7(4):S1-S2, 2008.

65. National Collegiate Athletic Association. *2009-10 NCAA banned drugs*. June 10, 2009.

66. Newell, ML, Wallis, GA, Hunter, AM, Tipton, KD, and Galloway, SDR. Metabolic responses to carbohydrate ingestion during exercise: Associations between carbohydrate dose and endurance performance. *Nutrients* 10(1):37, 2018.

67. Newsholme, EA and Blomstrand, E. Branched-chain amino acids and central fatigue. *J Nutr* 136:1 274S-276S, 2006.

68. Nieman, DC. Influence of carbohydrate on the immune response to intensive, prolonged exercise. *Exerc Immunol Rev* 4:64-76, 1998.

69. Noakes, TD. Fluid replacement during exercise. In *Exercise and Sport Sciences Reviews*. Holloszy, JO, ed. Baltimore: Williams & Wilkins, 297-330, 1993.

70. Ohtani, M, Sugita, M, and Maryuma, K. Amino acid mixture improves training efficiency in athletes. *J Nutr* 136:538S-543S, 2006.

71. Otukonyong, EE and Oyebola, DD. Electrolyte loss during exercise in apparently healthy Nigerians. *Cent Afr J Med* 40(3):74-77, 1994.

72. Paddon-Jones, D, Sheffield-Moore, M, Zhang, XJ, Volpi, E, Wolf, SE, Aarsland, A, Ferrando, AA, and Wolfe, RR. Amino acid ingestion improves protein synthesis in the young and elderly. *Am J Physiol Endocrinol Metab* 286:E321-E328, 2004.

73. Paik, IY, Jeong, MH, Jin, HE, Kim, YI, Suh, AR, Cho, SY, Roh, HT, Jin, CH, and Suh, SH. Fluid replacement following dehydration reduces oxidative stress during recovery. *Biochem Biophys Res Commun* 383(1):103-7, 2009.

74. Pederson, DL, Lessard, SJ, Coffey, VG, Churchley, EG, Wootton, AM, Ng, T, Watt, MH, and Hawley, JA. High rates of muscle glycogen resynthesis after exhaustive exercise when carbohydrate is coingested with caffeine. *J Appl Physiol* 105(1):7-13, 2008.

75. Rehrer, NJ. Fluid and electrolyte balance in ultra-aerobic endurance sport. *Sports Med* 31(10):701-715, 2001.

76. Requena, B, Zabala, M, Padial, P, and Feriche, B. Sodium bicarbonate and sodium citrate: Ergogenic aids? *J Strength Cond Res* 19(1):213-224, 2005.

77. Roberts, M, Lockwood, C, Dalbo, VJ, Tucker, P, Frye, A, Polk, R, Volek, J, and Kerksick, C. Ingestion of a high molecular weight modified waxy maize starch alters metabolic responses to prolonged exercise in trained cyclists. *FASEB* 23:1S, 2009.

78. Rosset, R, Egli, L, and Lecoultre, V. Glucose-fructose ingestion and exercise performance: The gastrointestinal tract and beyond. *Eur J Sport Sci* 17:7, 874-884, 2017.

79. Rowlands, DS, Thorp, RM, Rossler, K, Graham, DF, and Rockell, MJ. Effect of protein-rich feeding on recovery after intense exercise. *Int J Sport Nutr Exerc Metab* 17:521-543, 2007.

80. Sanders, B, Noakes, TD, and Dennis, SC. Water and electrolyte shifts with partial fluid replacement during exercise. *Eur J Appl Physiol* 80:318-323, 1999.

81. Sawka, MN, Burke, LM, Eichner, RE, Maughan, RJ, Montain, SJ, and Stachenfeld, NS. American College of Sports Medicine position stand: Exercise and fluid replacement. *Med Sci Sports Exerc* 39:377-390, 2007.

82. Seifert, J, Harmon, J, and DeClercq, P. Protein added to a sports drink improves fluid retention. *Int J Sport Nutr Exerc Metab* 16(4):420-429, 2006.

83. Shirreffs, SM, Aragon-Vargas, LF, Keil, M, Love, TD, and Phillips, S. Rehydration after exercise in the heat: A comparison of 4 commonly used drinks. *Int J Sport Nutr Exerc Metab* 17:244-258, 2007.

84. Shirreffs, SM and Maughan, RJ. Volume repletion after exercise-induced volume depletion in humans: Replacement of water and sodium losses. *Am J Physiol* 274:F868-F875, 1998.

85. Smith, A, Kendrick, A, Maben, A, and Salmon, J. Effects of breakfast and caffeine on cognitive performance, mood and cardiovascular functioning. *Appetite* 22(1):39-55, 1994.

86. Struder, HK, Hollman, W, Platen, P, Wöstmann, R, Ferrauti, A, and Weber, K. Effect of exercise intensity on free tryptophan to branched-chain amino acids ratio and plasma prolactin during aerobic endurance exercise. *Appl Physiol Nutr Metab* 22(3):280-291, 1997.

87. Tarnopolsky MA. Caffeine and creatine use in sport. *Ann Nutr Metab* 57(Suppl 2):1-8, 2010.

88. Tipton, KD and Wolfe, RR. Exercise-induced changes in protein metabolism. *Acta Physiol* 162:377-387, 1998.

89. Tipton, KD and Wolfe, RR. Protein and amino acids for athletes. *J Sports Sci* 22:65-79, 2004.

90. Turinsky, J and Long, CL. Free amino acids in muscle: Effect of muscle fiber population and denervation. *Am J Physiol* 258:E485-E491, 1990.

91. U.S. Anti-Doping Agency. n.d. DRO drug reference online. www.usada.org/dro/search/search.aspx.

92. Van Hall, G, Raaymakers, JS, Saris, WH, and Wagenmakers, AJ. Ingestion of branched-chain amino acids and tryptophan during sustained exercise in man: Failure to affect performance. *J Physiol* 486(Pt 3):789-94, 1995.

93. Van Hall, G, Shirreffs, SM, and Calbet, JA. Muscle glycogen resynthesis during recovery from cycle exercise: No effect of additional protein ingestion. *J Appl Physiol* 88(5): 1631-1636, 2000.

94. Van Nieuwenhoven, MA, Brummer, RB, and Brouns, F. Gastrointestinal function during exercise: Comparison of water, sports drink, and sports drink with caffeine. *J Appl Physiol* 89:1079-1085, 2000.

95. Vist, GE and Maughan, RJ. Gastric emptying of ingested solutions in man: Effect of beverage glucose concentration. *Med Sci Sports Exerc* 10:1269-1273, 1994.

96. Witard, OC, Turner, JE, Jackman, SR, Kies, AK, Juekendrup, AE, Bosch, JA, and Tipton, KD. High dietary protein restores overreaching induced impairments in leukocyte trafficking and reduces the incidence of upper respiratory tract infection in elite cyclists. *Brain Behav Immun* 39:211-219, 2014.

97. Wolfe, RR. Branched-chain amino acids and muscle protein synthesis in humans: Myth or reality? *J Int Soc Sports Nut* 14:30, 2017.

98. Wolfe, RR, Wolfe, MH, Nadel, ER, and Shaw, JH. Isotopic determination of amino acid-urea interactions in exercise in humans. *J Appl Physiol* 56:221-229, 1984.

99. Yeo, SE, Jentjens, RL, Wallis, GA, and Jeukendrup, AE. Caffeine increases exogenous carbohydrate oxidation during exercise. *J Appl Physiol* 99:844-850, 2005.

Chapter 10

1. Andersen, LL, Tufekovic, G, Zebis, MK, Crameri, RM, Verlaan, G, Kjaer, M, Suetta, C, Magnusson, P, and Aagaard, P. The effect of resistance training combined with timed ingestion of protein on muscle fiber size and muscle strength. *Metabolism: Clinical and Experimental* 54:151-156, 2005.

2. Aragon, AA and Schoenfeld, BJ. Nutrient timing revisited: Is there a post-exercise anabolic window? *J Int Soc Sports Nutr* 10:5, 2013.

3. Baty, JJ, Hwang, H, Ding, Z, Bernard, JR, Wang, B, Kwon, B, and Ivy, JL. The effect of a carbohydrate and protein supplement on resistance exercise performance, hormonal response, and muscle damage. *J Strength Cond Res* 21:321-329, 2007.

4. Beelen, M, Koopman, R, Gijsen, AP, Vandereyt, H, Kies, AK, Kuipers, H, Saris, WH, and van Loon, LJ. Protein coingestion stimulates muscle protein synthesis during resistance-type exercise. *Am J Physiol Endocrinol Metab* 295:E70-77, 2008.

5. Berardi, JM, Noreen, EE, and Lemon, PW. Recovery from a cycling time trial is enhanced with carbohydrate-protein supplementation vs. isoenergetic carbohydrate supplementation. *J Int Soc Sports Nutr* 5:24, 2008.

6. Berardi, JM, Price, TB, Noreen, EE, and Lemon, PW. Postexercise muscle glycogen recovery enhanced with a carbohydrate-protein supplement. *Med Sci Sports Exerc* 38: 1106-1113, 2006.

7. Bergstrom, J, Hermansen, L, Hultman, E, and Saltin, B. Diet, muscle glycogen and physical performance. *Acta Physiologica Scandinavica* 71:140-150, 1967.

8. Bergstrom, J and Hultman, E. Muscle glycogen synthesis after exercise: An enhancing factor localized to the muscle cells in man. *Nature* 210:309-310, 1966.

9. Biolo, G, Tipton, KD, Klein, S, and Wolfe, RR. An abundant supply of amino acids enhances the metabolic effect of exercise on muscle protein. *Am J Physiol* 273:E122-129, 1997.

10. Bird, SP, Tarpenning, KM, and Marino, FE. Effects of liquid carbohydrate/ essential amino acid ingestion on acute hormonal response during a single bout of resistance exercise in untrained men. *Nutrition* 22:367-375, 2006.

11. Bird, SP, Tarpenning, KM, and Marino, FE. Independent and combined effects of liquid carbohydrate/essential amino acid ingestion on hormonal and muscular adaptations following resistance training in untrained men. *Eur J Appl Physiol* 97:225-238, 2006.

12. Bird, SP, Tarpenning, KM, and Marino, FE. Liquid carbohydrate/essential amino acid ingestion during a short-term bout of resistance exercise suppresses myofibrillar protein degradation. *Metabolism: Clinical and experimental* 55:570-577, 2006.

13. Boirie, Y, Dangin, M, Gachon, P, Vasson, MP, Maubois, JL, and Beaufrere, B. Slow and fast dietary proteins differently modulate postprandial protein accretion. *Proc Natl Acad Sci U S A* 94:14930-14935, 1997.

14. Borsheim, E, Cree, MG, Tipton, KD, Elliott, TA, Aarsland, A, and Wolfe, RR. Effect of carbohydrate intake on net muscle protein synthesis during recovery from resistance exercise. *J Appl Physiol* 96:674-678, 2004.

15. Borsheim, E, Tipton, KD, Wolf, SE, and Wolfe, RR. Essential amino acids and muscle protein recovery from resistance exercise. *Am J Physiol Endocrinol Metab* 283:E648-657, 2002.

16. Bosch, AN, Dennis, SC, and Noakes, TD. Influence of carbohydrate loading on fuel substrate turnover and oxidation during prolonged exercise. *J Appl Physiol* 74:1921-1927, 1993.

17. Bucci, L and Unlu, L. Proteins and amino acid supplements in exercise and sport. In *Energy-Yield Macronutrients and Energy Metabolism in Sports Nutrition*. Driskell, J, Wolinsky, I, eds. Boca Raton, FL: CRC Press, 191-212, 2000.

18. Burke, LM, Cox, GR, Culmmings, NK, and Desbrow, B. Guidelines for daily carbohydrate intake: Do athletes achieve them? *Sports Med* 31:267-299, 2001.

19. Burke, LM, Loucks, AB, and Broad, N. Energy and carbohydrate for training and recovery. *J Sports Sci* 24: 675-685, 2006.

20. Bussau, VA, Fairchild, TJ, Rao, A, Steele, P, and Fournier, PA. Carbohydrate loading in human muscle: An improved 1 day protocol. *Eur J Appl Physiol* 87:290-295, 2002.

21. Candow, DG, Burke, NC, Smith-Palmer, T, and Burke, DG. Effect of whey and soy protein supplementation combined with resistance training in young adults. *Int J Sport Nutr Exerc Metab* 16:233-244, 2006.

22. Candow, DG, Forbes, SC, Chilibeck, PD, Cornish, SM, Antonio, J, and Kreider, RB. Variables Influencing the Effectiveness of Creatine Supplementation as a Therapeutic Intervention for Sarcopenia. *Front Nutr* 6:124, 2019.

23. Coburn, JW, Housh, DJ, Housh, TJ, Malek, MH, Beck, TW, Cramer, JT, Johnson, GO, and Donlin, PE. Effects of leucine and whey protein supplementation during eight weeks of unilateral resistance training. *J Strength Cond Res* 20:284-291, 2006.

24. Conlee, RK, Lawler, RM, and Ross, PE. Effects of glucose or fructose feeding on glycogen repletion in muscle and liver after exercise or fasting. *Annals of nutrition & metabolism* 31:126-132, 1987.

25. Coyle, EF, Coggan, AR, Hemmert, MK, and Ivy, JL. Muscle glycogen utilization during prolonged strenuous exercise when fed carbohydrate. *J Appl Physiol* 61:165-172, 1986.

26. Coyle, EF, Coggan, AR, Hemmert, MK, Lowe, RC, and Walters, TJ. Substrate usage during prolonged exercise following a preexercise meal. *J Appl Physiol* 59:429-433, 1985.

27. Cribb, PJ and Hayes, A. Effects of supplement timing and resistance exercise on skeletal muscle hypertrophy. *Med Sci Sports Exerc* 38:1918-1925, 2006.

28. Cribb, PJ, Williams, AD, and Hayes, A. A creatine-protein-carbohydrate supplement enhances responses to resistance training. *Med Sci Sports Exerc* 39:1960-1968, 2007.

29. Cribb, PJ, Williams, AD, Stathis, CG, Carey, MF, and Hayes, A. Effects of whey isolate, creatine, and resistance training on muscle hypertrophy. *Med Sci Sports Exerc* 39:298-307, 2007.

30. Currell, K and Jeukendrup, AE. Superior endurance performance with ingestion of multiple transportable carbohydrates. *Med Sci Sports Exerc* 40:275-281, 2008.

31. Dalton, RA, Rankin, JW, Sebolt, D, and Gwazdauskas, F. Acute carbohydrate consumption does not influence resistance exercise performance during energy restriction. *Int J Sport Nutr* 9:319-332, 1999.

32. Dangin, M, Boirie, Y, Garcia-Rodenas, C, Gachon, P, Fauquant, J, Callier, P, Ballevre, O, and Beaufrere, B. The digestion rate of protein is an independent regulating factor of postprandial protein retention. *Am J Physiol Endocrinol Metab* 280:E340-348, 2001.

33. Dennis, SC, Noakes, TD, and Hawley, JA. Nutritional strategies to minimize fatigue during prolonged exercise: Fluid, electrolyte and energy replacement. *J Sports Sciences* 15:305-313, 1997.

34. Earnest, CP, Lancaster, SL, Rasmussen, CJ, Kerksick, CM, Lucia, A, Greenwood, MC, Almada, AL, Cowan, PA, and Kreider, RB. Low vs. high glycemic

index carbohydrate gel ingestion during simulated 64-km cycling time trial performance. *J Strength Cond Res* 18:466-472, 2004.

35. Erickson, MA, Schwarzkopf, RJ, and McKenzie, RD. Effects of caffeine, fructose, and glucose ingestion on muscle glycogen utilization during exercise. *Med Sci Sports Exerc* 19:579-583, 1987.

36. Esmarck, B, Andersen, JL, Olsen, S, Richter, EA, Mizuno, M, and Kjaer, M. Timing of postexercise protein intake is important for muscle hypertrophy with resistance training in elderly humans. *J Physiol* 535:301-311, 2001.

37. Febbraio, MA, Chiu, A, Angus, DJ, Arkinstall, MJ, and Hawley, JA. Effects of carbohydrate ingestion before and during exercise on glucose kinetics and performance. *J Appl Physiol* 89:2220-2226, 2000.

38. Febbraio, MA, Keenan, J, Angus, DJ, Campbell, SE, and Garnham, AP. Pre-exercise carbohydrate ingestion, glucose kinetics, and muscle glycogen use: Effect of the glycemic index. *J Appl Physiol* 89:1845-1851, 2000.

39. Febbraio, MA and Stewart, KL. CHO feeding before prolonged exercise: Effect of glycemic index on muscle glycogenolysis and exercise performance. *J Appl Physiol* 81: 1115-1120, 1996.

40. Fielding, RA, Costill, DL, Fink, WJ, King, DS, Hargreaves, M, and Kovaleski, JE. Effect of carbohydrate feeding frequencies and dosage on muscle glycogen use during exercise. *Med Sci Sports Exerc* 17:472-476, 1985.

41. Foster, C, Costill, DL, and Fink, WJ. Effects of preexercise feedings on endurance performance. *Med Sci Sports Exerc* 11:1-5, 1979.

42. Fujita, S, Dreyer, HC, Drummond, MJ, Glynn, EL, Volpi, E, and Rasmussen, BB. Essential amino acid and carbohydrate ingestion before resistance exercise does not enhance postexercise muscle protein synthesis. *J Appl Physiol* 106:1730-1739, 2009.

43. Gleeson, M, Nieman, DC, and Pedersen, BK. Exercise, nutrition and immune function. *J Sports Sci* 22:115-125, 2004.

44. Goforth, HW, Laurent, D, Prusaczyk, WK, Schneider, KE, Petersen, KF, and Shulman, GI. Effects of depletion exercise and light training on muscle glycogen supercompensation in men. *Am J Physiol Endocrinol Metab* 285:1304-1311, 2003.

45. Haff, GG, Koch, AJ, Potteiger, JA, Kuphal, KE, Magee, LM, Green, SB, and Jakicic, JJ. Carbohydrate supplementation attenuates muscle glycogen loss during acute bouts of resistance exercise. *Int J Sport Nutr Exerc Metab* 10:326-339, 2000.

46. Hargreaves, M, Costill, DL, Coggan, A, Fink, WJ, and Nishibata, I. Effect of carbohydrate feedings on muscle glycogen utilization and exercise performance. *Med Sci Sports Exerc* 16:219-222, 1984.

47. Hartman, JW, Tang, JE, Wilkinson, SB, Tarnopolsky, MA, Lawrence, RL, Fullerton, AV, and Phillips, SM. Consumption of fat-free fluid milk after resistance exercise promotes greater lean mass accretion than does consumption of soy or carbohydrate in young, novice, male weightlifters. *Am J Clin Nutr* 86:373-381, 2007.

48. Harty, PS, Zabriskie, HA, Erickson, JL, Molling, PE, Kerksick, CM, and Jagim, AR. Multi-ingredient pre-workout supplements, safety implications, and performance outcomes: A brief review. *J Int Soc Sports Nutr* 15:41, 2018.

49. Hawley, JA, Bosch, AN, Weltan, SM, Dennis, SC, and Noakes, TD. Glucose kinetics during prolonged exercise in euglycaemic and hyperglycaemic subjects. *Pflugers Arch* 426:378-386, 1994.

50. Hawley, JA and Burke, LM. Effect of meal frequency and timing on physical performance. *Br J Nutr* 77 Suppl 1:S91-103, 1997.

51. Hawley, JA, Schabort, EJ, Noakes, TD, and Dennis, SC. Carbohydrate-loading and exercise performance. An update. *Sports Med* 24:73-81, 1997.

52. Hoffman, JR, Ratamess, NA, Tranchina, CP, Rashti, SL, Kang, J, and Faigenbaum, AD. Effect of protein-supplement timing on strength, power, and body-composition changes in resistance-trained men. *Int J Sport Nutr Exerc Metab* 19:172-185, 2009.

53. Impey, SG, Hearris, MA, Hammond, KM, Bartlett, JD, Louis, J, Close, GL, and Morton, JP. Fuel for the work required: A theoretical framework for carbohydrate periodization and the glycogen threshold hypothesis. *Sports Med* 48:1031-1048, 2018.

54. Ivy, JL. Glycogen resynthesis after exercise: Effect of carbohydrate intake. *Int J Sports Med* 19 Suppl 2: S142-145, 1998.

55. Ivy, JL, Goforth, HW, Jr., Damon, BM, McCauley, TR, Parsons, EC, and Price, TB. Early postexercise muscle glycogen recovery is enhanced with a carbohydrate-protein supplement. *Journal of applied physiology* (Bethesda, MD: 1985) 93:1337-1344, 2002.

56. Ivy, JL, Res, PT, Sprague, RC, and Widzer, MO. Effect of a carbohydrate-protein supplement on endurance performance during exercise of varying intensity. *Int J Sport Nutr Exerc Metab* 13:382-395, 2003.

57. Jentjens, R and Jeukendrup, A. Determinants of post-exercise glycogen synthesis during short-term recovery. *Sports Med* 33:117-144, 2003.

58. Jentjens, R and Jeukendrup, AE. High exogenous carbohydrate oxidation rates from a mixture of glucose and fructose ingested during prolonged cycling exercise. *Brit J Nutr* 93:485-492, 2005.

59. Jentjens, R, Shaw, C, Birtles, T, Waring, RH, Harding, LK, and Jeukendrup, AE. Oxidation of combined ingestion of glucose and sucrose during exercise. *Metab Clin and Experimental* 54:610-618, 2005.

60. Jentjens, R, van Loon, L, Mann, CH, Wagenmakers, AJM, and Jeukendrup, AE. Addition of protein and amino acids to carbohydrates does not enhance postexercise muscle glycogen synthesis. *J Appl Physiol* 91:839-846, 2001.

61. Jentjens, R, Venables, MC, and Jeukendrup, AE. Oxidation of exogenous glucose, sucrose, and maltose during prolonged cycling exercise. *J Appl Physiol* 96:1285-1291, 2004.

62. Jentjens, RL and Jeukendrup, AE. High rates of exogenous carbohydrate

oxidation from a mixture of glucose and fructose ingested during prolonged cycling exercise. *Br J Nutr* 93:485-492, 2005.

63. Jentjens, RL, Moseley, L, Waring, RH, Harding, LK, and Jeukendrup, AE. Oxidation of combined ingestion of glucose and fructose during exercise. *J Appl Physiol* 96:1277-1284, 2004.

64. Jeukendrup, AE. Carbohydrate intake during exercise and performance. *Nutrition* 20: 669-677, 2004.

65. Jeukendrup, AE and Jentjens, R. Oxidation of carbohydrate feedings during prolonged exercise: Current thoughts, guidelines and directions for future research. *Sports Med* 29: 407-424, 2000.

66. Jeukendrup, AE, Jentjens, RL, and Moseley, L. Nutritional considerations in triathlon. *Sports Med* 35:163-181, 2005.

67. Karlsson, J and Saltin, B. Diet, muscle glycogen, and endurance performance. *J Appl Physiol* 31:203-206, 1971.

68. Kavouras, SA, Troup, JP, and Berning, JR. The influence of low versus high carbohydrate diet on a 45-min strenuous cycling exercise. *Int J Sport Nutr Exerc Metab* 14:62-72, 2004.

69. Keizer, H, Kuipers, H, and van Kranenburg, G. Influence of liquid and solid meals on muscle glycogen resynthesis, plasma fuel hormone response, and maximal physical working capacity. *Int J Sports Med* 8:99-104, 1987.

70. Kerksick, C, Harvey, T, Stout, J, Campbell, B, Wilborn, C, Kreider, R, Kalman, D, Ziegenfuss, T, Lopez, H, Landis, J, Ivy, JL, and Antonio, J. International Society of Sports Nutrition position stand: Nutrient timing. *J Int Soc Sports Nutr* 5:17, 2008.

71. Kerksick, CM, Arent, S, Schoenfeld, BJ, Stout, JR, Campbell, B, Wilborn, CD, Taylor, L, Kalman, D, Smith-Ryan, AE, Kreider, RB, Willoughby, D, Arciero, PJ, VanDusseldorp, TA, Ormsbee, MJ, Wildman, R, Greenwood, M, Ziegenfuss, TN, Aragon, AA, and Antonio, J. International society of sports nutrition position stand: Nutrient timing. *J Int Soc Sports Nutr* 14:33, 2017.

72. Kerksick, CM, Rasmussen, C, Lancaster, S, Starks, M, Smith, P, Melton, C, Greenwood, M, Almada, A, and Kreider, R. Impact of differing protein sources and a creatine containing nutritional formula after 12 weeks of resistance training. *Nutrition* 23:647-656, 2007.

73. Kerksick, CM, Rasmussen, CJ, Lancaster, SL, Magu, B, Smith, P, Melton, C, Greenwood, M, Almada, AL, Earnest, CP, and Kreider, RB. The effects of protein and amino acid supplementation on performance and training adaptations during ten weeks of resistance training. *J Strength Cond Res* 20:643-653, 2006.

74. Koopman, R, Pannemans, DL, Jeukendrup, AE, Gijsen, AP, Senden, JM, Halliday, D, Saris, WH, van Loon, LJ, and Wagenmakers, AJ. Combined ingestion of protein and carbohydrate improves protein balance during ultra-endurance exercise. *Am J Physiol Endocrinol Metab* 287:E712-720, 2004.

75. Kraemer, WJ, Hatfield, DL, Spiering, BA, Vingren, JL, Fragala, MS, Ho, JY, Volek, JS, Anderson, JM, and Maresh, CM. Effects of a multi-nutrient supple-

ment on exercise performance and hormonal responses to resistance exercise. *Eur J Appl Physiol* 101:637-646, 2007.

76. Kreider, RB. Effects of creatine supplementation on performance and training adaptations. *Mol Cell Biochem* 244:89-94, 2003.

77. Kreider, RB, Kalman, DS, Antonio, J, Ziegenfuss, TN, Wildman, R, Collins, R, Candow, DG, Kleiner, SM, Almada, AL, and Lopez, HL. International Society of Sports Nutrition position stand: Safety and efficacy of creatine supplementation in exercise, sport, and medicine. *J Int Soc Sports Nutr* 14:18, 2017.

78. Kulik, JR, Touchberry, CD, Kawamori, N, Blumert, PA, Crum, AJ, and Haff, GG. Supplemental carbohydrate ingestion does not improve performance of high-intensity resistance exercise. *J Strength Cond Res* 22:1101-1107, 2008.

79. McConell, G, Snow, RJ, Proietto, J, and Hargreaves, M. Muscle metabolism during prolonged exercise in humans: Influence of carbohydrate availability. *J Appl Physiol* 87: 1083-1086, 1999.

80. Miller, SL, Tipton, KD, Chinkes, DL, Wolf, SE, and Wolfe, RR. Independent and combined effects of amino acids and glucose after resistance exercise. *Med Sci Sports Exerc* 35:449-455, 2003.

81. Moseley, L, Lancaster, GI, and Jeukendrup, AE. Effects of timing of pre-exercise ingestion of carbohydrate on subsequent metabolism and cycling performance. *Eur J Appl Physiol* 88:453-458, 2003.

82. Neufer, PD, Costill, DL, Flynn, MG, Kirwan, JP, Mitchell, JB, and Houmard, J. Improvements in exercise performance: Effects of carbohydrate feedings and diet. *J Appl Physiol* 62:983-988, 1987.

83. Nicholas, CW, Green, PA, and Hawkins, RD. Carbohydrate intake and recovery of intermittent running capacity. *Int J Sport Nutr* 7:251-260, 1997.

84. Nicholas, CW, Williams, C, Lakomy, HK, Phillips, G, and Nowitz, A. Influence of ingesting a carbohydrate-electrolyte solution on endurance capacity during intermittent, high-intensity shuttle running. *J Sports Sci* 13:283-290, 1995.

85. Pascoe, DD, Costill, DL, Fink, WJ, Robergs, RA, and Zachwieja, JJ. Glycogen resynthesis in skeletal muscle following resistive exercise. *Med Sci Sports Exerc* 25:349-354, 1993.

86. Patterson, SD and Gray, SC. Carbohydrate-gel supplementation and endurance performance during intermittent high-intensity shuttle running. *Int J Sport Nutr Exerc Metab* 17:445-455, 2007.

87. Paul, GL. The rationale for consuming protein blends in sports nutrition. *J Am Coll Nutr* 28 Suppl:464S-472S, 2009.

88. Phillips, SM, Tipton, KD, Ferrando, AA, and Wolfe, RR. Resistance training reduces the acute exercise-induced increase in muscle protein turnover. *Am J Physiol* 276:E118-124, 1999.

89. Pitkanen, HT, Nykanen, T, Knuutinen, J, Lahti, K, Keinanen, O, Alen, M, Komi, PV, and Mero, AA. Free amino acid pool and muscle protein balance after resistance exercise. *Med Sci Sports Exerc* 35:784-792, 2003.

90. Rasmussen, BB, Tipton, KD, Miller, SL, Wolf, SE, and Wolfe, RR. An oral essen-

tial amino acid-carbohydrate supplement enhances muscle protein anabolism after resistance exercise. *J Appl Physiol* 88:386-392, 2000.

91. Reed, MJ, Brozinick, JT, Jr., Lee, MC, and Ivy, JL. Muscle glycogen storage postexercise: Effect of mode of carbohydrate administration. *J Appl Physiol* 66:720-726, 1989.

92. Robergs, RA, Pearson, DR, Costill, DL, Fink, WJ, Pascoe, DD, Benedict, MA, Lambert, CP, and Zachweija, JJ. Muscle glycogenolysis during differing intensities of weight-resistance exercise. *J Appl Physiol* 70:1700-1706, 1991.

93. Rodriguez, NR, Di Marco, NM, and Langley, S. American College of Sports Medicine position stand. Nutrition and athletic performance. *Med Sci Sports Exerc* 41:709-731, 2009.

94. Saunders, MJ, Kane, MD, and Todd, MK. Effects of a carbohydrate-protein beverage on cycling endurance and muscle damage. *Med Sci Sports Exerc* 36:1233-1238, 2004.

95. Saunders, MJ, Luden, ND, and Herrick, JE. Consumption of an oral carbo-hydrate-protein gel improves cycling endurance and prevents postexercise muscle damage. *J Strength Cond Res* 21:678-684, 2007.

96. Schoenfeld, BJ, Aragon, A, Wilborn, C, Urbina, SL, Hayward, SE, and Krieger, J. Pre- versus post-exercise protein intake has similar effects on muscular adaptations. *PeerJ* 5: e2825, 2017.

97. Schoenfeld, BJ, Aragon, AA, and Krieger, JW. The effect of protein timing on muscle strength and hypertrophy: A meta-analysis. *J Int Soc Sports Nutr* 10:53, 2013.

98. Sherman, WM, Brodowicz, G, Wright, DA, Allen, WK, Simonsen, J, and Dernbach, A. Effects of 4 h preexercise carbohydrate feedings on cycling performance. *Med Sci Sports Exerc* 21:598-604, 1989.

99. Sherman, WM, Costill, DL, Fink, WJ, Hagerman, FC, Armstrong, LE, and Murray, TF. Effect of a 42.2-km footrace and subsequent rest or exercise on muscle glycogen and enzymes. *J Appl Physiol* 55:1219-1224, 1983.

100. Sherman, WM, Costill, DL, Fink, WJ, and Miller, JM. Effect of exercise-diet manipulation on muscle glycogen and its subsequent utilization during per-formance. *Int J Sports Med* 2:114-118, 1981.

101. Staples, AW, Burd, NA, West, DW, Currie, KD, Atherton, PJ, Moore, DR, Rennie, MJ, Macdonald, MJ, Baker, SK, and Phillips, SM. Carbohydrate does not augment exercise-induced protein accretion versus protein alone. *Med Sci Sports Exerc* 43:1154-1161, 2011.

102. Stecker, RA, Harty, PS, Jagim, AR, Candow, DG, and Kerksick, CM. Timing of ergogenic aids and micronutrients on muscle and exercise performance. *J Int Soc Sports Nutr* 16:37, 2019.

103. Tang, JE, Moore, DR, Kujbida, GW, Tarnopolsky, MA, and Phillips, SM. Inges-tion of whey hydrolysate, casein, or soy protein isolate: Effects on mixed muscle protein synthesis at rest and following resistance exercise in young men. *J Appl Physiol* 107: 987-992, 2009.

104. Tarnopolsky, MA, Bosman, M, Macdonald, JR, Vandeputte, D, Martin, J, and Roy, BD. Postexercise protein-carbohydrate and carbohydrate supplements increase muscle glycogen in men and women. *J Appl Physiol* 83:1877-1883, 1997.

105. Tarnopolsky, MA, Gibala, M, Jeukendrup, AE, and Phillips, SM. Nutritional needs of elite endurance athletes. Part I: Carbohydrate and fluid requirements. *Eur J Sport Sci* 5: 3-14, 2005.

106. Tarnopolsky, MA, Parise, G, Yardley, NJ, Ballantyne, CS, Olatinji, S, and Phillips, SM. Creatine-dextrose and protein-dextrose induce similar strength gains during training. *Med Sci Sports Exerc* 33:2044-2052, 2001.

107. Tipton, KD, Elliott, TA, Cree, MG, Aarsland, AA, Sanford, AP, and Wolfe, RR. Stimulation of net muscle protein synthesis by whey protein ingestion before and after exercise. *Am J Physiol Endocrinol Metab* 292:E71-76, 2007.

108. Tipton, KD, Elliott, TA, Cree, MG, Wolf, SE, Sanford, AP, and Wolfe, RR. Ingestion of casein and whey proteins result in muscle anabolism after resistance exercise. *Med Sci Sports Exerc* 36:2073-2081, 2004.

109. Tipton, KD, Ferrando, AA, Phillips, SM, Doyle, D, Jr., and Wolfe, RR. Postexercise net protein synthesis in human muscle from orally administered amino acids. *Am J Physiol* 276:E628-634, 1999.

110. Tipton, KD, Rasmussen, BB, Miller, SL, Wolf, SE, Owens-Stovall, SK, Petrini, BE, and Wolfe, RR. Timing of amino acid-carbohydrate ingestion alters anabolic response of muscle to resistance exercise. *Am J Physiol Endocrinol Metab* 281:E197-206, 2001.

111. Tipton, KD and Wolfe, RR. Exercise, protein metabolism, and muscle growth. *Int J Sport Nutr Exerc Metab* 11:109-132, 2001.

112. van Loon, LJ, Saris, WH, Kruijshoop, M, and Wagenmakers, AJ. Maximizing postexercise muscle glycogen synthesis: Carbohydrate supplementation and the application of amino acid or protein hydrolysate mixtures. *Am J Clin Nutr* 72:106-111, 2000.

113. Wallis, GA, Rowlands, DS, Shaw, C, Jentjens, R, and Jeukendrup, AE. Oxidation of combined ingestion of maltodextrins and fructose during exercise. *Med Sci Sports Exerc* 37:426-432, 2005.

114. White, JP, Wilson, JM, Austin, KG, Greer, BK, St John, N, and Panton, LB. Effect of carbohydrate-protein supplement timing on acute exercise-induced muscle damage. *J Int Soc Sports Nutr* 5:5, 2008.

115. Widrick, JJ, Costill, DL, Fink, WJ, Hickey, MS, McConell, GK, and Tanaka, H. Carbohydrate feedings and exercise performance: Effect of initial muscle glycogen concentration. *J Appl Physiol* 74:2998-3005, 1993.

116. Wilkinson, SB, Tarnopolsky, MA, Macdonald, MJ, Macdonald, JR, Armstrong, D, and Phillips, SM. Consumption of fluid skim milk promotes greater muscle protein accretion after resistance exercise than does consumption of an isonitrogenous and isoenergetic soy-protein beverage. *Am J Clin Nutr* 85:1031-1040, 2007.

117. Willoughby, DS, Stout, JR, and Wilborn, CD. Effects of resistance training

and protein plus amino acid supplementation on muscle anabolism, mass, and strength. *Amino Acids* 32:467-477, 2007.

118. Wright, DA, Sherman, WM, and Dernbach, AR. Carbohydrate feedings before, during, or in combination improve cycling endurance performance. *J Appl Physiol* 71:1082-1088, 1991.

119. Yaspelkis, BB, Patterson, JG, Anderla, PA, Ding, Z, and Ivy, JL. Carbohydrate supplementation spares muscle glycogen during variable-intensity exercise. *J Appl Physiol* 75:1477-1485, 1993.

120. Zawadzki, KM, Yaspelkis, BB, 3rd, and Ivy, JL. Carbohydrate-protein complex increases the rate of muscle glycogen storage after exercise. *J Appl Physiol* 72:1854-1859, 1992.

Chapter 11

1. Amabile, TM. Motivational synergy: Toward new conceptualizations of intrinsic and extrinsic motivation in the workplace. *Hum Resour Manag Rev* 3:185-201, 1993.

2. Antonio, J, Gann, M, Kalman, D, Katch, F, Kleiner, S, Kreider, R, and Willoughby, D. ISSN roundtable: FAQs about the ISSN. *JISSN* 2:1-3, 2005.

3. Aschbacher, K, Rodriguez-Fernandez, M, van Wietmarschen, H, Tomiyama, AJ, Jain, S, Epel, E, Doyle III, FJ, and van der Greef, J. The hypothalamic-pituitary-adrenal-leptin axis and metabolic health: A systems approach to resilience, robustness and control. *Interface Focus* 4:20140020, 2014.

4. Bandura, A. Self-efficacy mechanism in human agency. *Am Psychol* 37:122, 1982.

5. Bandura, A. *Social Foundations of Thought and Action*. Englewood Cliffs, NJ, 1-617, 1986.

6. Baum, A. Eating disorders in the male athlete. *Sports Med* 36:1-6, 2006.

7. Becker, CB, Bull, S, Schaumberg, K, Cauble, A, and Franco, A. Effectiveness of peer-led eating disorders prevention: A replication trial. *J Consult Clin Psychol* 76:347, 2008.

8. Bonci, CM, Bonci, LJ, Granger, LR, Johnson, CL, Malina, RM, Milne, LW, Ryan, RR, and Vanderbunt, EM. National Athletic Trainers' Association position statement: Preventing, detecting, and managing disordered eating in athletes. *J Athl Train* 43:80-108, 2008.

9. Britt, TW and Jex, SM. *Thriving Under Stress: Harnessing Demands in the Workplace*. New York: Oxford University Press, 1-240, 2015.

10. Dionne, MM and Yeudall, F. Monitoring of weight in weight loss programs: A double-edged sword? *JNEB* 37:315-318, 2005.

11. Duckworth, A. *Grit: The Power of Passion and Perseverance*. New York: Scribner, 1-352, 2016.

12. Duckworth, AL, Peterson, C, Matthews, MD, and Kelly, DR. Grit: Perseverance and passion for long-term goals. *J Pers Soc Psychol* 92:1087, 2007.

13. Gagné, M and Deci, EL. Self-determination theory and work motivation. *J Organ Behav* 26:331-362, 2005.

14. Galli, N and Vealey, RS. "Bouncing back" from adversity: Athletes' experiences of resilience. *J Sport Exerc Psychol* 22:316-335, 2008.

15. Glazer, JL. Eating disorders among male athletes. *CSMR* 7:332-337, 2008.

16. Holladay, CL and Quinones, MA. Practice variability and transfer of training: The role of self-efficacy generality. *J Appl Soc Psychol* 88:1094, 2003.

17. Lacey, K and Pritchett, E. Nutrition care process and model: ADA adopts road map to quality care and outcomes management. *J Acad Nutr Diet* 103:1061-1072, 2003.

18. Linke, J, Kirsch, P, King, AV, Gass, A, Hennerici, MG, Bongers, A, and Wessa, M. Motivational orientation modulates the neural response to reward. *Neuroimage* 49: 2618-2625, 2010.

18a. Louisiana Board of Examiners in Dietetics and Nutrition. 2019. Rules and regulations title 46, professional and occupational standards part LXIX: Registered dietitians/ nutritionists. www.lbedn.org/assets/docs/RULES.Finalwith cover.3.2019.pdf.

19. Mageau, GA and Vallerand, RJ. The coach-athlete relationship: A motivational model. *J Sports Sci* 21:883-904, 2003.

20. McArdle, WD, Katch, FI, and Katch, VL. *Exercise physiology: Nutrition, Energy, and Human Performance.* Baltimore: Lippincott Williams & Wilkins, 765-786, 2010.

21. Mountjoy, M, Sundgot-Borgen, J, Burke, L, Carter, S, Constantini, N, Lebrun, C, Meyer, N, Sherman, R, Steffen, K, and Budgett, R. The IOC consensus statement: Beyond the female athlete triad—Relative Energy Deficiency in Sport (RED-S). *Br J Sports Med* 48: 491-497, 2014.

22. Pekmezi, D, Barbera, B, and Marcus, BH. Using the transtheoretical model to promote physical activity. *ACSMs Health Fit J* 14:8-13, 2010.

23. Prochaska, J, Norcross, J, and DiClemente, C. *Changing for Good: A Revolutionary Six-Stage Program for Overcoming Bad Habits and Moving Your Life Positively Forward.* New York: Morrow, 1-304, 1994.

24. Rosenbloom, C. Sports nutrition: Applying ADA's nutrition care process and model to achieve quality care and outcomes for athletes. *SCAN Pulse* 24:10-17, 2005.

25. Russell, E. *Restoring Resilience: Discovering Your Clients' Capacity for Healing.* New York: Norton, 1-384, 2015.

26. Ryan, RM and Deci, EL. Self-determination theory and the facilitation of intrinsic motivation, social development, and well-being. *Am Psychol* 55:68, 2000.

27. Sandoval, WM, Heller, KE, Wiese, WH, and Childs, DA. Stages of change: A model for nutrition counseling. *Top Clin Nutr* 9:64-69, 1994.

28. Sundgot-Borgen, J and Torstveit, MK. Prevalence of eating disorders in elite athletes is higher than in the general population. *Clin J Sport Med* 14:25-32, 2004.

29. Thiel, A, Gottfried, H, and Hesse, F. Subclinical eating disorders in male athletes: A study of the low weight category in rowers and wrestlers. *Acta Psychiatrica Scandinavica* 88: 259-265, 1993.

30. Thirlaway, K and Upton, D. *The Psychology of Lifestyle: Promoting Healthy Behaviour.* New York: Routledge, 1-336, 2009.

31. Thomas, DT, Erdman, KA, and Burke, LM. Position of the Academy of Nutrition and Dietetics, Dietitians of Canada, and the American College of Sports Medicine: Nutrition and athletic performance. *J Acad Nutr Diet* 116:501-528, 2016.

32. Uher, R and Rutter, M. Classification of feeding and eating disorders: Review of evidence and proposals for ICD-11. *World Psychiatry* 11:80-92, 2012.

33. Zawila, LG, Steib, C-SM, and Hoogenboom, B. The female collegiate cross-country runner: Nutritional knowledge and attitudes. *J Athl Train* 38:67, 2003.

Index

Note: The italicized *f* and *t* following page numbers refer to figures and tables, respectively.

About the Editor

Bill I. Campbell, PhD, CSCS, FISSN, is a professor of exercise science and the director of the performance and physique enhancement laboratory at the University of South Florida, a research laboratory dedicated to innovation in sport nutrition and physique enhancement research. As a researcher and author, Campbell has published more than 200 scientific abstracts and papers in these areas. He is a paid consultant for professional sport team organizations and sport entertainment corporations. He has lectured to audiences all over the world and given interviews on various topics related to sport nutrition and

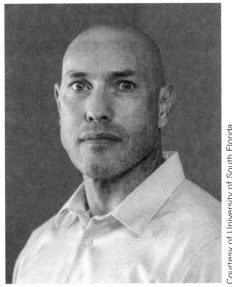

physique enhancement. In addition, he is a litigation consultant who provides expert testimony related to dietary supplementation.

Campbell is the former president and a current fellow of the International Society of Sports Nutrition. Campbell is also an active member of the National Strength and Conditioning Association and has earned their Certified Strength and Conditioning Specialist credential.

He received his PhD in exercise, nutrition, and preventive health from Baylor University in 2007. During that same year, he also received the Outstanding Doctoral Student Award for research and teaching. He is active on social media and can be followed on Instagram via @billcampbellphd.

About the NSCA

The National Strength and Conditioning Association (NSCA) is the world's leading organization in the field of sport conditioning. Drawing on the resources and expertise of the most recognized professionals in strength training and conditioning, sport science, performance research, education, and sports medicine, the NSCA is the world's trusted source of knowledge and training guidelines for coaches and athletes. The NSCA provides the crucial link between the lab and the field.

About the Contributors

Shawn M. Arent, PhD, CSCS*D, FISSN, FNAK, is a professor and chair of the Department of Exercise Science and director of the Sport Science Lab at the University of South Carolina. Dr. Arent's work has focused on physiological responses to training-related stressors and nutritional interventions and their contribution to optimal performance and recovery. He was named the 2017 Outstanding Sports Scientist of the Year by the NSCA and is a fellow in the National Academy of Kinesiology, American College of Sports Medicine, and the International Society of Sports Nutrition. He has worked with several professional, collegiate, and youth teams and athletes.

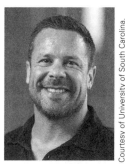

Laurent Bannock, DProf, MSc, CSCS, FISSN, RNutr, SENr, is the founder and director of the Institute of Performance Nutrition in London, UK, which specializes in the training, education, and continuing professional development of sport and exercise nutritionists. He has 28 years of professional experience as a practitioner and consultant with a diverse range of clients including many elite professional soccer and rugby teams, the military, boxers, MMA fighters, racing car drivers, tennis players, and endurance athletes. Recent notable roles include being the lead nutritionist to Great Britain fencing for the 2016 Olympics, and the Egyptian national soccer team for the FIFA 2018 World Cup.

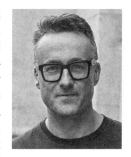

David Barr, CSCS, PPSC*M, CISSN, TSAC-F, RSCC, has spent more than 2 decades optimizing human performance across numerous domains. His experience has spanned from protein molecules to professional athletes, including his research for NASA at the Johnson Space Center, and work for both the NSCA and American College of Sports Medicine. He has innovated for *T-Nation*, *Bodybuilding.com*, and *EliteFTS*. He also published four books and four textbook chapters. David is revered throughout the world for his frequent use of hyperbole.

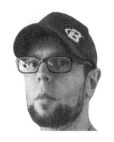

Ann Brown, PhD, CISSN, is an assistant professor and director of the Human Performance Laboratory in the Department of Movement Sciences at the University of Idaho in Moscow, Idaho. Her research focuses on interactions between metabolism, body composition, and performance, and includes the effects of protein supplementation on body composition, performance, and health. Dr. Brown's unique background in dance is a featured aspect of her research where she contributes to the growing body of literature in dance science, specifically in the realm of dance nutrition.

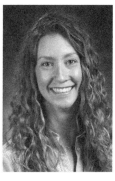

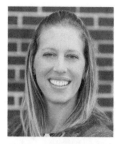

Jennifer Bunn, PhD, is an associate dean in the College of Health Sciences at Same Houston State University. Her areas of expertise in teaching include exercise physiology, sport and exercise nutrition, research methods, and exercise testing and prescription. Her research interests are centered on wearable technology and performance monitoring in athletic populations.

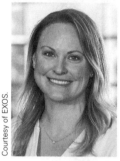

Courtesy of EXOS.

Amanda Carlson-Phillips, MS, RD, CSSD, is the senior vice president of Strategic Partnerships and Insights, and a leader on the EXOS Performance Innovation Team. Carlson-Phillips coordinates the company's strategic partnerships, performance research, and analytics team. She holds a master's degree in both sports/clinical nutrition and exercise physiology. She has worked with professional sports teams, elite athletes, military operators and forward-thinking organizations to optimize their human performance systems. Carlson-Phillips speaks and writes about the importance of improving nutrition for performance and overall health, and she now serves as an ambassador to the Collegiate and Professional Sports Dietitians Association after serving on their Board of Directors for six years.

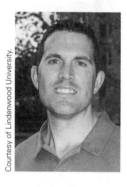

Courtesy of Lindenwood University.

Chad Kerksick, PhD, FNSCA, FISSN, CSCS*D, NSCA-CPT*D, is currently an associate professor in the exercise science department of the School of Health Sciences at Lindenwood University. He currently serves as the director of the Exercise and Performance Nutrition Laboratory (www.lindenwood.edu/epnl) and the Master of Science in Health Sciences program at Lindenwood University. His primary research interests include sport nutrition as well as the biochemical, cellular, and molecular adaptations relative to various forms of exercise and nutrition interventions, primarily those that promote muscle hypertrophy, prevent muscle atrophy, and promote health and recovery in healthy and clinical populations.

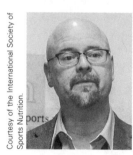

Courtesy of the International Society of Sports Nutrition.

Lonnie Lowery, PhD, RD, LD, FISSN, is an exercise physiologist, licensed nutritionist, and consulting business owner. He served on the exercise physiology and nutrition-dietetics faculty at four institutions, currently he is in the Department of Exercise, Sport & Nutrition Sciences at the University of Mount Union. His doctoral work centered on uncommon dietary fats; he currently studies coffee, dietary protein, and health. He is a long-time podcaster (IronRadio.org) and has written for over 100 nutrition or fitness publications. Dr. Lowery is past president of the American Society of Exercise Physiologists, and a fellow of the International Society of Sports Nutrition.

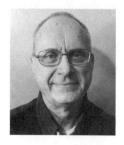

Henry Lukaski, PhD, FSLAN, is a retired senior scientist and research leader at the USDA-ARS, Grand Forks Human Nutrition Research Center, and currently adjunct professor at the University of North Dakota. He is an international authority on the interaction of diet (micronutrients) on body structure and function, and an international leader in methods to assess body composition. His scientific contributions include extensive publications in peer-reviewed literature, book chapters, books on sports nutrition and body composition; consultant to national and international scientific groups; a past and current member of editorial boards of scientific journals. He made hundreds of invited presentations at academic, governmental, and policy-making organizations worldwide.

JohnEric W. Smith, PhD, CSCS*D, CISSN, is an associate professor and applied physiology laboratory director at Mississippi State University with interests in carbohydrate and training for performance enhancement. Prior to his arrival at Mississippi State University, he was a research scientist for the Gatorade Sports Science Institute with a focus in carbohydrate metabolism and performance. He earned his master's and doctoral degrees at Auburn University focusing on thermoregulation and performance. Dr. Smith actively contributes to the scientific field through research publications and presentations while also contributing to sports and exercise by assisting multiple elite and professional sports.

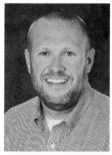

Courtesy of Mississippi State University.

Marie Spano, MS, RD, LD, CSCS, CSSD, is one of the country's leading sports nutritionists. Spano is the consulting major league sports dietitian for the Atlanta Braves and Atlanta Hawks. She previously worked for the Atlanta Falcons, Atlanta Thrashers and Blackzillians. Spano the lead author of *Nutrition for Sport, Exercise and Health* and co-editor of the first edition of *NSCA's Guide to Exercise and Sport Nutrition.* She has appeared on CNN as well as NBC, ABC, Fox and CBS affiliates, and authored hundreds of magazine articles and trade publication articles, and written book chapters and marketing materials. Find her on Twitter and Instagram @mariespano.

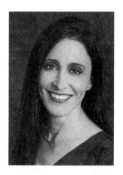

Colin Wilborn, PhD, FNSCA, CSCS, FISSN, is the executive dean of the Mayborn College of Health Sciences at the University of Mary Hardin-Baylor. He has published over 200 peer reviewed articles, abstracts, and book chapters on the effects of sport supplements and exercise on body composition, metabolism, and performance. Colin was the recipient of the NSCA's 2015 GNC Nutritional Research Award. He is a fellow and two-time vice president for the NSCA. He is also a fellow and former vice president of the International Society of Sports Nutrition, associate editor for the JISSN, and a senior associate editor for the JSCR.

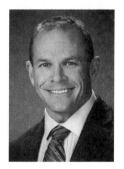

Tim N. Ziegenfuss, PhD, CSCS, FISSN, is a renowned sports nutrition and exercise scientist with graduate degrees from Purdue and Kent State University. He is a past president and fellow of the International Society of Sports Nutrition and CEO of the Center for Applied Health Sciences. As an exercise scientist, his client list includes current and former Olympic track and field athletes, professional MMA fighters, NFL, MLB, NHL, high school and NCAA athletes, firefighters, police, Department of Homeland Security personnel, and the US Military including the army, Navy Seals, and Secret Service.

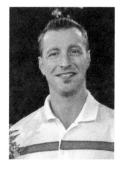

Contributors to the Previous Edition

Amanda Carlson Phillips, MS, RD, CSSD

Bill I. Campbell, PhD, CSCS, FISSN

Bob Seebohar, MS, RD, CSCS, CSSD

Chad M. Kerksick, PhD; ATC; CSCS*D; NSCA-CPT,*D

Colin Wilborn, PhD, ATC, CSCS, FISSN

Donovan L. Fogt, PhD

Henry C. Lukaski, PhD, FCASN

Jose Antonio, PhD, CSCS, FISSN, FNSCA

Lonnie Lowery, PhD, RD, LD

Marie A. Spano, MS, RD, LD, CSCS, CSSD, FISSN

Paul LaBounty, PhD, MPT, CSCS

Richard B. Kreider, PhD, FISSN

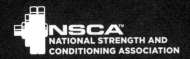
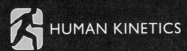

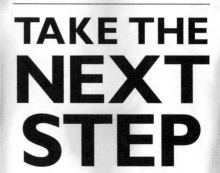
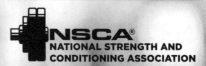
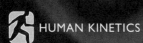